The
Thorax

To Cliff Fowler and Erl Pettman

Cliff and Erl are two manual therapy leaders in Canada who were among my first mentors and taught me to trust my hands and to always 'look for the criminal and treat more than the victim.'

I was, and still am, inspired by their clinical reasoning and curiosity for life-long learning.

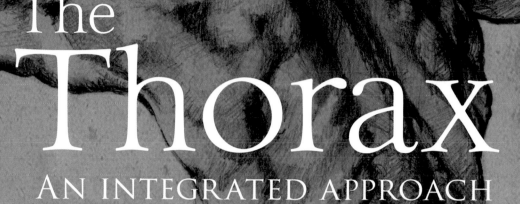

The Thorax

AN INTEGRATED APPROACH

Diane Lee

Foreword by Gregory S. Johnson PT, FFMT, FAAOMPT

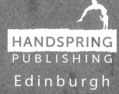

HANDSPRING
PUBLISHING
Edinburgh

HANDSPRING PUBLISHING LIMITED
The Old Manse, Fountainhall,
Pencaitland, East Lothian
EH34 5EY, Scotland
Tel: +44 1875 341 859
Website: www.handspringpublishing.com

First published 2018 in the United Kingdom by Handspring Publishing

ISBN 978-1-912085-05-7

British Library Cataloguing in Publication Data
A catalogue record for this book is available from the British Library

Library of Congress Cataloguing in Publication Data
A catalog record for this book is available from the Library of Congress

Notice
Neither the Publisher nor the Authors assume any responsibility for any loss or injury and/or damage to persons or property arising out of or relating to any use of the material contained in this book. It is the responsibility of the treating practitioner, relying on independent expertise and knowledge of the patient, to determine the best treatment and method of application for the patient.

Commissioning Editor Mary Law
Project Manager Morven Dean
Copy-editor Sally Davies
Designer Bruce Hogarth
Indexer Aptara, India
Typesetter DSM Soft, India
Printer Finidr, Czech Republic

The
Publisher's
policy is to use
paper manufactured
from sustainable forests

Copyright notice – illustrations

The illustrations listed below are the copyright of Diane G. Lee Physiotherapist Corp.

Chapter 1

Figures 1.2, 1.16, 1.24, 1.25, 1.26 1.28, 1.38, 1.39, 1.40, 1.41, 1.42, 1.50

Chapter 2

Figures 2.1, 2.3, 2.6, 2.12, 2.17, 2.19, 2.23

Chapter 3

Figures 3.2, 3.4A & B, 3.16, 3.25A, 3.28, 3.29, 3.51, 3.73, 3.75, 3.79, 3.81

Chapter 6

Figures 6.37A & B, 6.38A & B, 6.48A–D

Chapter 7

Figures 7.8, 7.21A & B, 7.22, 7.24A–D, 7.25, 7.29, 7.30, 7.31, 7.32, 7.33, 7.34, 7.37, 7.38, 7.40A–C, 7.42A–E, 7.43A–C, 7.44A–C, 7.45A & B, 7.46A–D, 7.47A–C, 7.48A & B, 7.49A–C, 7.50A–C

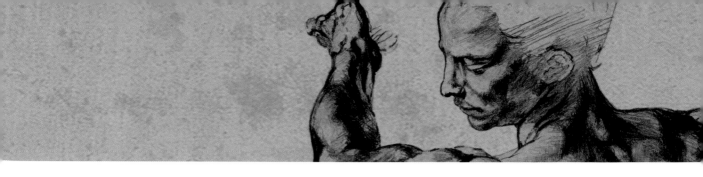

In 2003, when Diane Lee's earlier book on the thorax was released, the content of that work was instrumental in enhancing my knowledge of the thoracic cage. In preparing for writing this foreword, I returned to my original book to find it well-worn with many loose pages, secondary to extensive study by our Fellows-in-training. I am delighted to report that this new book demonstrates extensive evolution in thought and organization.

Every major profession, to progress and define itself, must have visionaries who propel the present state of knowledge to a new level. Diane Lee is one of those visionaries. This book presents a unique paradigm of evaluation and treatment (The Integrated Systems Model) that has the potential to transform our profession. The existing science and extensive clinical knowledge are melded into a guide for others to better understand the human body, and how to manage their patient's physical complaints. This book is not only about the thoracic cage, but one that explores the interconnections between the thoracic cage and the rest of the body. To quote from the text, as Diane expresses the concepts so well:

Today we understand that the thorax is part of many integrated and interdependent systems, including the musculoskeletal, neurological, respiratory, cardiovascular, digestive, and urogynecological systems. As such, it should not be considered in isolation from the rest of the body, but rather in relation to it...Sueki et al. (2013) refer to this as regional interdependence, a concept that suggests 'the function and health of one region of the body could potentially affect the function of another'.

The Integrated Systems Model is described as:

...an evidence-informed, clinical-reasoning, biopsychosocial approach. It is a framework, not a classification, that considers all three dimensions of the patient's experience (sensorial, cognitive, emotional) and the barriers that each may present to the recovery process for both acute and persistent conditions. The body or person can no longer be considered as individual parts or problems in either assessment or treatment.

Most tasks involve the whole body; therefore, assessment must include an analysis of the relationship between the body regions and the impact and interplay of each.

This well-organized book begins with an in-depth analysis of the anatomy of the thoracic cage including a guide to surface anatomy palpation.

Chapter 2 Biomechanics of the thorax

The second chapter, on biomechanics, begins with the following statement:

The thorax plays a critical role in multiple conditions since it is part of many integrated, and interdependent, systems including the musculoskeletal, respiratory, cardiovascular, digestive, and urogynecological systems.

This chapter highlights the current state of research evidence, as well as clinical observations pertaining to the biomechanics (osteokinematics and arthrokinematics) of the various regions of the thorax.

Chapter 3 Assessment of the thorax and its relationship to the whole body

Assessment and treatment of the whole person (body, mind and spirit) require an understanding of the relationship between, and the contribution of, various body regions, systems, thoughts, beliefs, and social behaviors or contexts that are ultimately manifesting as cognitive, emotional or sensorial dissonance or altered performance.

One of the brilliant breakthroughs that the book presents is the organized assessment to identify the primary drivers (body regions) to more effectively manage physical problems.

Chapter 4 Individualized treatment program

The goal of treatment is to motivate a change in the patient's physical, cognitive and emotional behavior to improve the strategies they use for function and well-being.

Treatment is presented as an integrated system of manual therapy, motor facilitation, releases for the neural and dural systems, and a home program in a biopsychosocial model.

Chapter 5 Case reports on the relationship of the thorax to the whole body

Well-organized and presented case studies illuminate the concepts of the integrated approach.

Chapter 6 Release techniques for system impairments

This great chapter which presents a step by step approach to treatment techniques begins with the following overview:

The Integrated Systems Model (ISM) helps the clinician to organize all the information from the assessment to develop prescriptive, individual treatment programs. The ISM acronym for treatment is RACM: Release, Align, Connect and Control, Move. ISM treatment is initially directed toward the driver or drivers and each session contains components of techniques, exercises, and education to release and align the driver (region of the body that when corrected has the biggest impact on the function of other regions).

Chapter 7 Motor learning and movement training

The final chapter wraps up the treatment approach with progressive training of the motor system (motor control)

and includes movement training exercises drawn from yoga and Pilates. Diane opens with the following paragraph:

The final and critical part of each treatment session is to train better strategies for function and performance, which requires motor learning and movement training. The aim is to build and use new and better 'brain maps' and movement strategies that share loads and control excessive canister pressures (cranial, thoracic, abdominal, pelvic) in a way that sustains tissue structure, blood flow and drainage, function, and overall health.

This is a ground-breaking text that can significantly contribute to the physical therapy profession.

The following quote says a lot about the author:

Every patient has a story to tell and it is a privilege to be given the opportunity to listen to that story and to try to illuminate a path to change that will result in improved quality of life.

Gregory S. Johnson PT, FFMT, FAAOMPT
Co-Director & Co-Founder, Institute of Physical Art, Inc.
Vice President, Functional Manual Therapy Foundation
Director, FMT Fellowship Program
Colorado, USA
2018

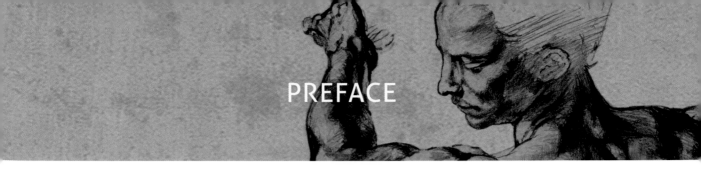

PREFACE

It has been over 30 years since Erl Pettman introduced the 'Quadrant Approach' for assessment and treatment of musculoskeletal disorders (Pettman 1981, 1984). This approach considered in part how suboptimal movement patterns, or biomechanics, of the thorax contributed to a wide variety of pain states and altered function of the neck, jaw, low back, shoulder girdle, and upper and lower extremities. Pettman's Quadrant Approach inspired the clinical enquiry, that continues today, of the role of the thorax in multiple conditions. Many Canadian physio therapists have contributed to the clinical knowledge and expertise highlighted in this text including Erl Pettman, Cliff Fowler, John Oldham, Janet Lowcock, Carol Kennedy, Laurie McLaughlin, Linda-Joy Lee, Cathy Rogers, Calvin Wong, Tamarah Nerreter and myself.

Today we understand that the thorax is part of many integrated and interdependent systems, including the musculoskeletal, neurological, respiratory, cardiovascular, digestive, and urogynecological systems. As such, it should not be considered in isolation from the rest of the body, but rather in relation to it. Sueki et al. (2013) refer to this as regional interdependence, a concept that suggests 'the function and health of one region of the body could potentially affect the function of another' and note this concept is not novel. In Canada, this has been the fundamental principle of our national, postgraduate, orthopedic manual therapy education for over 40 years. Recently, I have taught an integrated systems approach to the thorax under the name, the Integrated Systems Model (ISM) (Lee D 2011, Lee L-J & Lee D 2011). The ISM is an evolving, evidence-informed, clinical reasoning, biopsychosocial approach. While the focus of this text will be on the thorax, its relationship to the rest of the body and person will become clear through the long and short case reports throughout the text. The emphasis in this text is on the biocomponent of a biopsychosocial model and the psychological and social factors to be considered on an individual basis are recognized.

I am a clinician, educator and life-long student. I have learned from every mentor, associate, instructor and patient who has crossed my path and for that I am truly grateful. I am a synthesizer and knowledge translator. I enjoy reading chapter compilations of research (rather than the original studies, but I do read them) and testing proposed theories and evidence in the clinic. The clinic is my laboratory, my truth. Manual therapy, education and exercise have long been used to help those with musculoskeletal pain and the mechanisms as to 'how they work, or not,' have evolved over the 40 years I've been in clinical practice. I admit that I do not need to know the mechanisms, or exactly why someone is getting better; it is often more complex than can be simply explained. One thing is clear though, each patient is an individual and no single modality approach offers all the answers for everyone. Determining what to offer to whom is the current research challenge, and has long been the clinical one. Every patient has a story to tell and it is a privilege to be given the opportunity to listen to that story and to try to illuminate a path to change that will result in improved quality of life.

Diane Lee BSR, FCAMT, CGIMS
Lead Instructor, Learn with Diane Lee
Adjunct Professor, Physical Therapy, Faculty of Medicine, University of British Columbia,
Diane Lee & Associates, South Surrey, BC, Canada
2018

www.learnwithdianelee.com

ACKNOWLEDGMENTS

In addition to being grateful to every individual from whom I've learned anything, there are those who directly contributed to the content of this book and deserve my thanks. Frank Crymble (medical illustrator) has drawn images to explain the biomechanics of the thorax for me since 1993 and is always willing to take on another project for visual learners. He is responsible for all the biomechanical drawings in this text. Some are new, many are almost 25 years old. In 1994, he did the pencil drawing we have used for the cover of this book. Thank you, Frank, for your patience and willingness to go back to the digital drawing board and 'get it just right.'

Special thanks are due to Linda-Joy Lee (LJ). LJ and I worked together clinically from 1999 to 2004, and taught together from the early 2000s until 2013. We co-developed the Integrated Systems Model and many of the ISM-specific terms used in this text come from our hours of discussions. LJ's PhD focused on motor control in the thorax, her scientific work is included in this text and referenced appropriately. However, several of her novel, unpublished clinical concepts and techniques are also included in this text (Lee L-J 2004–2013). I have done my best to reference, and acknowledge, her clinical contributions within this work, and thank her immensely for our learning, and time, together.

Melanie Coffey-Prentice, Noelle Trotter, Jill Irvine, Tamarah Nerreter, Kjersti Malinsky, Chelsea Lee, and Leigh Fortuna volunteered to be models for several photo shoots that have spanned two-and-a-half decades. Thank you for all the hours of modeling and the many things I put you through – I have drawn from my extensive inventory of photos for this text. Stephen Scheibel masterfully captured many new photos for this text and not one edit was required after the proofs were received. It is truly a delight to work with Stephen, Lawrence Weiss, and their company, Info2Grow, which developed my online education platform: www.learnwithdianelee.com.

While my postgraduate physiotherapy training is primarily in the field of manual therapy and dry needling, I have completed a 200-hour yoga teacher training with Leanne Kitteridge, of Shibui Yoga. I now integrate ISM and yoga for movement training where applicable. My daughter, Chelsea Lee, is also a yoga therapist and integrates ISM principles into all her sessions, and yoga therapy teacher trainings. Yoga is not new, but yoga as therapy, in conjunction with physiotherapy, is. Both Leanne and Chelsea offer yoga therapy in our clinic in South Surrey to bridge the gap between rehab and the community. I'm inspired by how both Chelsea and Leanne work with the physiotherapists at Diane Lee & Associates to create movement programs that get patients back into community classes and more. Chelsea put together the yoga sequences in Chapter 7 originally for my book *Diastasis Rectus Abdominis A Clinical Guide for Those Who Are Split Down the Middle*.

Prior to my yoga training, I was introduced to Pilates by Karen Angelucci, and then collaborated clinically for many years sharing patients with Angela Stevenson. Both Karen and Ange could adapt traditional Pilates 'protocols' and develop movement programs suitable for less abled patients, particularly those with difficulty loading through their thorax or pelvis. Recently, I have met, and now train with, Lori Thompson of Mindful Movement Pilates. I met Lori at a time when I couldn't do yoga anymore due to severe degeneration of my left hip (OA). While preparing for surgery, Lori helped me improve my strength and conditioning, physically, mentally and emotionally through Pilates as well as meditation. A lot of my movement training has come from personal experiences in the gym and in yoga and Pilates studios. You will see these various forms of movement training in Chapter 7.

And now, acknowledgments and thanks to those who helped put this book together. Calvin Wong and Tamarah Nerreter are senior associates at Diane Lee & Associates with special interest in both women's and men's health and have contributed two of their patient's stories to Chapter 5. Thank you so much for highlighting the role of the whole body (including the thorax) on pelvic floor pain and impairments.

Thanks also to the multiple students from the autumn 2017 teaching tour to Europe, USA, Canada and Japan who agreed to share their stories scattered throughout the text. The longer case reports are from patients in our clinic – the place where you really must make a difference, and not just have an opinion. Thank you for granting permission to share your stories.

Gail Wetzler, physiotherapist and director of the Barral Institute of Advanced Manual Therapy, has embraced the ISM approach and has hosted the ISM Series twice (California 2015, Denver 2018). It is always an incredible opportunity for me to learn with her. We consolidated the terminology around 'listening' so that the two approaches (ISM and Visceral) were consistent. I am grateful for her collaboration, open mind and endless curiosity, even when she can 'hear' that vector faster than I can figure it out!

Many thanks to Cathy Rogers, senior associate and senior assistant for the ISM Series. Cathy edited every chapter of this text, offered many ideas for clarity and ensured consistency of language for both ISM and the book. Cathy has a highly organized, GABA brain, and pays phenomenal attention to the details that matter. ISM has evolved, in part, from our discussions in writing, teaching, and co-consulting in the clinic.

And last, but not least, my heartfelt thanks to Mary Law, Andrew Stevenson and the team at Handspring Publishers for putting this all together. Mary and I go back to the very first writing contract I signed for the first edition of *The Pelvic Girdle* published by Elsevier in 1986. Thank you both for believing there was a need for this book, *The Thorax – An Integrated Approach.*

Diane Lee BSR, FCAMT, CGIMS
Lead Instructor, Learn with Diane Lee
Adjunct Professor, Physical Therapy, Faculty of Medicine,
University of British Columbia
Diane Lee & Associates, South Surrey, BC, Canada
2018

www.learnwithdianelee.com

This book includes images and figures that correspond to the materials being discussed. There are times, however, when pictures alone do not convey the entire concept. This is why we have included access to online videos. You can access the videos by scanning a code with a smartphone or tablet, or directly from the website (no special device required).

QR codes

As each video reference is mentioned you will see a QR code that you can scan and be taken straight to the appropriate video. The first step is to make sure you can scan these codes and then to test this you will scan the following code to gain access to the videos.

https://learnwithdianelee.com/
course-code/thx-e7m75HLarR/

iPad or iPhone

If you are using an iPad or iPhone running the latest software (iOS 11 or higher) then no additional app is required. Simply follow these steps to test with the QR code above.

1. Open your camera app.

2. Point it at the code (no need to take a picture).

3. A notification should pop down from the top.

4. Tap that and you will be taken to the access form.

If that works, you're ready! If not, you need an app.

QR scanning app

Not all scanning apps are created equal. Some work better with our website than others. For up to date recommendations on apps that have been tested by our web team please visit https://learnwithdianelee.com/qr-codes/

Follow these steps to get started and try it out:

1. Once the app is installed, open it. The app needs to have access to your camera so click yes or accept.

2. Once the app opens you should see a view similar to when you take a photo. If not, you may need to click Scan.

3. Hold your device over the QR code so that it is clearly visible and in focus within your smartphone's screen.

4. Two things can happen when you correctly hold your smartphone over a QR code:

   • The phone automatically scans the code.

   • On some readers, you have to press a button to snap a picture, not unlike the button on your smartphone camera.

5. After a successful scan your mobile web browser should open to a page on the Learn with Diane Lee website.

Creating an account

The online videos are only accessible to those who have purchased this book. In order to access them you need to first set up an account on the Learn with Diane Lee website and use a special code to gain access to the videos.

To do this, scan the QR code above or type the associated link into a web browser. Careful with capital letters as this is case sensitive. If you already have an account you still need to scan the code or visit the link. From there you can sign in and the form data will populate itself.

Website

You can use the QR codes, the website or a combination of both. To access the videos on the website you still need to create an account on the Learn with Diane Lee website (or log in if you already have one). You must visit the previous link to get access to the videos (it is case sensitive so please copy it exactly).

Once you fill out the information and submit you will find *The Thorax* videos listed as a 'course under courses' in your profile menu (top right).

Support

If you experience problems signing up or accessing the materials please visit https://learnwithdianelee.com/help/ and fill out the support form at the bottom of the page.

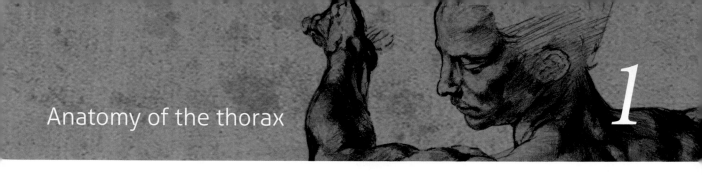

Note to reader: The main anatomical information for this chapter comes from the 40th edition of *Gray's Anatomy* (Standring 2008). When content comes from an alternate source it is referenced accordingly.

The thorax contributes approximately 20 per cent to the overall length of the body compared to 12 per cent from the lumbar spine and 8 per cent from the cervical spine. While the anatomy of the thorax is highly variable between individuals, there are general similarities that are fundamental to understanding the biomechanics, assessment, and treatment of this large part of the trunk and body. There are four regions of the thorax, differentiated by the anatomy and consequential biomechanics: the vertebromanubrial, vertebrosternal, vertebrochondral, and thoracolumbar (Fig. 1.1A & B). Except for the thoracolumbar, each region is comprised of a variable number of thoracic rings (Fig. 1.2).

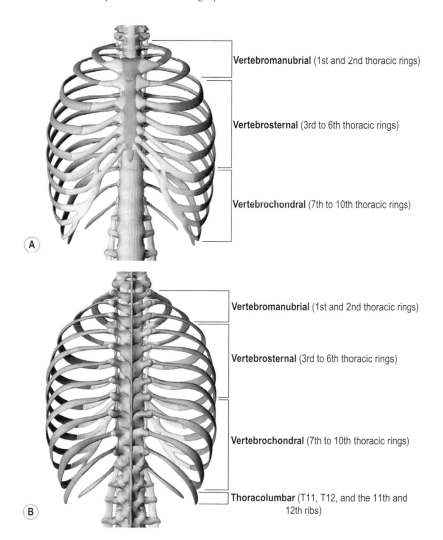

Vertebromanubrial (1st and 2nd thoracic rings)

Vertebrosternal (3rd to 6th thoracic rings)

Vertebrochondral (7th to 10th thoracic rings)

(A)

Vertebromanubrial (1st and 2nd thoracic rings)

Vertebrosternal (3rd to 6th thoracic rings)

Vertebrochondral (7th to 10th thoracic rings)

Thoracolumbar (T11, T12, and the 11th and 12th ribs)

(B)

Figure 1.1

(A) Three regions of the thorax are evident from the anterior aspect; the vertebromanubrial (upper thoracic rings 1 and 2), the vertebrosternal (middle thoracic rings 3 to 6) and the vertebrochondral (lower thoracic rings 7 to 10). (B) The fourth region, the thoracolumbar, does not contain 'rings' since the 11th and 12th ribs do not attach to the sternum.

Reproduced from Essential Anatomy 5 3D4Medical with permission.

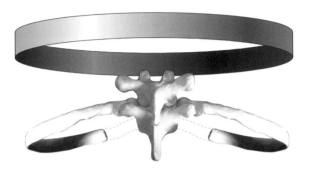

Figure 1.2

A thoracic ring as defined by Lee (Lee D 1994) consisting of the left and right ribs of the same number, the inferior half of the top vertebra and the superior half of the bottom vertebra, the left and right costocartilages, and the manubrium or sternum. There are 13 joints in each typical thoracic ring.

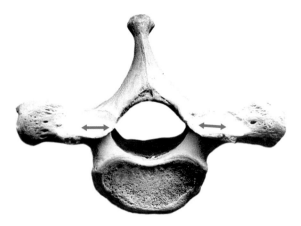

Figure 1.3

The superior aspect of the 1st thoracic vertebra. The zygapophyseal joints lie in the coronal plane.

A thoracic ring (Lee D 1994) is derived from one embryological somite which divides into a sclerotome, myotome and dermatome, and consists of the following:

- Left and right ribs which are derived from the costal element of two adjacent sclerotomes (one half from each).

- Adjacent thoracic vertebrae and the intervening intervertebral discs. Each thoracic vertebra develops from two adjacent sclerotomes; therefore, the proper definition of a thoracic ring would include the inferior half of the superior vertebra and the superior half of the inferior vertebra and the intervening intervertebral disc to which these two ribs attach.

- Left and right costocartilages.

- Manubrium or sternum.

Therefore, the 4th thoracic ring consists of the left and right 4th ribs and the associated costocartilages, the bottom half of the 3rd and the top half of the 4th thoracic vertebrae, and the sternum. Because the ribs in the thoracolumbar region do not attach anteriorly to the sternum, they are not considered part of a thoracic ring.

Regions and osteology of the thorax

Vertebromanubrial region

There are two thoracic rings in the vertebromanubrial region (upper thorax) and both have a direct attachment to the manubrium. This region contains the 1st and 2nd thoracic vertebrae, the 1st and 2nd ribs, and the manubrium.

The 1st thoracic vertebra has a large, nonbifid spinous process and the superior aspect of this process is in the same transverse plane as the T1–T2 zygapophyseal joints (Fig. 1.1B). The facets on the superior articular processes, which articulate with C7, are in the coronal plane (Fig. 1.3) while those on the inferior articular process, which articulate with T2, present a slight curve in both the transverse and sagittal planes (Fig. 1.4). The transverse processes of T1 are long and thick and are located between the superior and inferior articular processes at the dorsal aspect of the pedicle. On the ventral aspect of each transverse process there is a deep concave facet which articulates with a convex facet on the 1st rib to form the 1st costotransverse joint (Fig. 1.5). In the normal upright posture, the orientation of this joint is anteroinferior.

The superior aspect of the vertebral body of T1 is concave in the coronal plane (Fig. 1.5). This concavity is formed by the uncinate process at each posterolateral corner of the

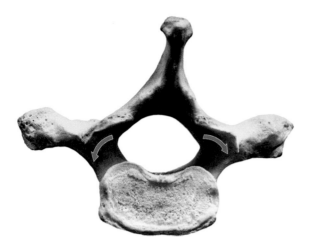

Figure 1.4

The inferior aspect of the 1st thoracic vertebra. The zygapophyseal joints are gently convex in both the transverse and sagittal planes. The ventral aspect of the transverse process contains a concave facet for articulation with the 1st rib.

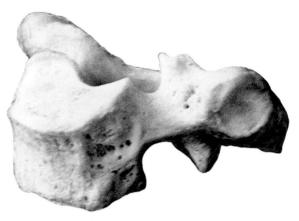

Figure 1.5

Anterolateral view of the 1st thoracic vertebra. The uncinate process at each posterolateral corner creates a concavity on the superior aspect of the vertebral body. There is a full facet at the superolateral aspect of the vertebral body for the head of the 1st rib. A demifacet on the inferolateral aspect of the vertebral body articulates with the head of the 2nd rib in the 2nd decade of life. Note the concave facet on the transverse process for articulation with the 1st rib.

vertebral body. These processes articulate with the inferior aspect of the body of C7 to form a nonsynovial, uncovertebral joint. There are two ovoid facets on either side of the vertebral body for articulation with the head of the 1st rib. The inferior aspect of the vertebral body of T1 is flat and contains a small facet at each posterolateral corner for articulation with the head of the 2nd rib (Fig. 1.4). This articulation is incomplete until early adolescence when a secondary ossification center appears to complete the formation of the head of the rib. In children, the head of the 2nd rib only articulates with T2.

The 1st rib (Figs 1.1A, Fig. 1.6) is the shortest and broadest at its anterior end. The 1st sternochondral joint is unique in that it is fibrous rather than synovial. The 1st costocartilage is the shortest and this, together with the fibrous sternochondral joint, contributes to passive control (form closure) of the 1st thoracic ring. The convex head of the 1st rib articulates with the body of T1 at the costovertebral joint. The neck of the rib is located between the head and the tubercle. The articular portion of the tubercle is convex and directed posterosuperiorly when the head and neck are in the normal upright posture (Fig. 1.1B). The 2nd

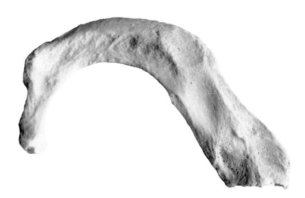

Figure 1.6

Superior aspect of the 1st rib.

rib is approximately twice the length of the 1st and its features are like the vertebrosternal region described below. Anteriorly, the costocartilage of the 2nd thoracic ring articulates with both the manubrium and the sternum at the manubriosternal symphysis (Fig. 1.1A).

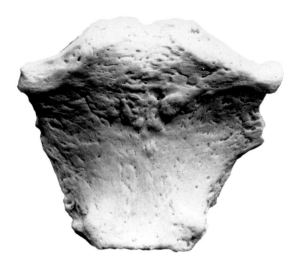

Figure 1.7

The manubrium. Note the shallow concave surface for articulation with the clavicles.

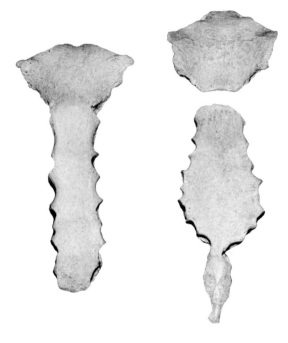

Figure 1.8

The manubriosternal symphysis is usually maintained through life; however, ossification can occur. The eight full concave facets articulate with the costocartilages of the 3rd to 6th ribs.

The manubrium (Fig. 1.7) is a broad triangular shaped bone, which articulates with the clavicles and the costocartilage of the 1st and 2nd ribs. The manubriosternal symphysis remains separate throughout life although ossification can occur (Fig. 1.8).

Vertebrosternal region

The vertebrosternal region (middle thorax) contains the thoracic rings that attach directly and individually to the sternum. The costotransverse joints in this region have a concavo-convex orientation. This region includes the bottom half of the 2nd thoracic vertebra to the top half of the 6th thoracic vertebra, the 3rd to 6th ribs, and the sternum.

The vertebrosternal vertebrae have long, thin, overlapping spinous processes. The tip of the spinous process can be three finger widths inferior to the transverse process of the same vertebra and frequently deviates from the midline. The facets on both the superior and inferior articular processes present a slight curve in both the transverse and sagittal planes (Fig. 1.9). This orientation permits multidirectional movement. A model of the zygapophyseal joints can be simulated by placing two circular bowls inside one another (Fig. 1.10). The top bowl can rotate forward, backward, sideways, and around the bottom bowl. Translation of the top bowl meets immediate resistance. The coronal orientation of the superior articular processes resists posteroanterior translation of the superior vertebra on the vertebra below.

The transverse processes, located at the dorsal aspect of the pedicle between the superior and inferior articular processes, are ideally situated for palpation of intervertebral joint motion. In this region, the ventral aspect of the transverse process contains a deep, concave facet for articulation with the rib of the same number (Fig. 1.11). This curvature (Fig. 1.12) influences the conjunct rotation that occurs when the rib glides in a superoinferior direction (see Costal arthrokinematics in Chapter 2). In the normal upright posture, the orientation of the facet on the transverse process is anterolateral.

The posterolateral corners of both the superior and inferior aspects of the vertebral body contain an ovoid

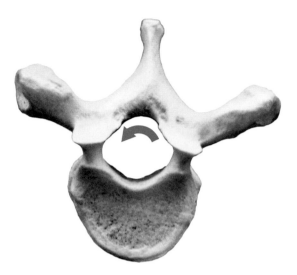

Figure 1.9

The superior aspect of the 4th thoracic vertebra. The zygapophyseal joint is gently convex in both the transverse and sagittal planes. The ventral aspect of the transverse process contains a concave facet for articulation with the 4th rib.

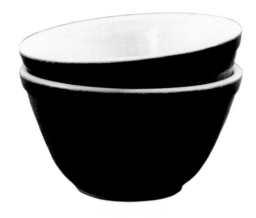

Figure 1.10

Two mixing bowls model the potential biomechanics of the zygapophyseal joints in the thorax.

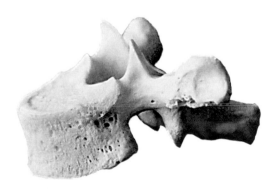

Figure 1.11

Anterolateral view of the 4th thoracic vertebra. Note the concave facet on the transverse process for articulation with the 4th rib as well as the two demifacets on the lateral aspect of the vertebral body for articulation with the heads of the 4th and 5th ribs.

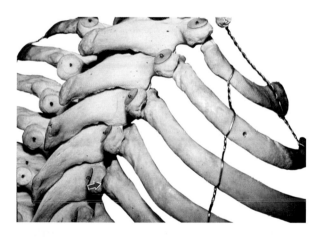

Figure 1.12

Posterolateral view of the articulated thorax in the vertebrosternal region. Note the curvature of the costotransverse joint in this region (arrow).

demifacet for articulation with the head of the rib. Development of the superior costovertebral joint is delayed until early adolescence accounting for the flexibility of the young thorax. The shaft of the rib is long and thin and twists to a variable degree at the posterior angle (Fig. 1.13).

The sternum (Figs 1.1A, 1.8) has eight full concave facets which articulate with the costocartilages of the 3rd to 6th ribs. Superiorly, the 2nd rib (part of the vertebromanubrial region) articulates with the sternum at a demifacet; inferiorly, the 7th rib (part of the vertebrochondral region) articulates with both the xyphoid and the sternum.

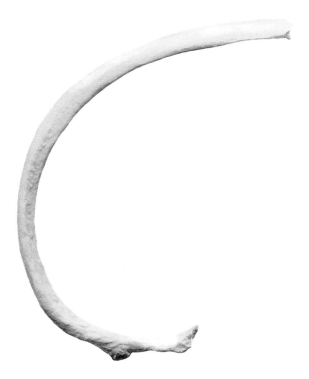

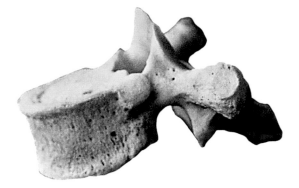

Figure 1.14

Anterolateral view of the 8th thoracic vertebra. Note the planar facet on the transverse process for articulation with the 8th rib as well as the large superior demifacet for articulation with the head of the 8th rib and the small demifacet for articulation with the head of the 9th rib.

Figure 1.13

The 4th rib. Note the convex articular tubercle, which articulates with the concave facet on the transverse process to form the costotransverse joint.

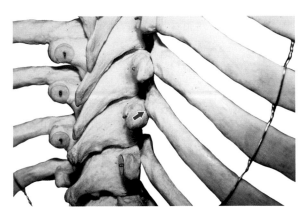

Figure 1.15

Posterolateral view of the articulated thorax, vertebrochondral region. Note the planar orientation of the 9th costotransverse joint (arrow).

Vertebrochondral region

All thoracic rings in this region (lower thorax) have an indirect attachment to the sternum via a common cartilaginous bar (Fig. 1.1A). The bottom half of the 6th to the 10th thoracic vertebrae, and the 7th to 10th ribs are included in the vertebrochondral region.

The vertebrae in this region (Fig. 1.14) (T7, T8, T9, T10) differ from those in the vertebrosternal region. The spinous process is shorter, although still directed inferiorly such that the tip lies close to the transverse plane of the transverse processes of the inferior vertebra (Fig. 1.1B). The facet on the transverse process is flat and faces anterolaterally and superiorly (Fig. 1.15). Therefore, when the tubercle of the rib glides superiorly, it also glides posteromedially with minimal conjunct rotation (Fig. 1.16). When the tubercle of the rib glides inferiorly, it also glides anterolaterally following the plane of the costotransverse joint (see Costal arthrokinematics in Chapter 2). The orientation of the facet for the costotransverse joint accommodates greater loading from the upper limb and thorax (Singer & Goh 2000). At both T2 (vertebromanubrial region) and T5 (vertebrosternal region), the facet on the transverse process faces anteroinferiorly when the thorax is viewed in a normal upright posture. At T9 (vertebrochondral region), the facet on the transverse process faces superolaterally such that the rib rests on top of the transverse process (Fig. 1.15).

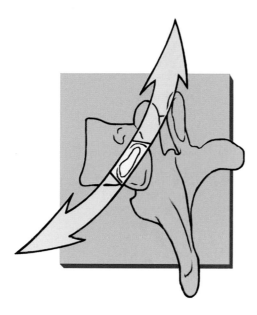

Figure 1.16

The direction of the arthrokinematic glide of the rib relative to the transverse process in the vertebrochondral region. This direction is posteromediosuperior and occurs when the rib anteriorly rotates and anterolateroinferior when the rib posteriorly rotates.

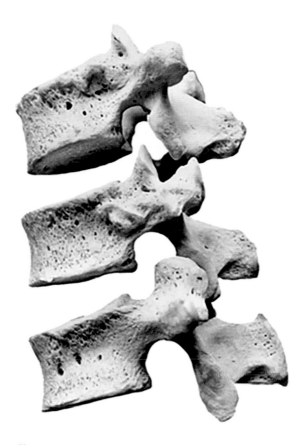

Figure 1.17

The 11th and 12th thoracic and the 1st lumbar vertebrae. Note the orientation of the zygapophyseal joints.

T7, T8 and T9 have four demifacets on the vertebral body for articulation with the head of the 7th, 8th and 9th ribs. T10 is variable. Often, there is only a small articulation between the superior aspect of the head of the 10th rib and the inferior aspect of the vertebral body of T9. Occasionally, the 10th rib will articulate only with T10 at the base of the pedicle via an unmodified ovoid joint.

Anteriorly, the 8th to 10th ribs articulate indirectly with the sternum via a series of cartilaginous bars which blend to attach to the xyphoid and sternum (Fig. 1.1A). There are a variable number of synovial joints between the costocartilages (interchondral joints) and this arrangement permits greater flexibility for motion coupling in this region of the thorax.

Thoracolumbar region

The thoracolumbar region (Fig. 1.1B) is the lowest part of the thorax and includes the 11th and 12th vertebrae and the 11th and 12th ribs. These ribs do not attach directly to the sternum.

The T11 and T12 spinous processes are short, stout, and contained entirely within the lamina of their own vertebrae (Fig. 1.17). The facets on the articular processes of T11 (Fig. 1.18) resemble those of both the vertebrosternal and vertebrochondral regions. The facets on the inferior articular process of T12 resemble the lumbar region. They have a coronal and sagittal component and when articulated with L1 restrict axial rotation. The orientation of T11–T12 does not restrict axial rotation.

Laterally, the transverse processes are small tubercles (Fig. 1.19) and the mammillary processes are larger and more superficial. The spinous process is a more reliable point for palpating intervertebral motion in this region.

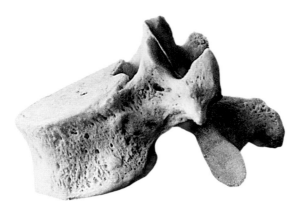

Figure 1.18

Lateral view of the 12th thoracic vertebra. Note the change in direction of the facets on the superior and inferior articular processes. There is one facet on the lateral aspect of the vertebral body for articulation with the head of the 12th rib. There is no facet on the small transverse process, there is no costotransverse joint.

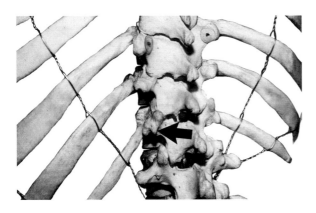

Figure 1.19

The transverse processes of the 12th thoracic vertebrae are small tubercles (arrow) and cannot be used for palpating intervertebral motion.

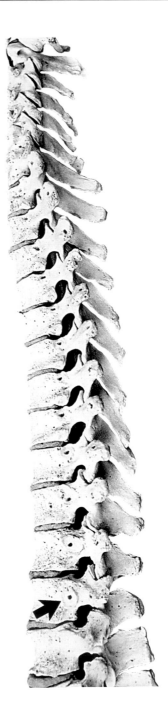

Figure 1.20

Lateral view of the thoracic spine. Note the unmodified ovoid facet for the head of the 12th rib (arrow).

The heads of the 11th and 12th ribs articulate only with the vertebral body at the base of the pedicle via an unmodified ovoid joint (Fig. 1.20). There is no costotransverse joint in this region. The ribs do not have a neck and do not twist significantly. They remain detached from the rest of the thorax anteriorly (Fig. 1.1B) and provide attachment for

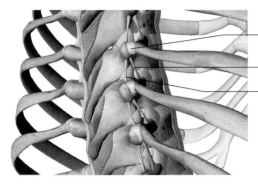

Lateral costotransverse ligament

Superior costotransverse ligament

Intertransverse ligament

Figure 1.21

The ligaments of the costotransverse joint: the lateral costotransverse, superior costotransverse and intertransverse.

Reproduced from Essential Anatomy 5 3D4Medical with permission.

the diaphragm and trunk musculature. The shape of the costovertebral joint facilitates multidirectional movement of the vertebral body even when the large muscles contract and fix the 11th and 12th ribs. The 11th segment (T11, T12, 11th ribs) is the most flexible in the thorax.

Assessment and treatment of the thoracolumbar region is more related to the lumbar spine than the rest of the thorax and will not be included in this text other than to describe the landmarking.

Arthrology of the thorax

Zygapophyseal joints

The zygapophyseal joints of the thorax are synovial and, like other synovial joints, contain small intra-articular folds comprised of fibrous or fibro-fatty tissue (Giles & Singer 2000). These folds originate medially from within the joint space and extend a variable distance into the joint cavity. The capsule of the zygapophyseal joint is supported by the ligamentum flavum medially and the rotatores muscle laterally (Bogduk 1997). The deepest fibers of the rotatores insert directly into the joint capsule.

Costal joints

The costotransverse joints are synovial and contain small intra-articular folds (Giles & Singer 2000). The lateral costotransverse ligament (Fig. 1.21) supports the lateral aspect of the joint and is transversely oriented. It attaches to the tip of the transverse process and inserts into the nonarticular portion of the tubercle of the rib. The superior costotransverse ligament has a variable number of bands that run in a superoinferior direction from the inferior aspect of the transverse process to the neck of the rib below.

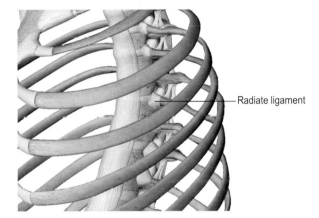

Radiate ligament

Figure 1.22

The radiate ligament of the costovertebral joint.

Reproduced from Essential Anatomy 5 3D4Medical with permission.

The neurovascular elements of the thoracic segment emerge between the bands of this ligament and can be compromised when a thoracic ring is held in a translated and rotated position (see Axial rotation of the trunk in Chapter 2).

The 2nd to 9th, and variably the 10th, costovertebral joints are divided into two synovial cavities; each cavity is separated by an intra-articular ligament. The capsule is supported by the radiate ligament (Fig. 1.22) which has fibers extending from the head of the rib both anteriorly and posteriorly to blend with the vertebral body of the level above, the intervertebral disc, and the vertebral body of the level below. The costotransverse ligament connects the neck of the rib to the ventral aspect of the adjacent transverse process. The 1st, 11th and 12th, and sometimes the

10th, costovertebral joints contain a single facet located at the base of the pedicle. They are essentially unmodified ovoid in shape.

Except for the 1st joint, the sternocostal joints are all synovial. The lateral costochondral joints are fibrous and the periosteum and perichondrium are continuous with one another. The 2nd sternocostal joint has two joint cavities (one part of the cartilage attaching to the manubrium and the other to the sternum) and is separated by an intra-articular ligament.

Intervertebral discs

The intervertebral discs of the thoracic spine are narrower than those in the cervical and lumbar regions and constitute approximately one-sixth of the length of the thoracic vertebral column. Since the ratio of the height of the disc to the vertebral body is 1:5, motion between the segments of the thorax is small. There is a linear increase in the cross-sectional area of the disc in the lower thorax reflecting an increase in the weight-bearing function of these levels.

Manubriosternal symphysis

The joint between the manubrium and the sternum is complex. The bones are covered by hyaline cartilage and the two surfaces joined by fibrocartilage that may ossify later in life (Fig. 1.8) (Ehara 2010).

Sternoclavicular joint

The sternoclavicular joint contains a circular intra-articular disc that divides the joint connecting the medial end of the clavicle to the manubrium into two compartments. The medial end of the clavicle is convex in the craniocaudal plane and much larger than the concave surface of the manubrium. The inferior part of the medial end of the clavicle also articulates with the costocartilage of the 1st rib. The manubrium and the medial end of the clavicle are covered with a fibrin-infused hyaline cartilage, which makes this joint well suited for compression loading. Several ligaments provide passive control for the joint including the interclavicular ligament, capsular (superior) ligament, and the costoclavicular ligaments.

Myology of the thorax

The muscles of the thorax can be divided into deep and superficial. In general, the deeper muscles of the posterior thorax are segmental and thought to play a significant role in controlling motion and/or informing about motion between the thoracic rings. The superficial muscles of the thorax tend to span several segments and function to move the thorax relative to the lumbar spine, pelvis, and hip. Recruitment strategies of the deep and superficial muscles of the thorax are task dependent (Lee L-J et al. 2005, 2009, 2011).

Deeper muscles of the thorax

The deeper muscles relevant to the thorax include the transversus thoracis, transversus abdominis, diaphragm, rotatores thoracis, multifidus, levator costarum brevis and longus, and the internal and external intercostal muscles.

Transversus thoracis

This muscle is just beneath the sternum arising from its lower third, the xyphoid process, and the costocartilages of the 6th to 3rd ribs (Fig. 1.23A & B). The fibers diverge to insert into the lower borders of the costocartilages of the 2nd to 6th ribs. The lower fibers are horizontal and continuous with the uppermost fibers of the transversus abdominis and the diaphragm. The obliquity of the fiber orientation increases such that the uppermost fibers are almost vertical.

Transversus abdominis

The transversus abdominis (Figs 1.24, 1.25) is the deepest of the lateral abdominal muscles and arises bilaterally from the thoracolumbar fascia via the common transversus abdominis tendon (Fig. 1.26) (Schuenke et al. 2012), the anterior three-quarters of the inner lip of the iliac crest, the costocartilage of the lower six ribs (interdigitating with the diaphragm), and the lateral third of the inguinal ligament. The upper and middle fibers are oriented transversely and become aponeurotic to form the dorsal sheath of the rectus abdominis above the infraumbilical transition region and then the intermediate zone of the linea alba (Axer et al. 2001a, 2001b). Below the transition region, the aponeurosis of the lower fibers of the transversus abdominis

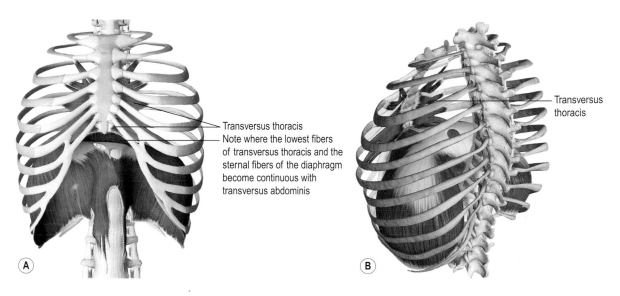

Transversus thoracis
Note where the lowest fibers of transversus thoracis and the sternal fibers of the diaphragm become continuous with transversus abdominis

Transversus thoracis

(A)

(B)

Figure 1.23 A & B

The transversus thoracis is located inside the skeletal thorax. The lowest fibers are continuous with the transversus abdominis and the diaphragm.

Reproduced from Essential Anatomy 5 3D4Medical with permission.

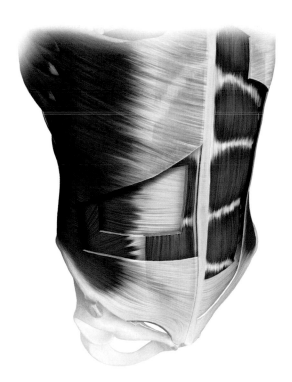

Figure 1.24

The abdominal wall. Note the orientation of the muscular fibers in each layer. The external oblique muscle fibers run inferior, anterior and medial interdigitating with the serratus anterior laterally. The aponeurosis of the external oblique passes anterior to the rectus abdominis forming part of the rectus sheath and then the linea alba. The internal oblique runs superior and medial, the posterior fibers attach to the 11th and 12th ribs, the aponeurosis of the intermediate portion splits to contribute to both the ventral and dorsal rectus sheaths as well as the linea alba. The most anterior fibers that arise from the inguinal ligament (not visible in this drawing) run horizontally and the aponeurosis passes ventral to the rectus abdominis contributing only to the ventral sheath. The deepest lateral abdominal is the transversus abdominis. The fibers run transversely and the aponeurosis passes dorsally to the rectus abdominis forming the dorsal rectus sheath and then the linea alba. The rectus abdominis is contained within the aponeuroses of the lateral abdominals and connected to each other via the linea alba.

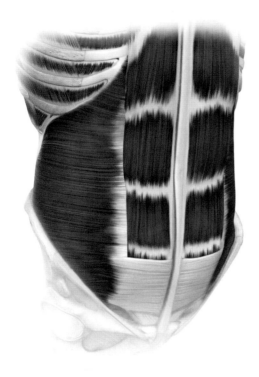

Figure 1.25

The transversus abdominis (TrA) is the deepest abdominal and plays an important role in increasing fascial tension both anteriorly and posteriorly as well as increasing intra-abdominal pressure – two mechanisms known to enhance lumbopelvic control. The fascial connections of TrA link it to the pelvic floor, quadratus lumborum, the erector spinae, and the diaphragm.

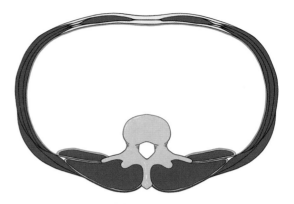

Figure 1.26

Note the continuity of the aponeuroses of the lateral abdominals to the anterior and posterior muscles of the trunk.

contributes to the ventral sheath of the rectus abdominis (along with the aponeurosis of the external oblique and internal oblique) before forming the intermediate zone of the linea alba (Fig. 1.27A–C). These lower fibers of the transversus abdominis curve inferomedially together with the internal oblique to form the inguinal ligament.

The fascial envelopes of these three layers of lateral abdominal muscles (external oblique, internal oblique, and transversus abdominis) are separated by a thin layer of loose connective tissue that facilitates gliding of the layers with movement and activation (Guimberteau & Armstrong 2015,

Stecco 2015). The three layers are connected by this same fibrillar network that facilitates transference of force both linearly along the length of the aponeuroses and in parallel (Brown & McGill 2009, Guimberteau & Armstrong 2015).

In addition,

'[the] connective tissue supporting the various attachments to the muscles of the anterior abdominal wall take on a complex arrangement that allow them to deform in complex manners, notably simultaneous expansion or contraction along multiple axes, to conform to the different forces acting throughout the system.' (Brown & McGill 2008)

'Some of the force can be transmitted from sarcomere to sarcomere in parallel, and subsequently, through a shear linkage mechanism, outwards through fascial or connective tissue attachments between muscles. Force and stiffness generated by the abdominal wall were reduced when the transverse abdominis aponeurosis was disrupted.' (Brown & McGill 2009)

Urquhart et al. (2005) describe three distinct (although connected) regions of the transversus abdominis: upper, middle, and lower (Fig. 1.28). The upper region is from the 6th costal cartilage to the inferior border of the rib cage; the middle region is between the inferior border of the rib cage and a line connecting the superior borders of the iliac crest; and the lower region from a line connecting

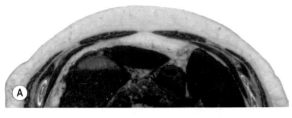

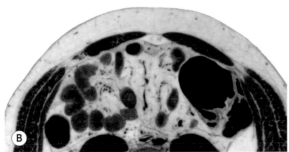

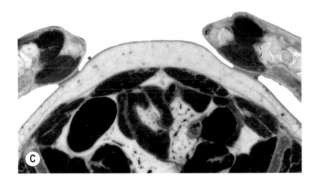

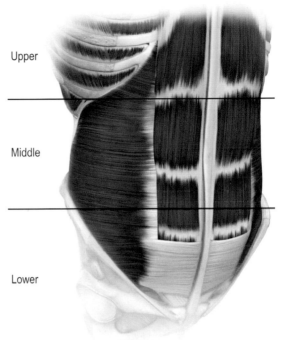

Upper

Middle

Lower

Figure 1.28

The three regions of the transversus abdominis as described by Urquhart et al. (2005).

Figure 1.27

(A) The upper fibers of the transversus abdominis interdigitate with the diaphragm laterally and the aponeuroses form the dorsal rectus sheath. (B) The aponeuroses of the middle fibers of the transversus abdominis form the posterior rectus sheath. The aponeuroses of the internal oblique splits to contribute to both the anterior and posterior rectus sheaths and this anatomy can be variable between sides as is seen here. (C) Below the transition zone of the linea alba the aponeuroses of all three lateral abdominals form the ventral rectus sheath; the posterior rectus sheath is derived only from the transversalis fascia of the parietal peritoneum in this region. Note how narrow the inter-recti distance is in this region.

Reproduced with permission from the Visible Human Project, US National Library of Medicine.

the anterior superior iliac spines and the level of the pubic symphysis. A consistent septum of connective tissue was found that differentiated the upper from the middle and lower regions (Fig. 1.29). Variations in the anatomy of the transversus abdominis were also noted including:

- complete and partial detachment of the transversus abdominis from the iliac crest,

- abrupt change in fascicle orientation between the lower and middle regions,

- absence of fascicles below the iliac crest,

- passage of the iliohypogastric and ilioinguinal nerves through the septa, and

- fusion of the lower fascicles with the internal oblique.

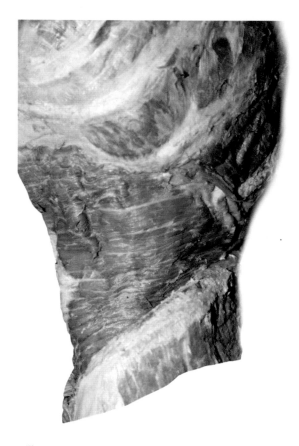

Figure 1.29

Note the connective tissue septum dividing the upper and middle fibers of the transversus abdominis.

Courtesy of Carl DeRosa and Jim Porterfield.

Diaphragm

The diaphragm (Figs 1.23, 1.30, 1.31) separates the thoracic cavity from the abdominal canister and its anatomy and function can impact both compartments. It is comprised of two domes (cupolae), which on forced exhalation ascend as high as the 4th costocartilage on the right and the 5th on the left. On full inhalation, they can descend as much as 10 cm to reach the tip of the 6th rib on the right. The domes are higher in supine lying than in erect standing.

Anatomically, the diaphragm is considered to have three parts: sternal, costal (anterior and posterior), and lumbar.

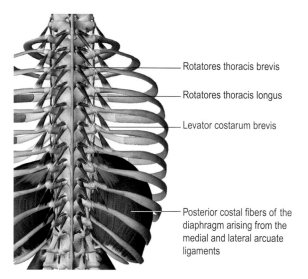

Rotatores thoracis brevis

Rotatores thoracis longus

Levator costarum brevis

Posterior costal fibers of the diaphragm arising from the medial and lateral arcuate ligaments

Figure 1.30

The posterior costal fibers of the diaphragm and the levator costarum brevis. The rotatores thoracis brevis and longus are deep to the multifidus and impossible to distinguish with palpation.

Reproduced from Essential Anatomy 5 3D4Medical with permission.

The sternal portion arises from the back of the xyphoid, and the costal portion arises from the internal surfaces of the lower six costocartilages and ribs and interdigitates with the transversus abdominis in the interval between the sternal and costal origins. The lumbar part arises from the anterior aspect of the lumbar vertebra and the medial and lateral arcuate ligaments that arch over the psoas and the quadratus lumborum. The right lumbar crura descends to L3, the left lumbar crura to L2, and both crura blend with the anterior longitudinal ligament. The medial borders of the left and right crura form an arch that crosses over the aorta, thoracic duct, and lymphatic trunks at the level of the T12–L1 intervertebral disc slightly to the left of midline.

These distal attachments merge to form the central tendon of the diaphragm. The anterior sternal fibers are short and run horizontally. The costal fibers are initially oriented vertically and then curve toward the central tendon. The lateral crural fibers from the lumbar portion diverge to reach the central tendon, while the medial fibers of both sides cross and then encircle the esophagus, gastric nerves,

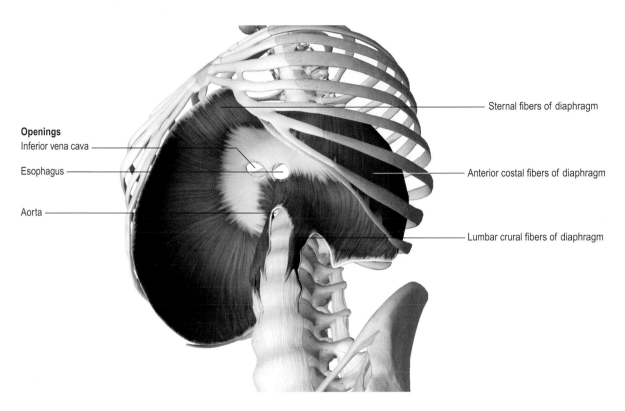

Openings

Inferior vena cava

Esophagus

Aorta

Sternal fibers of diaphragm

Anterior costal fibers of diaphragm

Lumbar crural fibers of diaphragm

Figure 1.31

The diaphragm. Note the location of the apertures for the inferior vena cava, esophagus, and aorta.

Reproduced from Essential Anatomy 5 3D4Medical with permission.

and esophageal vessels forming a sphincter of support at the level of T10. The inferior vena cava, together with some branches of the phrenic nerve, passes through the central tendon at the level of the intervertebral disc between T8 and T9. Although, Pak et al. (2016) note that:

'There were also discrepancies between the Iranian population and commonly-referenced medical textbooks and recent evidence-based literature concerning the vertebral levels of the diaphragmatic openings of the esophagus, aorta, and inferior vena cava. Much of our current knowledge of surface anatomy is based on older studies of cadavers rather than living people, and does not take ethnic and individual variations into consideration.'

The pericardium of the heart is firmly attached to the superior aspect of the diaphragm (Fig. 1.32).

Rotatores thoracis

The eleven pairs of rotatores thoracis brevis and longus (Fig. 1.30) arise from the inferior border and lateral surface of the lamina of the thoracic vertebra and run inferolaterally to insert onto the superoposterior aspect of the base of the transverse process of the subjacent segment (brevis) and two segments below (longus). These muscle fibers attach to the capsule of the zygapophyseal joint.

Levator costarum

The levator costarum brevis (Fig. 1.30) is found from C7 to T11 and arises from the tip of the transverse process. The short fibers pass inferolaterally to insert onto the subjacent rib between the tubercle and the angle; this muscle is segmental. The levator costarum longus is comprised of four muscular slips which arise from the transverse processes

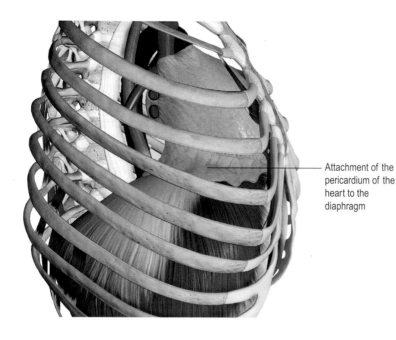

Figure 1.32

The pericardium firmly connects the heart to the diaphragm.

Reproduced from Essential Anatomy 5 3D4Medical with permission.

Attachment of the pericardium of the heart to the diaphragm

of T7, T8, T9, and T10 (vertebrochondral region only). The fibers are longer than those of the levator costarum brevis and pass inferolaterally to insert between the tubercle and angle of the rib two segments below their origin; this muscle is multisegmental.

Multifidus

Multifidus (Fig. 1.33) overlies the rotatores thoracis between the spinous process and the base of the transverse processes. The deepest fibers of multifidus arise from the lateral aspect of the spinous process and pass inferolaterally to attach to the base of the transverse process. These deep fibers are segmental, while the superficial fibers of multifidus span two to four vertebral segments.

All fascicles arising from the spinous process of a given vertebra are innervated by the medial branch of the dorsal ramus of that segment (Bogduk 1997) regardless of the length or depth of the muscle.

Internal and external intercostals

The intercostal muscles (internal and external) (Fig. 1.34A & B) fill the gap between adjacent ribs and although their action is facilitated with expiration (internal) and inspiration (external) respectively (Wilson et al. 2001), their main

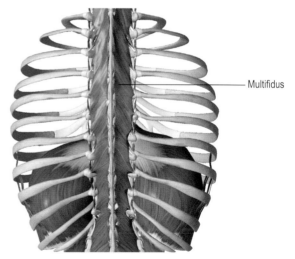

Multifidus

Figure 1.33

The multifidus has deep segmental and superficial multisegmental fibers in the thorax similar to the lumbar region.

Reproduced from Essential Anatomy 5 3D4Medical with permission.

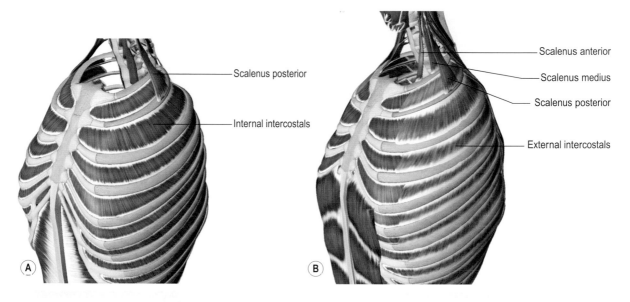

Scalenus posterior

Internal intercostals

Scalenus anterior

Scalenus medius

Scalenus posterior

External intercostals

(A)

(B)

Figure 1.34

(A) The internal intercostals, scalenus posterior, and transversus abdominis. (B) The external intercostals, rectus abdominis, scalenus posterior, scalenus medius, and scalenus anterior.

Reproduced from Essential Anatomy 5 3D4Medical with permission.

function is to stiffen the chest wall during respiration. The internal intercostal muscle lies deep to the external intercostal muscle and arises from the subcostal groove and costal cartilage, and passes inferolaterally and anteriorly, and inferomedially and posteriorly. The external intercostal muscle arises from the lower border of the rib inferolaterally in the posterior aspect of the thorax, and inferomedially in the anterior aspect of the thorax until the costochondral joint. Beyond this point it continues to attach to the sternum as the external intercostal membrane.

Superficial muscles of the anterior thorax

The superficial muscles that influence the functioning of the thorax include the serratus anterior, pectoralis major, pectoralis minor, subclavius, external oblique, internal oblique, and rectus abdominis on the anterior aspect of the thorax, and the semispinalis thoracis, spinalis thoracis, longissimus thoracis, iliocostalis thoracis, and iliocostalis lumborum, serratus posterior superior and serratus posterior inferior on the posterior aspect. These muscles generate torque and function to produce direction-specific movements.

Serratus anterior

The serratus anterior consists of three divisions: upper, middle, and lower (Webb et al. 2018) (Fig. 1.35A–C). The upper fascicles arise from the 1st and 2nd ribs (superior aspect) and attach to the medial and superior borders of the scapula at the superior angle (Fig. 1.35B & C). The middle division arises from the inferior aspect of the 2nd and 3rd ribs and inserts all along the medial border of the scapula (Fig. 1.35B & C). The lower division is comprised of the fascicles arising from the 4th to 8th (9th) ribs and inserts at the inferior angle of the scapula. There are two distinct fascicles that arise from the 2nd rib, the superior fascicle inserts into the superior angle of the scapula while the inferior fascicle inserts into the entire medial border of the scapula.

Pectoralis major

The pectoralis major (Fig. 1.36) covers a large part of the anterior thorax arising from the anterior surface of the medial half of the clavicle. It covers half the width of the anterior manubrium and sternum, the 1st to 7th costocartilages,

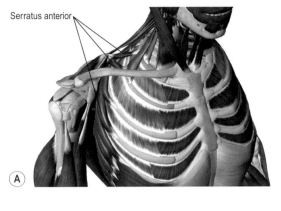

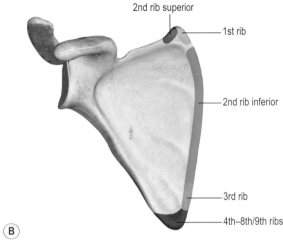

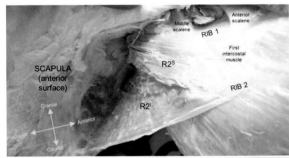

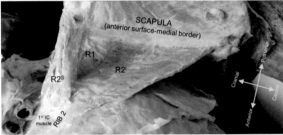

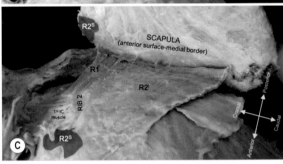

Figure 1.35

The serratus anterior. (A) This muscle arises from nine digitations from the first nine ribs and inserts into the medial border of the scapula. (B) There are two fascicles from the 2nd rib; the superior attaches to the superior angle of the scapula while the inferior inserts along the entire length of the medial border along with the fascicle from the 3rd rib. The fascicles from ribs 4 to 8 (or 9) insert into the inferior angle of the scapula. (C) Dissection of the serratus anterior clearly showing the attachments of the parts of this muscle to the scapula.

(A) is reproduced from Essential Anatomy 5 3D4Medical with permission. (B) and (C) are reproduced from Webb et al. 2018 with the permission of the Japanese Association of Anatomists.

and the aponeurosis of the external oblique. The fibers converge to insert via a flat tendon on the lateral lip of the sulcus of the humerus.

Pectoralis minor

This muscle lies deep to the pectoralis major arising from the upper margins of the 3rd to 5th ribs and from the fascia of the adjacent intercostals (Fig. 1.36). The fibers ascend from this origin to attach to the coracoid process of the scapula.

Subclavius

The subclavius (Fig. 1.37) arises from the junction of the 1st rib with its costocartilage anterior to the costoclavicular ligament. Fibers pass laterally to insert into the undersurface of the middle third of the clavicle.

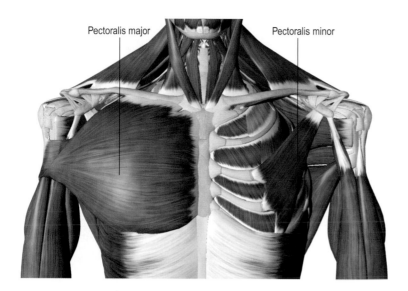

Pectoralis major   Pectoralis minor

Figure 1.36

The pectoralis major. The fascia of this muscle blends with that of the external oblique. The pectoralis minor is deep to the pectoralis major and attaches to the 3rd to 5th ribs.

Reproduced from Essential Anatomy 5 3D4Medical with permission.

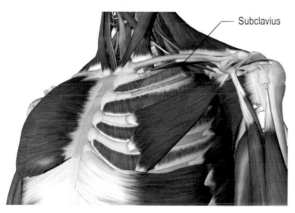

Subclavius

Figure 1.37

The subclavius.

Reproduced from Essential Anatomy 5 3D4Medical with permission.

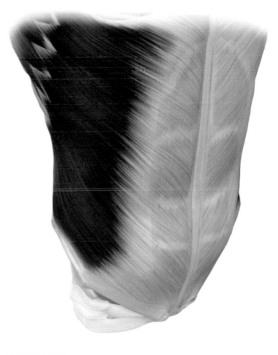

The information below is from the book *Diastasis Rectus Abdominis – A Clinical Guide for Those Split Down the Middle* (Lee D 2017b).

External oblique

The external oblique (Figs 1.24, 1.38) is the most superficial, or external, abdominal muscle on the lateral abdomen and has eight fascicles that arise from the 5th to 12th ribs. The upper attachments of the external oblique arise close

Figure 1.38

The external oblique is part of a continuous myofascial sling that links the neck and thorax to both the ipsilateral and contralateral pelvis through the fascial sheaths and linea alba. It is part of the superficial abdominal wall.

to the costochondral joints, the middle attachments to the body of the ribs and the lowest to the tip of the cartilage of the 12th rib. Bilaterally, the upper five fascicles (from the 5th to 9th ribs) interdigitate with the serratus anterior and thus create a continuous myofascial sling from the abdomen to the scapula. Posteriorly, this sling continues medially via the levator scapulae, rhomboids and middle trapezius muscles to reach the cervical and thoracic spines. The lower three fascicles (from the 10th to 12th ribs) interdigitate with the latissimus dorsi and run almost vertical to insert into the anterior half of the outer lip of the iliac crest. The middle and upper fascicles pass inferiorly, anteriorly and medially (obliquely) and become aponeurotic before contributing to the ventral sheath of the rectus abdominis and from there form the ventral zone of the linea alba (Axer et al. 2001a, 2001b). The aponeurosis of the external oblique forms the inguinal ligament that runs from the anterior superior iliac spine of the ilium to the pubic symphysis, which it crosses to insert on the contralateral side (Stecco 2015).

Internal oblique

The internal oblique (Figs 1.24, 1.39) forms the middle layer of the lateral abdominal wall. It is internal to the external oblique but external to the transversus abdominis. Bilaterally, it arises posteriorly from the thoracolumbar fascia via the common transversus abdominis tendon (Fig. 1.26) (Schuenke et al. 2012), the anterior two-thirds of the iliac crest and the lateral half of the inguinal ligament. The posterior fibers run superiorly and medially to insert on the inferior border of the 12th rib. The intermediate fibers run superomedially, of which some insert on the 11th and 10th ribs while others become aponeurotic. The medial extension of this aponeurosis appears variable in that it splits to contribute to both the ventral and dorsal sheaths of the rectus abdominis in some individuals, whereas in others it only contributes to the ventral sheath. This variation can occur between sides within the same subject. In the midline, the aponeurosis of the internal oblique fuses with that of the external oblique to form the ventral zone of the linea alba (Axer et al. 2001a, 2001b). The most anterior fibers of the internal oblique arise from the inguinal ligament and run horizontally arching inferomedially before becoming

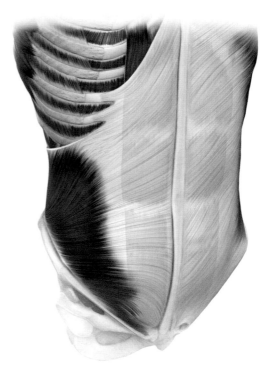

Figure 1.39

The internal oblique is also part of a continuous myofascial sling and although it is an intermediate layer it is considered part of the superficial abdominal wall. Due to its behavior in response to perturbations of the trunk, it is a direction-specific muscle.

aponeurotic to contribute to the ventral sheaths of the rectus abdominis.

Rectus abdominis

The most anterior and superficial abdominal muscle is the rectus abdominis (Figs 1.24, 1.40). Bilaterally, the rectus abdominis arises from the pubic symphysis, crest and tubercle and runs superiorly to attach to the xyphoid and costocartilage of the 5th to 7th ribs. It is contained within the ventral and dorsal rectus sheaths, which are derived from the aponeurosis of the external oblique, internal oblique and transversus abdominis muscles. Below the

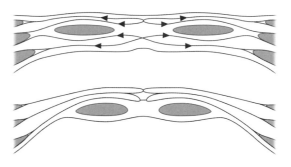

Figure 1.41

Williams (1995) suggests that above the transition zone, the aponeurosis of the transversus abdominis on one side becomes the aponeurosis of the internal oblique on the other. This anatomy is completely inaccurate.

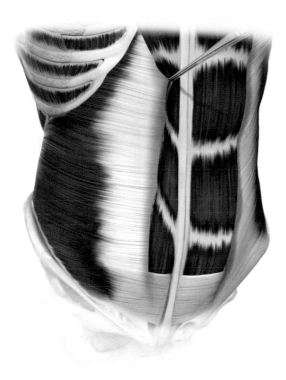

Figure 1.40

The rectus abdominis is divided into eight compartments by three bands of connective tissue.

infraumbilical transition zone, all three aponeuroses pass ventral to the rectus abdominis. Above this zone, the transversus abdominis forms the dorsal, or posterior, rectus sheath and the external oblique forms the ventral, or anterior, rectus sheath. The internal oblique is variable, sometimes splitting to contribute to both sheaths, while other times only contributing to the ventral sheath. There are three bands of connective tissue that traverse both the left and right rectus abdominis dividing it into eight compartments, four on each side.

The anterior fascial connections

The linea alba is commonly described as being formed from the aponeurotic continuations of the transversus abdominis, internal oblique and the external oblique muscles and

Williams (1995) suggests that the aponeurosis of the transversus abdominis blends with that of the internal oblique on the opposite side (Fig. 1.41). Later versions of *Gray's Anatomy* (Standring 2008) continue to suggest that the fibers of the three lateral abdominal aponeuroses: 'decussate anteroposteriorly, crossing from anterior sheath [rectus] to posterior sheath' (Standring 2008). This anatomy has been refuted by Axer et al. (2001a, 2001b) who studied the orientation of the collagen fibers of the medial aspect of the ventral and dorsal rectus sheaths and the linea alba using laser microscopy. While there was some individual variation, a general pattern of fibril orientation was found (Fig. 1.42). Essentially, the linea alba can be divided into three zones in its anteroposterior dimension and four regions in its craniocaudal dimension. Anteroposteriorly, there is a superficial ventral zone of obliquely arranged fibrils, an intermediate zone of transverse fibrils, and a thin dorsal zone of oblique fibrils. Craniocaudally, there are four different regions categorized according to the morphological characteristics of the collagen fibrils. The 1st, or supraumbilical, region has a fibril scheme as shown in Figure 1.43. The 2nd, or umbilical, region has circular collagen fibril bundles around the umbilicus, which interweave with the fibril bundles of the linea alba (Fig. 1.44). The 3rd, or infraumbilical, region is the transition area where oblique fibrils predominate and

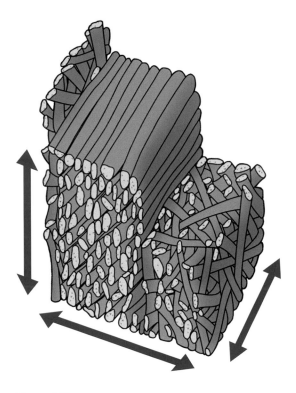

Figure 1.42

The linea alba is a highly organized fibrillar network and is derived from the aponeuroses of the lateral abdominals and the rectus sheaths. The superficial ventral zone of oblique fibers is derived from the aponeuroses of the external oblique and the internal oblique whereas the intermediate zone of transverse fibers comes from the aponeurosis of the transversus abdominis. The deepest dorsal zone is a thin layer of obliquely oriented fibers. This arrangement of fibers provides greater resistance to lateral forces while still permitting elongation in the craniocaudal dimension.

the layer of transverse fibrils is smaller (Fig. 1.45). The transition region corresponds to where the fibril bundles of the dorsal rectus sheath become distributed onto the ventral rectus sheaths. The 4th, or infra-arcuate, region is the most caudal and has the same fibril orientation as the supraumbilical region (Fig. 1.46).

Axer et al. (2001a, 2001b) found that the mean diameter (thickness) of the fibril bundles was smaller in the supraumbilical region (meaning the linea alba was thinner). The authors suggest this may be why primary hernias

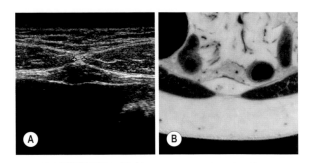

Figure 1.43

The anatomy of the supraumbilical region of the linea alba. The superficial ventral zone is comprised of obliquely arranged fibrils, the intermediate zone of transverse fibrils and the dorsal zone, which is thin and comprised of oblique fibrils. (A) Ultrasound image of the left and right rectus abdominis and linea alba in the supraumbilical region. (B) Transverse plane section of the same region.

(B) is reproduced with permission from the Visible Human Project, US National Library of Medicine.

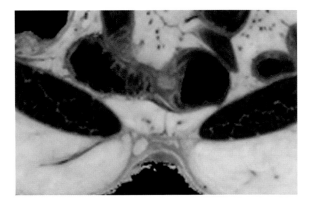

Figure 1.44

The anatomy of the umbilical region of the linea alba. The umbilical region contains circular collagen fibril bundles that interweave with the bundles of the linea alba.

Reproduced with permission from the Visible Human Project, US National Library of Medicine.

are found only in the supraumbilical and umbilical regions of the linea alba and not the infraumbilical region.

There are significant differences between men and women in the number of fibers in the linea alba regionally

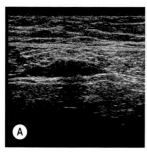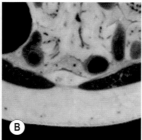

Figure 1.45

The anatomy of the infraumbilical transition zone of the linea alba, which is below the umbilicus and above the infra-arcuate region where all the aponeuroses pass ventral to the rectus abdominis. Anterior obliquely oriented fibrils predominate. The transverse fibril layer is smaller.
(A) Ultrasound image of the linea alba in this region.
(B) Transverse plane section of the same region.

(B) is reproduced with permission from the Visible Human Project, US National Library of Medicine.

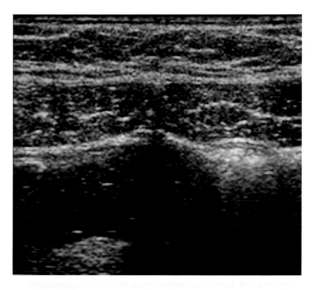

Figure 1.46

Ultrasound image of the anatomy of the infra-arcuate region of the linea alba. This region has the same fibril orientation as the supraumbilical region.

(Gräßel et al. 2005) and in the relative compliance in either of the transverse or oblique plane. Women have more transverse fibers relative to oblique fibers in the infraumbilical region (60.4% vs 39.6%) whereas men have more oblique fibers relative to transverse (62.5% vs 37.5%).

For both sexes, the highest compliance (i.e., least amount of stiffness) of the linea alba is in the longitudinal direction (craniocaudal) and the least (i.e., greatest amount of stiffness) in the transverse direction in the infraumbilical region. On compliance testing, the infraumbilical region of female subjects had the least compliance of all regions in the transverse plane. One female subject in Gräßel et al.'s 2005 study was nulliparous and her fiber orientation distribution and compliance in the transverse plane were like that of the male group. The authors hypothesize that the linea alba adapts to increases in intra-abdominal pressure during pregnancy by increasing both fiber size and number.

The aponeuroses of the external oblique, internal oblique and transversus abdominis muscles form the sheaths that envelop, and compartmentalize, the left and right rectus abominis muscles. Axer et al. (2001a, 2001b) did not investigate the lateral sheaths of the recti; therefore, the fibril orientation of the collagen is unknown here. They did, however, investigate the medial, ventral, and dorsal rectus sheaths and found an interesting orientation of collagen fibrils. Three different regions were described for the medial sheaths of the rectus abdominis: the supraumbilical, transition, and infra-arcuate. In the supraumbilical region, the medial ventral rectus sheath contains mainly obliquely orientated fibril bundles (from the external and internal oblique), which intermingle with each other, while the medial dorsal rectus sheath contains mainly fibrils that are oriented transversely (from the transversus abdominis). They do not note whether the internal oblique aponeurosis splits around the rectus abdominis in this region. In the second region, the transition zone (below the umbilicus), the dorsal transverse bundles from the transversus abdominis begin to move to the ventral side of the rectus sheath. This transition is not sudden but rather occurs over a few centimeters (Axer et al. 2001a, 2001b). In the infra-arcuate region, the dorsal sheath of the rectus contains only a few thin collagen fibers whereas the ventral sheath continuously becomes thicker. Axer et al. suggest that an arcuate line, or linea semicircularis, does not exist and that the line is a zone of transition of fibers with a high degree of variability.

While the work of Axer et al. (2001a, 2001b) and Gräßel et al. (2005) is extremely important, it is critical to note that these studies were done on cadavers and not living tissue. Guimberteau and Armstrong (2015) have shown that living fascia, or connective tissue, is quite different from dead tissue both anatomically and biomechanically when loaded and unloaded. Connective tissue is comprised of an adaptable fibrillar network of collagenous tubes filled with proteoglycans and water, the microvacuolar spaces between the fibrils are polyhedral and change shape according to the forces and loads imposed on them. They appear and disappear as the fibrils lengthen, slide and divide relative to one another (Guimberteau 2005).

Guimberteau and Armstrong (2015) did not directly study the aponeuroses of the abdominal muscles, yet they did confirm that these structures are comprised of the same connective tissue. This anatomy facilitates two important functions of the abdominal wall:

1. to be mobile and adaptable (move, slide, glide), and

2. to transfer force between the thorax, low back, and pelvis.

Width of the linea alba – the inter-recti distance

To define an abnormal width of the linea alba, it is critical to know what is average, or normal, in healthy nulliparous individuals. In 2009, Beer et al. used ultrasound imaging to investigate the width of the linea alba in 150 healthy, nulliparous women between the ages of 20 and 45. The inter-recti distance was measured at three points along the linea alba: at the xyphoid, 3 cm above the umbilicus and 2 cm below the umbilicus. They found high variability at all three levels and reported the mean width to be 7 mm ± 5 at the xyphoid, 13 mm ± 7 at a point 3 cm above the umbilicus and 8 mm ± 6 at a point 2 cm below the umbilicus. An inter-recti distance wider than these values is considered abnormal.

The posterior fascial connections

Posteriorly, the aponeuroses of external oblique, internal oblique and transversus abdominis merge to form a common tendon (Fig. 1.26) (Schuenke et al. 2012, Willard et al. 2012). After a short distance this aponeurotic tendon divides posteriorly to form the medial laminar and posterior laminar fibers of the thoracolumbar fascia. Between, and contained by, the medial and posterior laminar fibers are the multifidus, longissimus and iliocostalis muscles.

Superficial muscles of the posterior thorax

Semispinalis thoracis

The semispinalis thoracis is part of the transversospinalis group and is superficial to multifidus and deep to the spinalis thoracis (part of the erector spinae group). It arises from tendinous slips from the transverse processes of T6 to T10 and inserts cranially into the lateral aspect of the spinous processes of C6 to T4.

Spinalis thoracis

The spinalis thoracis (Fig. 1.47) (medial part of the erector spinae group) lies medial to the thoracic component of the longissimus thoracis and posterior to the thoracic component of semispinalis. It arises from the lateral aspect of the

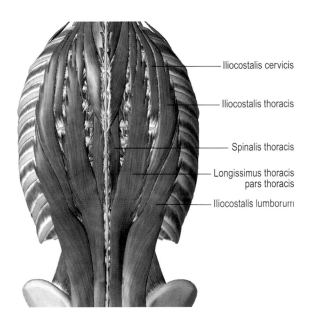

Iliocostalis cervicis

Iliocostalis thoracis

Spinalis thoracis

Longissimus thoracis pars thoracis

Iliocostalis lumborum

Figure 1.47

The component parts of the erector spinae.

Reproduced from Essential Anatomy 5 3D4Medical with permission.

spinous process from T11 to L2. From these four slips, it forms a small muscle which inserts cranially into the lateral aspect of the spinous processes of T1 to T8.

Longissimus thoracis

The thoracic component of the longissimus thoracis (Fig. 1.47) (longissimus thoracis pars thoracis) is the largest part of the erector spinae group in the thoracic spine and forms the bulk of the paravertebral muscle mass adjacent to the spine. It arises from the ribs (between the tubercle and angle of the rib) and transverse processes of T1 to T12 and descends to attach serially via the aponeurosis of the erector spinae to the spinous processes of the lumbar spine and sacrum (Fig. 1.48) (MacIntosh & Bogduk 1991). In the upper three segments the costal origin merges with that from the transverse process (Bogduk 1997).

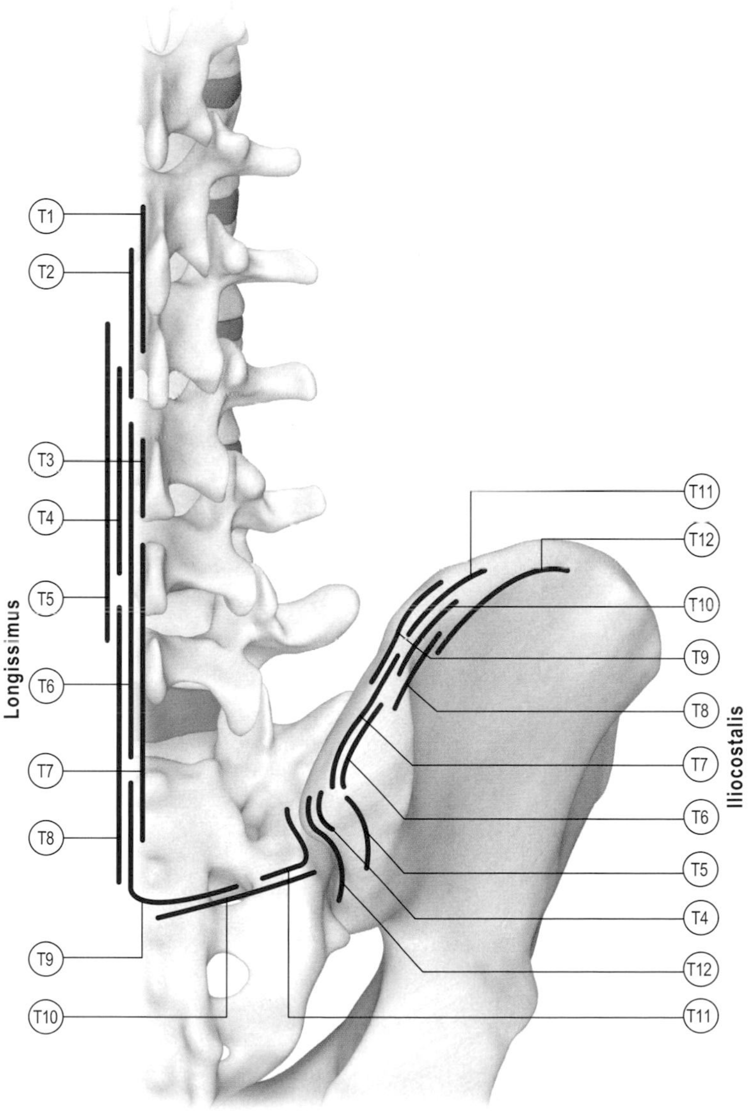

Figure 1.48

Each fascicle of the longissimus and iliocostalis has a specific point of insertion into the thoracolumbar fascia and thus into the lumbar spine, sacrum, and iliac crest (MacIntosh & Bogduk 1991).

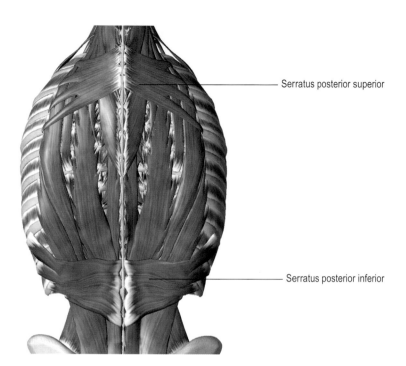

Serratus posterior superior

Serratus posterior inferior

Figure 1.49

Serratus posterior superior and inferior.

Reproduced from Essential Anatomy 5 3D4Medical with permission.

Iliocostalis thoracis

The iliocostalis thoracis (Fig. 1.47) (lateral part of the erector spinae) lies lateral to the longissimus (below the 7th rib) and medial to the thoracic component of iliocostalis lumborum. Between the 3rd and 7th thoracic rings the iliocostalis thoracis lies lateral to the iliocostalis cervicis, which ascends to insert into the transverse processes of C4 to C6. The iliocostalis thoracis arises from the superior border of the angle of the 7th to 12th ribs inserting into the superior border of the angle of the 1st to 6th ribs and the transverse process of C7. This muscle is contained entirely within the thorax.

Iliocostalis lumborum

The thoracic component of the iliocostalis lumborum is large and the most lateral part of the erector spinae muscle group. Fascicles from the inferior borders of the angles of the lower eight or nine ribs (i.e., the 4th to 12th ribs) originate laterally to the attachment of the iliocostalis thoracis and descend to attach to the iliac crest (Figs 1.47, 1.48), and together with the thoracic component of the longissimus thoracis form the aponeurosis of erector spinae.

Serratus posterior superior

This superficial muscle lies deep to the rhomboid and superficial to the erector spinae arising from the spinous processes of C7 to T3 and the intervening supraspinous ligaments (Fig. 1.49). Fibers descend laterally in four digitations to attach to the upper border of the 2nd to 5th ribs just lateral to the rib's angle.

Serratus posterior inferior

Arising from the spinous process of T11–L2 and the intervening supraspinous ligament, four digitations ascend to insert into the inferior border of the 9th to 12th ribs just lateral to the rib's angle (Fig. 1.49).

Neurology of the thorax

It is outside the scope of this text to describe the entire nervous system within the thorax; therefore, only pertinent nerves and plexi relevant to assessment and treatment will be covered.

Thoracic spinal nerves

There are 12 pairs of thoracic spinal nerves and the ventral rami remain segmental in their distribution. The first

11 pairs travel between the ribs and are called intercostal nerves (Fig. 1.50) and the 12th pair, the subcostal nerve, travels below the 12th rib. A large part of the 1st, and part of the 2nd, thoracic ventral rami pass into the brachial plexus. The 3rd to 6th thoracic ventral rami supply the thoracic wall and the 7th to 12th supply both the thoracic and abdominal walls. The thoracic dorsal rami have medial and lateral branches supplying the deep and superficial muscles of the thorax.

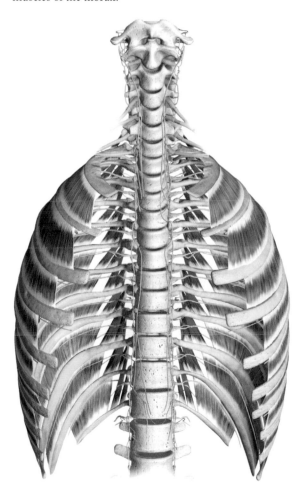

Figure 1.50

The intercostal nerves and their relationship to the sympathetic trunks, which lie directly in front of the heads of the ribs.

Sympathetic trunks

There are two sympathetic trunks that lie anterior to the heads of the ribs each containing 11 ganglia (Fig. 1.50). The first fuses with the inferior cervical ganglion to form the cervicothoracic ganglion. The gray and white rami communicantes connect each ganglion with its corresponding spinal nerve.

Surface anatomy – landmarking the thorax

Given the high variability in the anatomy of the individual thorax, it is important to have a consistent, structured approach to landmarking the ribs and thoracic vertebrae for accurate assessment and treatment of alignment, biomechanics, and control of each thoracic ring. It is not uncommon for clinicians to assume that ribs of the same number are directly across from one another as commonly depicted in anatomy applications (Fig. 1.1A & B). Clinically, this is often not the case. The angle of the rib from the transverse process to the midaxillary line is highly variable and assumptions often result in landmarking errors when trying to place two parts of the hand on one rib. For these reasons, it is imperative to describe a way of ensuring proper landmarking for the individual thoracic rings.

Thoracolumbar junction

Things to note: 11th and 12th ribs, spinous process of T11 and T12.

Patient position: Sitting.

Therapist: Standing behind the patient.

Landmarking the ribs and related vertebrae: With the fingers of both hands extended and palms flat, palpate the highest part of the iliac crest (Fig. 1.51). Then with the back of the hands, palpate the inferior aspect of the rib cage (Fig. 1.52). Specifically palpate the lowest rib and note if it has a sharp end (11th or 12th rib). If the rib continues around the front of the rib cage and connects to the common cartilaginous bar, it is the 10th rib. If it ends with a sharp point and there is another rib with a sharp end below it, you are on the 11th rib. If it ends with a sharp point and there is another rib with a sharp end above it, you are on the 12th rib. Place an X on the tip of the 12th rib (Fig. 1.53). Place your middle finger on the tip of this rib over the X and the thumb of the same hand immediately adjacent (Fig. 1.54). Then move the thumb along the rib, ensuring that you do

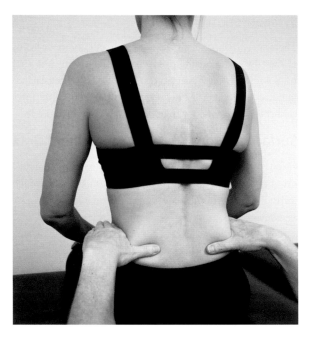

Figure 1.51

Placement of the hands for landmarking the highest part of the left and right iliac crest.

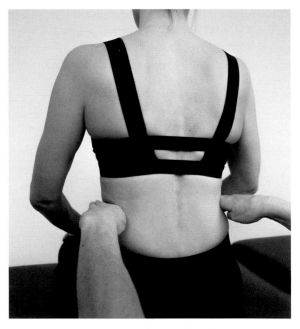

Figure 1.52

Placement of the hands for landmarking the inferior aspect of the rib cage.

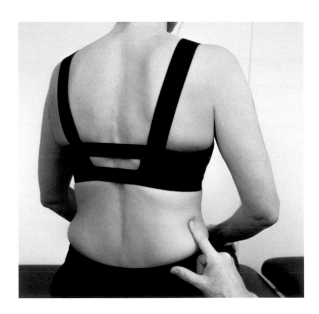

Figure 1.53

Landmarking the tip of the 12th rib, which is marked with an X.

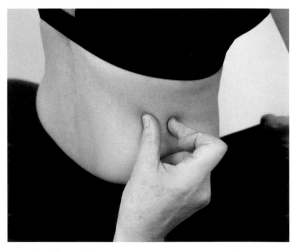

Figure 1.54

Accurate landmarking of two points of a rib is critical for analysis of position and motion. Begin by placing the middle finger over the tip of the 12th rib and the thumb immediately beside the middle finger.

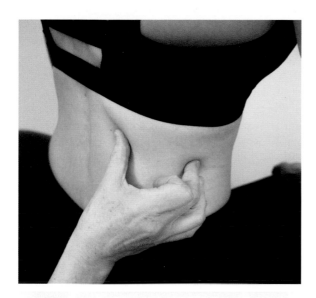

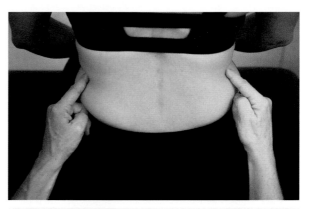

Figure 1.56

The left and right index fingers are marking the end of the left and right 12th ribs. Note that, in this individual, they do not lie in the same transverse plane.

Figure 1.55

To reach the medial aspect of the 12th rib, move your thumb medially ensuring you maintain contact with the bone and do not drift into the intercostal space.

not drift into the intercostal space above or below (Fig. 1.55), until you reach the spinous process; this will be the 12th thoracic vertebra. Repeat the process to landmark the 12th rib on the opposite side of the thorax. Note the level of the Xs at the tips of the ribs and whether they are in the same, or a different, transverse plane (Fig. 1.56).

Vertebrochondral region

Things to note: 7th to 10th ribs, transverse processes T7–T10.

Patient position: Sitting.

Therapist: Standing behind the patient.

Landmarking the ribs: Start by finding the lowest rib that continues around to the front of the rib cage and connects to the common cartilaginous bar to the sternum; this is the 10th rib. Note the difference in the density of the rib compared to that of the intercostal space above it. Stay in the midaxillary line and note, and count, the ribs and intercostal spaces up to the 8th rib. Mark the 8th rib with an X in the midaxillary line. Place your middle finger on the rib over the X and the thumb of the same hand immediately adjacent (Fig. 1.57). Then move the thumb along the rib, tracing its trajectory (orientation)

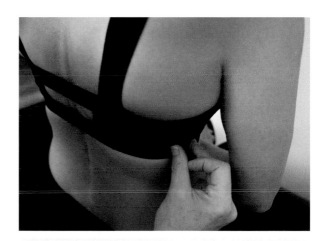

Figure 1.57

This is a critical step for accurately landmarking two points on the 8th rib. Begin by locating the rib in the midaxillary line. Place the middle finger here and the thumb adjacent.

back toward the transverse process of T8 ensuring that you do not drift into the intercostal space above or below. Put a second X on the back of the 8th rib as far medial as you can reliably feel and still be able to palpate the X in the midaxillary line. Put the thumb on the medial X and the middle finger on the lateral X; you are now palpating two points of the 8th rib (Fig. 1.58). Repeat the process and landmark the 8th rib on the opposite site. Note the level of the four Xs on the left and right 8th ribs

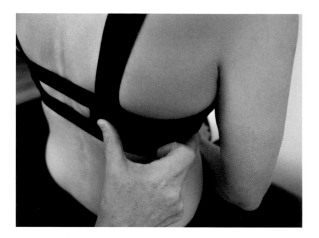

Figure 1.58

To reach the medial aspect of the 8th rib, move the thumb medially ensuring you maintain contact with the bone and do not drift into the intercostal space above or below. In this figure, the thumb and middle finger are palpating two points on the right 8th rib.

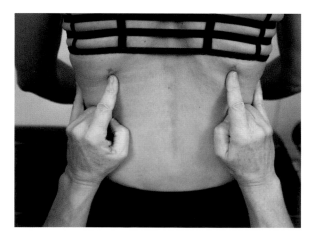

Figure 1.59

There are four Xs landmarking the left and right 8th rib. Only two can be seen in this image. Note how the left rib and right rib are not on the same transverse plane. This suggests that the thoracic ring is translated or rotated.

and whether they are in the same, or a different, transverse plane (Fig. 1.59). Palpate the left and right 8th ribs accurately (i.e., over the Xs); this is how you palpate the 8th thoracic ring for assessment and treatment of osteokinematic motion (see the sections on osteokinematics of inhalation and exhalation in Chapter 2) (Fig. 1.60A & B). Ask the patient to inhale and exhale. You should feel both ribs move symmetrically and equally; however, if the ribs are not in the same transverse plane you will likely feel asymmetric and/or unequal motion.

Landmarking the relative transverse process: From the medial X on the rib follow an imaginary trajectory back

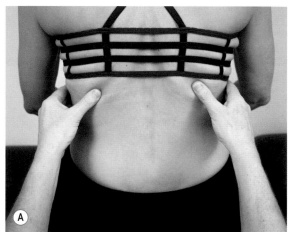

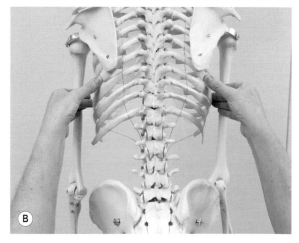

Figure 1.60

A & B Hand placement for accurate landmarking of the left and right 8th ribs for analysis of position and osteokinematic motion of the 8th thoracic ring.

toward the vertebral column. In the vertebrochondral region the transverse process, to which the rib articulates, is below the rib (Fig. 1.15). Find the transverse process of T8 below the 8th rib and mark it with an X. Place the thumb of one hand on the X on the T8 transverse process and the thumb and middle finger of the other hand on the two Xs on the 8th rib (Fig. 1.61A & B); this is how you palpate the 8th

costotransverse joint for assessment and treatment of arthrokinematic motion. Ask the patient to inhale and exhale. On the inhalation, you should feel the rib move anterolaterally and inferiorly relative to the transverse process and posteromedially and superiorly relative to the transverse process on the exhalation (see the sections on arthrokinematics of inhalation and exhalation in Chapter 2) (Fig. 1.62 A & B).

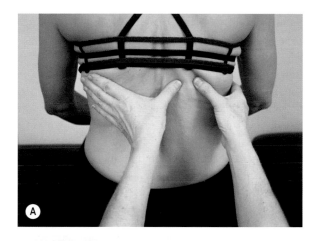
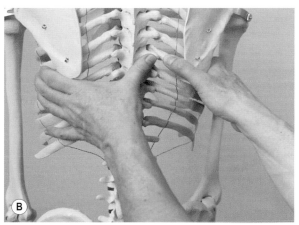

Figure 1.61

A & B Hand placement for accurate landmarking of the right transverse process of T8 and the right 8th rib for analysis of arthrokinematic motion of the right 8th costotransverse joint.

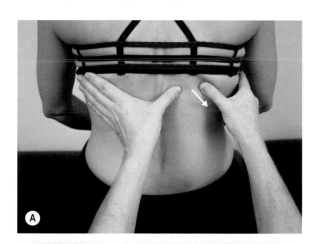
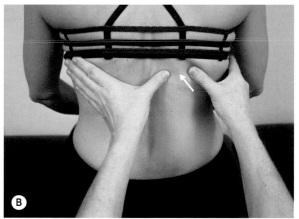

Figure 1.62

Arthrokinematic motion of the 8th costotransverse joint during respiration. (A) During inhalation, the right 8th rib should osteokinematically posteriorly rotate and the rib should glide arthrokinematically at the costotransverse joint in an anterolateroinferior direction (arrow). (B) During exhalation, the right 8th rib should osteokinematically anteriorly rotate and the rib should glide arthrokinematically at the costotransverse joint in a posteromediosuperior direction (arrow).

Vertebrosternal region

Things to note: 3rd to 6th ribs, transverse processes T3 to T6.

Patient position: Sitting.

Therapist: Standing behind the patient.

Landmarking the ribs: Find the 1st rib just lateral to the transverse process of T1. Note the density of this rib compared to the intercostal space below it. Continue to palpate inferiorly and note when the density hardens again, this is the posterior aspect of the 2nd rib, which is much easier to landmark for position and biomechanics on the anterior aspect of the chest (see Vertebromanubrial region below). Find the intercostal space between the 2nd and 3rd ribs, 3rd and 4th ribs, and 5th and 6th ribs. All the thoracic rings in the vertebrosternal region are overlapped by the scapula, the spine of which should be at the level of the 3rd rib. To find the posterior and midaxillary aspect of a rib in this region, pick one of the ribs between 3 and 6 medial to the scapula and lateral to the thoracic spine and place the tips of your index and middle fingers over the back of this rib. Place your other hand, oriented vertically in the midaxillary line, at the level of the vertebrosternal region (Fig. 1.63). Move the rib you have chosen in its posterior location and feel for the rib to respond to this force in the midaxillary line. Push the rib in the midaxillary line and feel for the response medial to the scapula. If you are on the rib of the same number you should feel it move both posteriorly and in the midaxillary line. Now find, and mark with an X, the left and right 4th rib in the midaxillary line (Fig. 1.64). With the pads of the index, middle and ring fingers, palpate the left and right 4th rib in the midaxillary line (Fig. 1.65A & B). Push the 4th thoracic ring medially with one hand and feel the response with the other. Be sure not to compress the ribs at the same time into the vertebral column as no interthoracic ring motion will occur if you do this. Repeat the motion with the opposite hand. If you are on the left and right 4th ribs, you should feel the entire thoracic ring move a small amount in the mediolateral plane in response to this pressure. You can now confirm that you are palpating the 4th thoracic ring in the midaxillary line; this is how you palpate the 4th thoracic ring for assessment and treatment of osteokinematic motion. Ask the patient to inhale and exhale. You should feel both ribs move symmetrically and equally. However, if the ribs are not in the same transverse plane you will likely feel asymmetric and/or unequal motion.

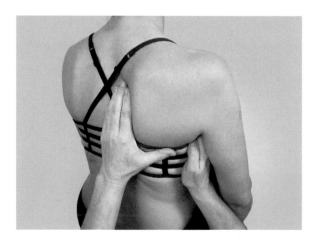

Figure 1.63

The index and middle fingers of the left hand are over the posterior aspect of the right 4th rib. The right hand is palpating the ribs in the vertebrosternal region in the midaxillary line.

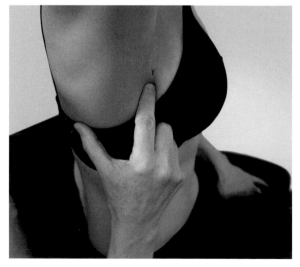

Figure 1.64

The X is marking the 4th rib in the midaxillary line.

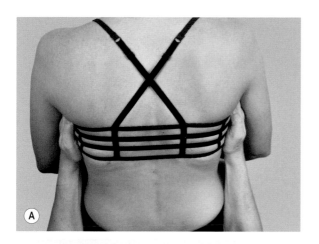

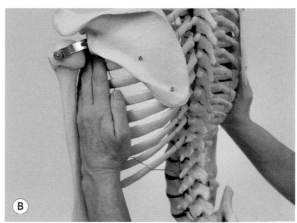

Figure 1.65

A & B The index, middle and ring fingers of both hands are palpating the body of the left and right 4th rib in the midaxillary line.

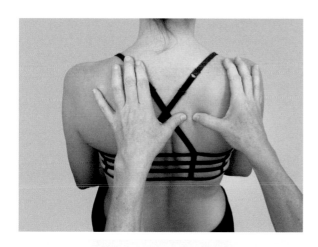

Figure 1.66

Hand placement for accurate landmarking of the right transverse process of T5 and the right 5th rib for analysis of arthrokinematic motion of the right 5th costotransverse joint.

Landmarking the relative transverse process: Find the posterior aspect of the 5th rib. Follow an imaginary trajectory back toward the vertebral column. In the vertebrosternal region the transverse process is level with the rib (Fig. 1.12). With your opposite thumb, palpate the

transverse process of T5; this is how you palpate the 5th costotransverse joint for assessment and treatment of arthrokinematic motion (Fig. 1.66). Ask the patient to inhale and exhale. On the inhale, you should feel the rib move inferiorly with a slight posterior roll relative to the transverse process and superiorly with a slight anterior roll relative to the transverse process on the exhale (see the sections on arthrokinematics of inhalation and exhalation in Chapter 2) (Fig. 1.67A & B).

Vertebromanubrial region

Things to note: 1st and 2nd ribs, transverse processes T1 to T2.

Patient position: Sitting.

Therapist: Standing in front of, or behind, the patient.

Landmarking the ribs: Begin by finding the manubriosternal symphysis (Fig. 1.68). Palpate the left and right sides of the manubrium and note its direction of rotation (Fig. 1.69A). The side that is most ventral (forward) informs the direction of rotation. If the right side is forward, the manubrium is rotated to the left. Move your fingers, or thumbs, laterally and note the difference in density between the 2nd costocartilage and the manubrium. Continue to trace the path and orientation of

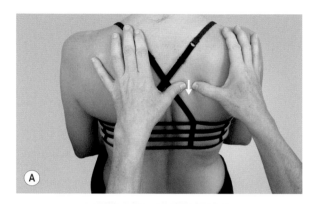
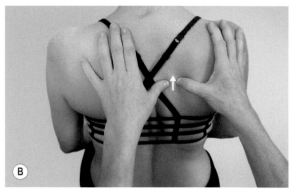

Figure 1.67

Arthrokinematic motion of the 5th costotransverse joint during respiration. (A) During inhalation, the right 5th rib should osteokinematically posteriorly rotate and the rib should glide arthrokinematically at the costotransverse joint in an inferior direction (arrow) with a slight posterior roll. (B) During the exhalation phase, the right 5th rib should osteokinematically anteriorly rotate and the rib should glide arthrokinematically at the costotransverse joint in a superior direction (arrow) with a slight anterior roll.

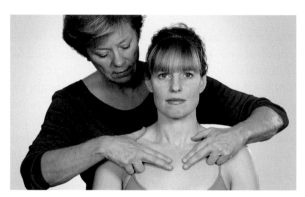

Figure 1.68

Landmarking the manubriosternal symphysis. This can be done by standing either behind or in front of the patient.

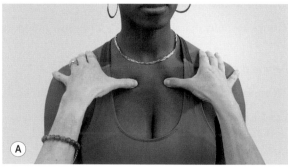
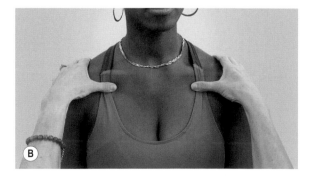

Figure 1.69

(A) This woman's manubrium is rotated to the left in the transverse plane. Note how the right side is more ventral than the left. (B) However, when palpating the left and right 2nd ribs, the 2nd thoracic ring is rotated to the right. The left rib is more ventral than the right. The 2nd ring has an intrathoracic ring biomechanical incongruence and this is consistent with a loss of articular integrity within the 2nd thoracic ring. Note the 'bump' at the right 2nd sternocostal joint. The woman had a compression injury to her thorax while playing rugby several years ago, sprained this joint and has noticed this tender bump ever since.

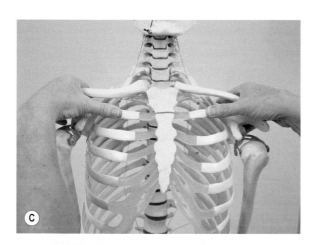

Figure 1.69 *continued*

(C) Note the palpation points for landmarking and analysis of position and motion of the left and right 2nd rib.

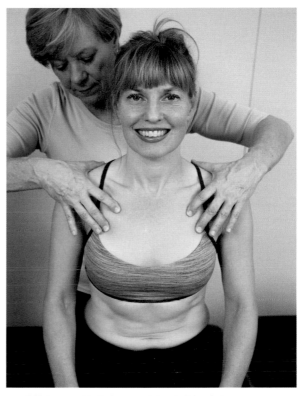

Figure 1.70

Landmarking the 2nd and 3rd ribs anteriorly while standing behind the patient. The index fingers are on the left and right 2nd rib, the middle fingers are on the left and right 3rd rib.

the left and right 2nd ribs up toward the clavicle and note how this thoracic ring hangs like a necklace on the anterior thorax. Place the thumbs over the left and right 2nd ribs halfway between the costocartilage and the clavicle and note any difference in the anteroposterior (Fig. 1.69B & C) and then the superoinferior position of the ribs; they should be level if the 2nd thoracic ring is in a neutral position.

Move your thumbs inferior to the 2nd ribs and note the change in density when you are in the intercostal space between the 2nd and 3rd ribs. The ribs of the 3rd thoracic ring can be landmarked anteriorly by palpating inferiorly, or laterally, to the 2nd rib (Fig. 1.70). Consistently being aware of when you are in the intercostal space and when you are on a rib will assist your landmarking accuracy in this region of the thorax.

Only a small part of the 1st rib can be palpated below the clavicle where it attaches to the short 1st costocartilage. It is more reliable to palpate the body of the 1st rib in the supraclavicular space between the clavicle and the scapula, anterior to the horizontal fibers of the upper trapezius muscle. Gently press into this space to contact the superior aspect of the left and right 1st ribs (Fig. 1.71A & B).

Palpate the left and right 2nd ribs anteriorly. Ask the patient to inhale and exhale. You should feel both ribs move symmetrically and equally. However, if the ribs are not in the same transverse plane you will likely feel asymmetric and/or unequal motion.

Landmarking the relative transverse process: Finding the transverse process of the thoracic rings in the vertebromanubrial region is identical to the process for the vertebrosternal region. See Figure 1.72A–D for how to landmark the costotransverse joint of the 2nd thoracic ring and its response to breathing.

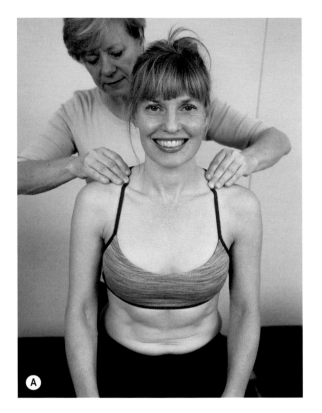

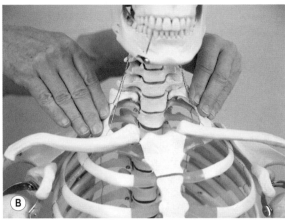

Figure 1.71 A & B

Hand placement for landmarking the left and right 1st ribs in the supraclavicular space.

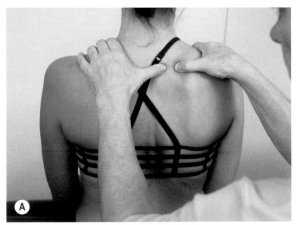

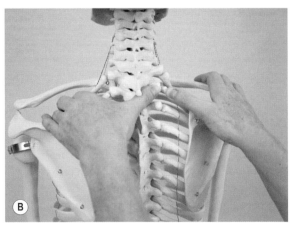

Figure 1.72

(A) Hand placement for accurate landmarking of the right transverse process of T2 and the right 2nd rib for analysis of arthrokinematic motion of the right 2nd costotransverse joint. (B) The same points on a skeleton.

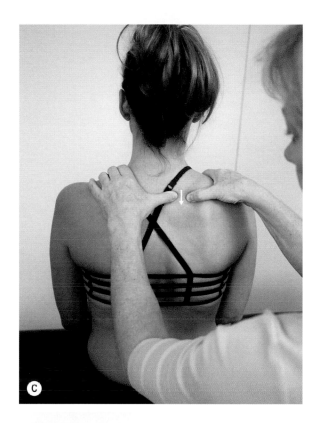

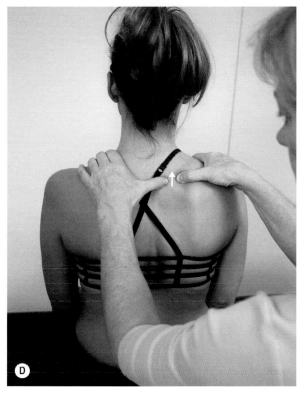

Figure 1.72 *continued*

(C) During inhalation, the right 2nd rib should osteokinematically posteriorly rotate and the rib should glide arthrokinematically at the costotransverse joint in an inferior direction (arrow) with a slight posterior roll. (D) During exhalation, the right 2nd rib should osteokinematically anteriorly rotate and the rib should glide arthrokinematically at the costotransverse joint in a superior direction (arrow) with a slight anterior roll.

Conclusion

Knowing the anatomy of the thorax helps to understand the regional biomechanics and improves reliability for landmarking the individual thoracic rings in both assessment and treatment. Anatomy (and motor control) underpins biomechanics, which is fundamental for optimal strategies for posture and performance of the entire body.

Biomechanics of the thorax

Introduction

The thorax plays a critical role in multiple conditions since it is part of many integrated, and interdependent, systems including the musculoskeletal, respiratory, cardiovascular, digestive, and urogynecological systems. As such, many health disciplines (orthopedic physiotherapists, manual therapists, respiratory therapists and respirologists, massage therapists, cardiac physiotherapists and cardiologists, gastroenterologists, etc.) assess and treat the thorax mainly through the lens of their training and experience. Across all disciplines a biopsychosocial approach is recommended.

The biopsychosocial model considers the influence of biological, psychological and sociological factors in the clinical presentation of the whole person. Biomechanics (the study of biology and mechanics) is part of the biological domain of the biopsychosocial model. Moseley and Butler (2017) emphatically state in their new book *Explain Pain Supercharged*:

'To iterate (because it is of fundamental importance to the rest of this book), the biopsychosocial model does reject the biomedical model because the biomedical model is not concerned with the person, but it does not reject the role of structural, biomechanical and functional disturbance of body tissue as potentially powerful DIMs [danger in me] that modulate an individual's wellbeing.'

The biomechanics of the thorax are fundamental to function and therefore relevant to all forms of treatment across multiple conditions. How movement patterns of the thorax are interpreted depends on one's understanding of optimal biomechanics in this region. Compared to the low back, there is little in vivo research on intrathoracic or interthoracic ring biomechanics to guide clinical interpretation of movement patterns. Perhaps the reason for this lack of research evidence is that the rib cage and its 13 joints per typical thoracic ring (Fig. 1.2) pose significant methodological challenges for investigating intrathoracic and interthoracic ring biomechanics. For this reason, the thorax is often modeled as a box. Many of the ex vivo studies investigating movement and/or control of a thoracic

ring use cadaveric specimens without an intact rib cage, and while this is occasionally seen in clinical practice (rib removal), it is not a common clinical presentation. Consequently, these studies are limited for application to clinical practice. Edmondston (2004) notes:

'A clearer understanding of thoracic spine mechanics has been achieved through the combined results of motion analysis studies of asymptomatic subjects in conjunction with clinical observation.'

Evidence-based practitioners are encouraged to consider the best research evidence, their clinical expertise and the patient's values when determining treatment for the individual patient (Sackett et al. 2000). An evidence-based practitioner:

- Informs themselves of the relevant research evidence relating to the topic and patient;

- Continues to develop clinical expertise (i.e., develop the skills needed to determine reliable findings and apply clinical reasoning to understand the relevance of the findings to the clinical picture); and

- Attempts to understand the patient's values and goals to provide meaningful treatment in the context of a biopsychosocial model.

This chapter will highlight the current state of research evidence, as well as observations from clinical experience, pertaining to the biomechanics of the thorax. Each section will include a detailed description of how to palpate the biomechanics described. It is encouraging to see more interest in the thorax (Henegan & Rushton 2016) and an acknowledgment that 'silent impairments' may underpin some common pain syndromes.

Terminology

To facilitate the subsequent discussion, the terminology used in this text requires definition (Table 2.1). Osteokinematics refers to the study of motion of bones regardless of the motion of the respective joints (MacConaill & Basmajian 1977). Angular motion is an osteokinematic motion and is named according to the axis about which the bone rotates. Flexion and extension occur about a coronal axis, anterior and posterior rotation about a paracoronal axis, side bending, or lateral flexion, about a sagittal axis and axial rotation about a vertical axis. A tilt (i.e., anterior, posterior, or lateral tilt) refers to motion of a group of bones collectively. For example, a thoracic tilt describes motion of either a thoracic ring, or the entire thorax (multiple rings) as a unit. Coupled motion refers to the combination of movements which occur because of an induced motion. Movement between bones (or body regions) that are congruent are moving in the same direction while those that are incongruent are moving in the opposite direction.

Linear motion, or translation, is named according to the axis along which the bone translates. Mediolateral translation occurs along a coronal axis; anteromedial and posterolateral translation occur along a paracoronal axis; traction and compression occur along a vertical axis; and anteroposterior translation occurs along a sagittal axis.

Arthrokinematics refers to the study of motion of joints regardless of the motion of the respective bones (MacConaill & Basmajian 1977). These movements are named according to the direction in which the joint surfaces glide.

Table 2.1
Terms used in the clinical biomechanical model for the thorax

TERM	DEFINITION
Osteokinematics	Study of the motion of bones regardless of the motion of the associated joints Angular motions are named according to the plane they occur in and the axis about which they rotate: • Sagittal plane and coronal axis: Flexion and extension • Parasagittal plane and paracoronal axis: Anterior and posterior rotation • Coronal plane and sagittal axis: Side bending or lateral flexion • Transverse plane and vertical axis: Axial rotation Linear motions are named according to the axis along which they translate: • Coronal axis: Mediolateral translation • Paracoronal axis: Anteromedial and posterolateral translation • Vertical axis: Distraction and compression • Sagittal axis: Anteroposterior translation Tilting: Motion of several bones that comprise a functional unit
Arthrokinematics	Study of the motion of joints regardless of the motion of the bones Motions are named according to the direction in which the joint surfaces glide relative to each other
Coupling	Coupling biomechanics is the rotation or translation of a bone about or along one axis that is consistently associated with the main rotation or translation on, or about, another axis
Translation	When movement is such that all particles in the body at a given time have the same direction of motion relative to a fixed coordinate system
Rotation	Rotation occurs as a spinning or angular displacement of the vertebral body around a particular axis of rotation

Research evidence

In vivo biomechanics of the thorax is difficult to investigate since no system can yet measure the various parameters of intrathoracic or interthoracic ring motion. Studies that investigate the motion of one thoracic ring with markers on the spinous process and related ribs without considering the relative motion of this thoracic ring to the one above or below cannot determine interthoracic ring biomechanics; only regional conclusions can be made. The methods and findings of six studies that investigated the regional biomechanics of the thorax under varying conditions are outlined in Table 2.2 (Hsu et al. 2008, Willems et al. 1996, Edmondston et al., 2007, Edmondston et al. 2012, Theodoridis & Ruston 2002, Delphinus & Sayers 2013). The variability of coupling in the thorax 'should warn clinicians against biasing selection of therapeutic movement techniques on purely theoretically derived

---

Table 2.2
Findings from six studies investigating the biomechanics of the thorax.

AUTHORS	METHOD	FINDINGS
Hsu et al. 2008	Surface sensors on spinous processes C7, T12, S1, and mid-thigh Electromagnetic tracking of sensors during movement in sagittal, coronal and transverse planes	Thorax contributed most to axial rotation; 60 per cent of motion came from thorax
Willems et al. 1996	Surface sensors on spinous processes T1, T4, and T8 Electromagnetic tracking of sensors during movement in sagittal, coronal, and transverse planes	Thorax contributed most to axial rotation; T4–T8 produced 50 per cent of total axial rotation Coupling of side bending and axial rotation highly variable
Edmondston et al. 2007	Reflective markers on transverse processes T6 and 6th ribs Investigated influence of flexion and extension on amplitude and pattern of coupling of axial rotation	Pattern of coupling was variable and influenced by posture Postulate variations in anatomy, soft tissue extensibility and/or motor control strategies influencing pattern variability
Edmondston et al. 2012	Reflective markers on spinous processes T1, T4, T8, and T12 Lateral radiographs and photographic image analysis of thorax during bilateral arm elevation	Thorax extends – lower region more than upper region
Theodoridis & Ruston 2002	Electromagnetic tracking of T2–T7 during unilateral arm elevation	Variable coupling of lateral flexion and axial rotation; most coupled ipsilaterally
Delphinus & Sayers 2013	Reflective markers on spinous processes C7, T10, suprasternal notch, xiphoid process, pelvis (anterior and posterior superior iliac spine), greater trochanters Eight-camera motion analysis system tracked 3D movements of thorax and pelvis during left and right axial rotation in neutral spine posture Four different trunk inclination positions with and without pelvic constraint	At 45 degrees of anterior trunk inclination the thorax contributed 54 per cent of the total trunk rotation Up to 30 degrees of anterior trunk inclination; the pelvis contributed more than 50 per cent of the total trunk rotation

Reproduced with permission Lee D G (2015) Biomechanics of the thorax – research evidence and clinical expertise. The Journal of Manual & Manipulative Therapy 23(3)128–138.

patterns' (Willems et al. 1996). Edmondston et al. (2007) agree and suggest that clinicians 'should not seek stereotypical patterns of coupled motion in the examination of spinal mobility.'

The biomechanical model of the thorax (Lee D G 1993) was derived principally from clinical observations and a review of the literature. The study that most influenced the development of this model was by Panjabi et al. (1976). Motion coupling of a *partial* thoracic ring was investigated in this study. The ribs were cut 3 cm from the costotransverse joint thus the anterior portion of the ribs, the sternum and the anterior costochondral and sternochondral joints were not considered part of the functional spinal unit in this study (Fig. 2.1). Therefore, knowledge gained from this study must be interpreted carefully since it is not representative of patients seen in clinical practice as most have complete thoracic rings. However, it is the only study that has reported on transverse plane translation

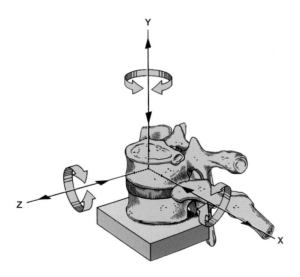

Figure 2.1

In an in vitro study by Panjabi et al. (1976), 396 load displacement curves were obtained for six degrees of motion at each thoracic segment noting both amplitude and coupling of motion for each. This is the only study that has described the transverse plane lateral translation that couples with axial rotation in the thorax.

being contralaterally coupled with axial rotation. No in vivo studies have yet measured the presence, or absence, of this coupled motion. The axis for thoracic rotation differs between the intact and non-intact thoracic ring in that the intact anatomy influences the biomechanics (Molnár et al. 2006). Therefore, all studies without an intact thoracic ring should be interpreted cautiously (Dickey & Kerr 2003).

Only one study has been found to date that has investigated in vivo, intact intrathoracic ring biomechanics. Beyer et al. (2014) used in vivo spiral computed tomography to determine the three-dimensional motion of the thoracic ring at full inhalation, full exhalation and a point somewhere in between. This study confirmed the clinical impression that ribs 1 to 7 posteriorly rotate in full inhalation and anteriorly rotate in full exhalation. The axis for anterior and posterior rotation of the ribs was not along the neck of the rib as Kapandji (1964) previously described. Rather, the axis ran anterolateral and inferior at approximately 45 degrees to the transverse plane. Between-subject variations of the axis at the lower levels were noted and the investigators postulate that different conditions (i.e., pulmonary, neuromusculoskeletal) may influence the kinematics observed. This study did not investigate the changes in rib cage motion that have been found to occur when breathing in different postures of the spine.

Lee L-J et al. (2010) investigated changes in chest wall shape, motion and volume in seven different seated postures (habitual posture, neutral, slump, thoracolumbar extension, full trunk rotation to the right, half-range trunk rotation to the right, lateral rib cage shift to the left) and found that while volumes did not differ between postures, subtle changes in sitting posture did alter chest wall shape and the amplitudes of motion in various parts of the chest. These results support the hypothesis that in the healthy chest postures 'predicted to reduce compliance in one region or dimension involve increased motion elsewhere in the chest wall' (Lee L-J et al. 2010).

Sizer et al. (2007) feel it is important to understand the three-dimensional spine coupling characteristics for treating patients with spinal pain. This systematic review analyzed 56 studies including in vivo, in vitro or mathematical modeling of coupled motion in the thoracic spine.

Six studies used trunk motion and two used upper extremity elevation to produce the coupling behavior in the thoracic spine. Included in this review were studies pertaining to either cadaveric specimens with non-intact thoracic rings and mathematical modeling studies that did not consider the role of the ribs or sternum (Panjabi et al. 1976, Oxland et al. 1992, Schultz et al. 1973, Scholten & Veldhuizen 1985). If these studies are eliminated due to their nonclinical applicability, only one remains to consider: the study by Willems et al. (1996). However, this study did not investigate segmental, interthoracic ring biomechanics and therefore no conclusions can be made about segmental coupling for an intact thoracic ring for lateral flexion or axial rotation.

Sizer et al. (2007) note that across all studies 'variations were reported in side-bending and rotation initiation and no consistent pattern was observed when comparing in vivo versus in vitro findings.'

In addition:

'In vivo studies are clinically applicable but lead to challenges in controlling extraneous variables that include motor and postural control, as well as tissue adaptation, anatomical and circadian variability, applied preload forces, the degree of thoracic kyphosis and scoliosis, and technical difficulty in measuring spinal coupling.'

However, these variables are the reality for clinicians. Practitioners are expected to interpret movement behavior with these variables in situ: 'The lack of a common coupling pattern may merit individual clinical assessment for each patient examined' (Sizer et al. 2007).

How should clinicians interpret the biomechanical findings? What are the normal, or optimal, biomechanics for the thorax? What is abnormal? To date, the highest ranked level of evidence does not provide clinicians with a biomechanical model against which to compare the patient's movement results.

Some insight for this noted variability of the biomechanics of the thorax across multiple studies comes from the anatomical study by Masharawi et al. (2004). The orientation of the facets of the zygapophyseal joints was measured in 240 specimens from T1–L5 in over 4,080 vertebrae. An asymmetric orientation (differences between the left and right sides) was found to be a 'normal characteristic in the thorax.' Andriacchi et al. (1974) suggest that the mechanical response of the costovertebral joint is strongly influenced by the joint's geometry; the same could be suggested for the zygapophyseal joints. Asymmetric anatomy may be a contributor to variability in motion coupling in the thorax.

Clinical expertise

A clinical model of in vivo biomechanics of the thorax was proposed in 1993 (Lee D G 1993). An updated proposal of the in vivo biomechanics follows with consideration given to both the current research evidence and clinical experience gained since 1993.

Forward bending of the trunk

The strategy used for forward bending of the trunk is variable and includes:

- a hip strategy in which either minimal movement occurs in the thoracolumbar spine or the thoracolumbar spine extends (Fig. 2.2A);
- a spinal strategy in which most movement occurs in the spine (Fig. 2.2B); or
- a combination of both (Fig. 2.2C).

In a combination strategy, the thorax anteriorly tilts, the amount of which varies between individuals and between the thoracic rings, the lumbar spine flexes, and the pelvis anteriorly tilts relative to the femurs. The least amount of motion occurs in the midthoracic region.

When the thoracic ring anteriorly tilts during forward bending of the trunk, the following biomechanics are proposed to be optimal (Fig. 2.3).

Thoracic spine osteokinematics

The superior vertebra flexes relative to the inferior vertebra in all four regions of the thorax. In the vertebrosternal (VS – 3rd to 6th thoracic rings) and vertebrochondral (VC – 7th to 10th thoracic rings) regions the superior articular process is inclined slightly anterior in the coronal plane; therefore, a small amount of anterior translation of the superior vertebra occurs in conjunction with flexion.

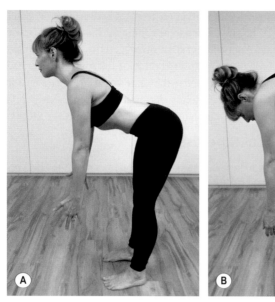
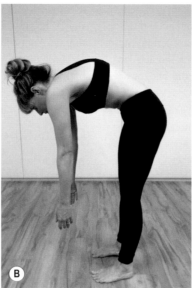
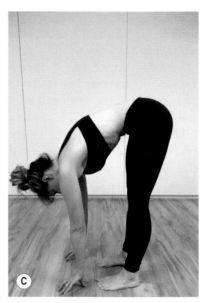

Figure 2.2

Forward bending of the trunk. (A) Hip strategy with minimal movement in the thoracolumbar spine. (B) Spinal strategy with most movement occurring in the spine. (C) Combination strategy with loads distributed between the thorax, lumbar spine, pelvis, and hips.

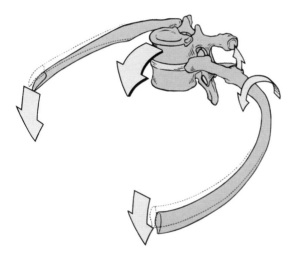

Figure 2.3

Osteokinematic and arthrokinematic motion of a thoracic ring in the vertebrosternal region during an anterior tilt.

Thoracic spine arthrokinematics

The inferior articular processes of the superior vertebra glide superiorly and slightly anteriorly following the joint's orientation, which may be variable both regionally and between sides of the same segment.

Palpation of the thoracic spinal osteokinematics and arthrokinematics

All regions of the thorax: With the index fingers and thumbs, palpate the four transverse processes of the thoracic ring (Fig. 2.4). Ask the patient to flex their neck and thorax to the level being palpated. Optimally, the index fingers should move away from the thumbs as the superior vertebra flexes and the inferior articular processes glide superiorly (Fig. 2.5).

Costal osteokinematics

The left and right ribs of the thoracic ring anteriorly rotate relative to their starting position (Fig. 2.3). The axis for this motion has not been determined. With increased age and/or stiffening of the thorax this motion is often lacking.

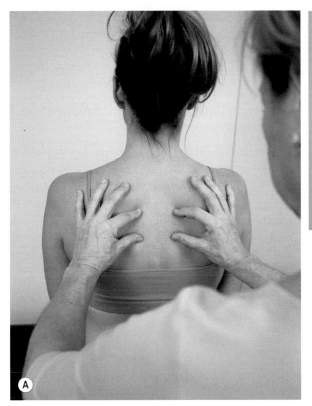

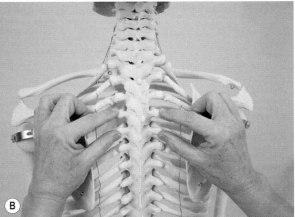

Figure 2.4 A & B

Position of index fingers and thumbs for motion analysis of the spinal component of a thoracic ring.

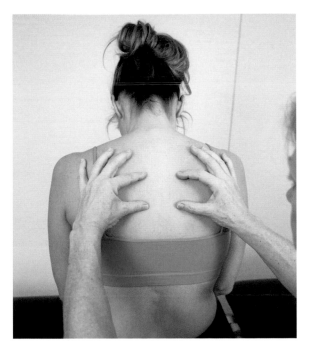

Figure 2.5

During flexion of the neck and thorax the superior thoracic vertebra should flex (osteokinematics) and the inferior articular processes should glide superiorly relative to the superior articular processes of the inferior vertebra (arthrokinematics). The motion should be symmetric between sides and the index fingers should move away from the thumbs an equal amount, unless there is a structural asymmetry in the anatomy.

Costal arthrokinematics

The shape of the costotransverse joint in both the vertebromanubrial (VM) and vertebrosternal regions is concavo-convex (Figs 1.5, 1.12); therefore, when the rib anteriorly rotates relative to the vertebra of the same number, the convex facet on the rib glides superiorly and rolls anteriorly relative to the facet on the transverse process (Fig. 2.3). This arthrokinematic motion depends on the strategy chosen (motor control) and any additional forces (force closure) potentially compressing the joint (relative flexibility).

The shape of the costotransverse joint in the vertebrochondral region is planar (Fig. 1.15) and the orientation of the joint plane is anterolateroinferior and posteromediosuperior (ALI and PMS) (Fig. 2.6). Thus, anterior rotation of ribs 7 to 10 relative to the transverse process requires a PMS glide of the joint's surfaces. Alternately, if the chosen motor control strategy significantly compresses the costotransverse joints, no motion may occur between the rib and the relevant transverse process when the thoracic ring anteriorly tilts during forward bending of the trunk.

Palpation of the thoracic costal osteokinematics and arthrokinematics

Vertebromanubrial and vertebrosternal regions: Palpate the rib just lateral to the tubercle and medial to the angle with your thumb. With your other thumb, palpate the transverse process of the same number as the rib (Fig. 2.7). Ask the patient to flex their neck and thorax to the level being palpated. Optimally, the thumb on the rib should move superiorly relative to the thumb on the transverse process (Fig. 2.8).

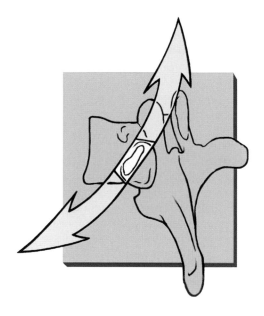

Figure 2.6

The plane of the costotransverse joint in the vertebrochondral region is anterolateroinferior and posteromediosuperior. When the rib anteriorly rotates, the facet on the rib glides in a posteromedial superior direction relative to the facet on the transverse process. When the rib posteriorly rotates, the facet on the rib glides in an anterolateral inferior direction relative to the facet on the transverse process.

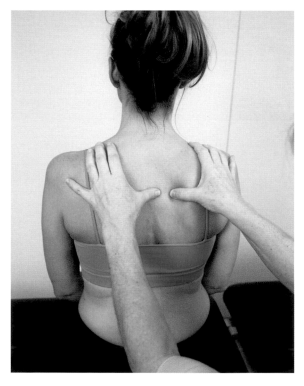

Figure 2.7

Position of the thumbs for arthrokinematic motion analysis of the costotransverse joint of the thoracic ring in the vertebromanubrial and vertebrosternal regions of the thorax.

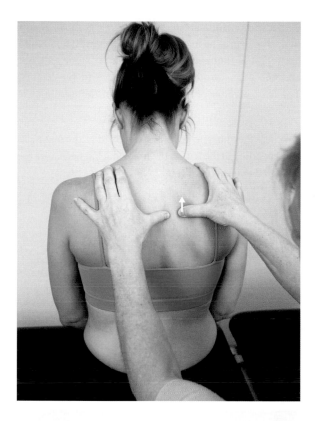

Figure 2.8

Vertebromanubrial and vertebrosternal regions: During flexion of the neck and thorax the rib should move superiorly (arrow) relative to the transverse process and the motion should be symmetric between sides, unless there is a structural asymmetry in the anatomy.

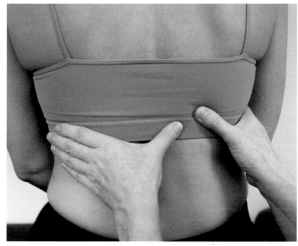

Figure 2.9

Position of the hands for arthrokinematic motion analysis of the costotransverse joint of the thoracic ring in the vertebrochondral region. Note that the thumb palpating the relative transverse process is inferior to that palpating the rib.

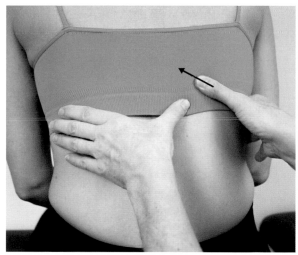

Figure 2.10

Vertebrochondral region: During flexion of the neck and thorax the rib should move in a posteromedial superior direction (arrow) relative to the transverse process and the motion should be symmetric between sides unless there is a structural asymmetry in the anatomy.

Vertebrochondral region: Palpate the rib just lateral to the tubercle with your thumb and the body of the rib with the middle finger of the same hand. With your other thumb, palpate the transverse process of the same number as the rib (Fig. 2.9). Remember that the rib is superior to the transverse process. Ask the patient to flex their neck and thorax to the level being palpated. Optimally, the rib should move in a posteromedial superior direction relative to the thumb on the transverse process (Fig. 2.10).

Backward bending of the trunk

The strategy used for backward bending of the trunk is variable and includes:

- a hip strategy in which either minimal movement occurs in the thoracolumbar spine (Fig. 2.11A);

- a spinal strategy in which most movement occurs in the thoracolumbar spine (Fig. 2.11B); or

- a combination of both (Fig. 2.11C).

In a combination strategy, the thorax posteriorly tilts (with the degree of tilt varying between individuals and between the thoracic rings), the lumbar spine extends, and the pelvis posteriorly tilts relative to the femurs. The least amount of motion occurs in the midthoracic region.

When the thoracic ring posteriorly tilts during backward bending of the trunk, the following biomechanics are proposed to be optimal (Fig. 2.12).

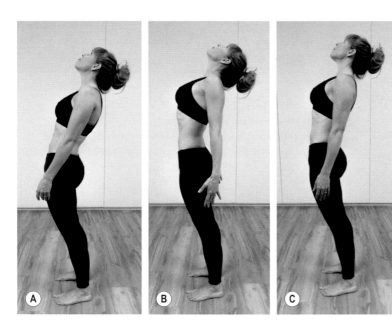

Figure 2.11

Backward bending of the trunk. (A) Hip strategy with minimal movement in the thoracolumbar spine. (B) Spinal strategy with most movement occurring in the spine. (C) Combination strategy with loads distributed between the thorax, lumbar spine, pelvis, and hips.

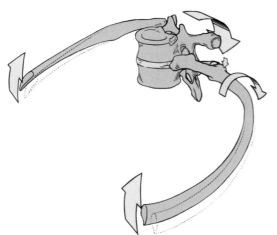

Figure 2.12

Osteokinematic and arthrokinematic motion of a thoracic ring in the vertebrosternal region during a posterior tilt.

Thoracic spine osteokinematics

The superior vertebra extends relative to the inferior vertebra in all four regions of the thorax. In the vertebrosternal and vertebrochondral regions the superior articular process is inclined slightly anterior in the coronal plane; therefore, a small amount of posterior translation of the superior vertebra occurs in conjunction with extension.

Thoracic spine arthrokinematics

The inferior articular processes of the superior vertebra glide inferiorly and slightly posteriorly following the joint's orientation, which may be variable both regionally and between sides of the same segment.

Palpation of the thoracic spinal osteokinematics and arthrokinematics

All regions of the thorax: With the index fingers and thumbs, palpate the four transverse processes of the thoracic ring (Fig. 2.4). Ask the patient to extend their thorax to the level being palpated. Optimally, the index fingers should move toward the thumbs as the superior vertebra extends and the inferior articular processes glide inferiorly (Fig. 2.13).

Costal osteokinematics

The left and right ribs of the thoracic ring posteriorly rotate relative to their starting position (VM, VS, and VC regions). The axis for this motion has not been determined. With increased age and/or stiffening of the thorax this motion is often lacking.

Costal arthrokinematics

The shape of the costotransverse joint in both the vertebromanubrial and vertebrosternal regions is concavo-convex (Figs 1.5, 1.12); therefore, when the rib posteriorly rotates relative to the vertebra of the same number, the convex facet on the rib glides inferiorly and rolls posteriorly relative to the facet on the transverse process (Fig. 2.12). This arthrokinematic motion depends on the strategy chosen (motor control) and any additional forces (force closure) potentially compressing the joint (relative flexibility).

The shape of the costotransverse joint in the vertebrochondral region is planar (Fig. 1.15) and the orientation

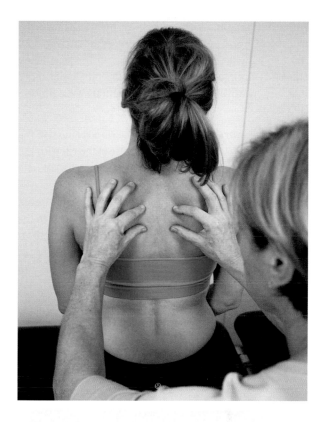

Figure 2.13

During extension of the neck and thorax the superior thoracic vertebra should extend and the inferior articular processes should glide inferiorly relative to the superior articular processes of the inferior vertebra. The motion should be symmetric between sides and the index fingers should move toward the thumbs an equal amount, unless there is a structural asymmetry in the anatomy.

of the joint is in the ALI and PMS plane (Fig. 2.6). Thus, posterior rotation of ribs 7 to 10 relative to the vertebra requires an ALI glide of the joint's surfaces. Alternately, if the chosen motor control strategy significantly compresses the costotransverse joints, no motion may occur between the rib and the relevant vertebra when the thoracic ring posteriorly tilts during forward bending of the trunk.

Palpation of the thoracic costal osteokinematics and arthrokinematics

Vertebromanubrial and vertebrosternal regions: Palpate the rib just lateral to the tubercle and medial to the angle with your thumb. With your other thumb, palpate the transverse process of the same number as the rib (Fig. 2.7). Ask the patient to extend their thorax to the level being palpated. Optimally, the thumb on the rib should move inferiorly relative to the thumb on the transverse process (Fig. 2.14).

Vertebrochondral region: Palpate the rib just lateral to the tubercle with your thumb and the body of the rib with the middle finger of the same hand. With your other thumb, palpate the transverse process of the same number as the rib (Fig. 2.9) (remember that the rib is superior to the transverse process). Ask the patient to extend their thorax to the level being palpated. Optimally, the rib should move in an

anterolateral inferior direction relative to the thumb on the transverse process (Fig. 2.15).

Given both regional and side-to-side variations in anatomy, asymmetry in the amplitude of motion should not be considered pathognomonic of suboptimal biomechanics for forward or backward bending. Other clinical considerations are required to determine the relevance of asymmetry.

Side bending of the trunk

Side bending of the trunk produces segmental lateral flexion of the thorax at all regions and a variety of coupling possibilities. Overall, a gentle even curve convex on the opposite side of the side bending should occur (Fig. 2.16). The ribs approximate on the ipsilateral side and separate on the contralateral side. Once side-bent, anterior or posterior tilting and rotation of the thorax become more limited.

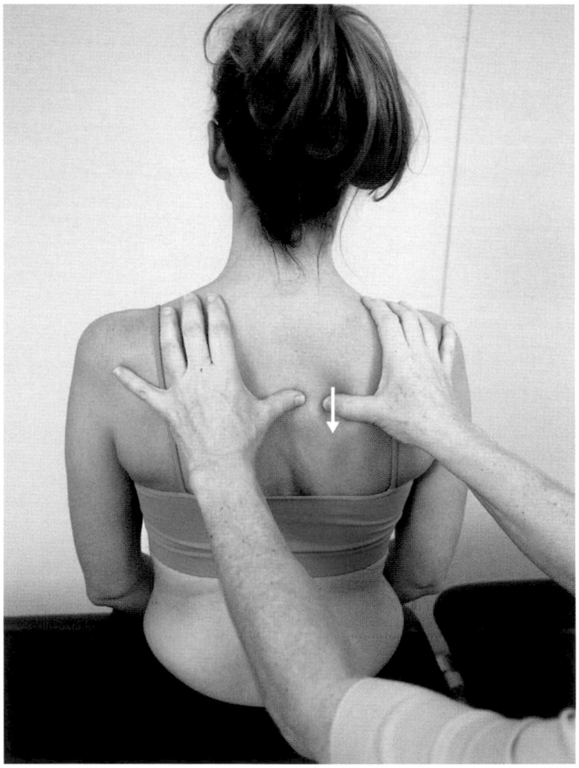

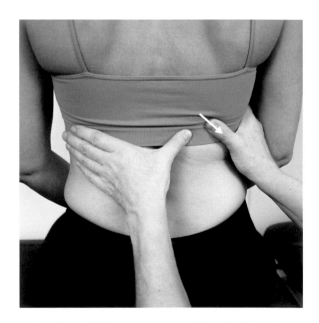

Figure 2.14

Vertebromanubrial and vertebrosternal regions: During extension of the neck and thorax the rib should move inferiorly (arrow) relative to the transverse process and the motion should be symmetric between sides unless there is a structural asymmetry in the anatomy.

Figure 2.15

Vertebrochondral region: During extension of the thorax the rib should move in an anterolateral inferior direction (arrow) relative to the transverse process and the motion should be symmetric between sides unless there is a structural asymmetry in the anatomy.

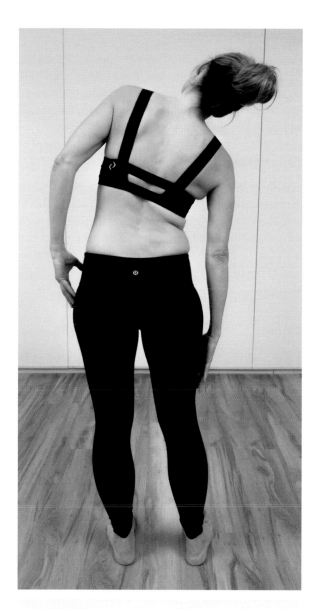

Figure 2.16

Side bending of the trunk should produce a smooth even curve of the entire spine which is convex on the contralateral side.

When the thoracic ring laterally flexes in side bending of the trunk, the following biomechanics are proposed to be optimal (Fig. 2.17).

Thoracic spine osteokinematics

The superior vertebra laterally flexes relative to the inferior vertebra in all four regions of the thorax and rotation may be coupled ipsilaterally or contralaterally. If the superior vertebra is free to follow the orientation of the zygapophyseal joints then the pattern is often ipsilateral.

Thoracic spine arthrokinematics

During right lateral flexion, the right inferior articular process of the superior vertebra glides inferiorly (and slightly posteriorly) and the left glides superiorly (and slightly anteriorly). The anteroposterior translation that couples with the arthro-

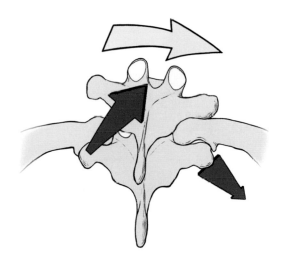

Figure 2.17

During side bending of the neck and thorax the superior vertebra should laterally flex (yellow arrow) to the ipsilateral side and the rotation that is coupled with this motion is variable. The red arrows depict the relative motion of the transverse process at the costotransverse joints (vertebrochondral region) as the vertebrae continue to laterally flex after all osteokinematic costal motion has ceased. The right transverse process glides in an anterolateral inferior direction to the right rib while the left transverse process glides in a posteromedial superior direction to the left rib.

kinematic glide likely depends on the amplitude, direction, and symmetry of inclination of the facets in the coronal plane.

Palpation of the thoracic spinal osteokinematics and arthrokinematics

All regions of the thorax: With the index fingers and thumbs, palpate the four transverse processes of the thoracic ring (Fig. 2.4). Ask the patient to side-bend the thorax to the level being palpated. Optimally, the index finger should move toward the thumb on the ipsilateral side and away from the thumb on the contralateral side as the superior vertebra laterally flexes and the inferior articular process of the superior vertebra glides inferiorly on the ipsilateral side and superiorly on the contralateral side (Fig. 2.18A & B).

Costal osteokinematics

During right side bending, the ribs approximate on the right and separate on the left in the VM, VS, and VC regions (Fig. 2.19). What happens at the end of the range depends on the motor control strategy chosen for the task and the degree of articular compression (stiffness).

Costal arthrokinematics

Vertebromanubrial and vertebrosternal regions: When the ribs stop moving the thoracic spine may still be able to laterally flex to the right. If so, the right transverse process will glide inferiorly and roll around the convex articular surface of the right rib while the left transverse process will glide

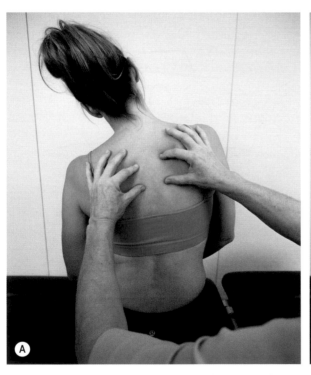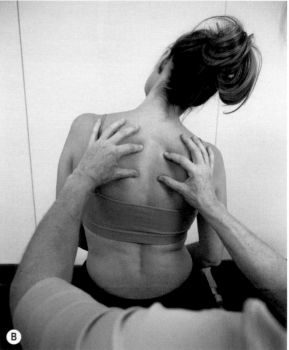

Figure 2.18

Arthrokinematic palpation of the thoracic spine. (A) During left lateral flexion of the thoracic ring the index finger and thumb on the left transverse processes should approximate while those on the right should move apart. The spinous processes should form a gentle C-curve which is convex to the right. (B) Note how in this individual during right side bending, the right index finger does not move closer to the right thumb, the left index finger does not move away from the left thumb, and the spinous processes remain straight. This suggests a right lateral flexion restriction at this segment.

superiorly and roll around the convex articular surface of the left rib facilitating further right (ipsilateral) rotation of the superior vertebra *in space*. However, the resultant *segmental*

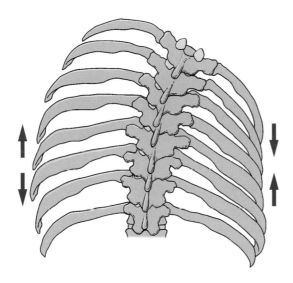

Figure 2.19

As the thorax side-bends to the right, the ribs on the right approximate and the ribs on the left separate at their lateral margins.

coupling of spinal osteokinematics depends on what the inferior vertebra does (relative biomechanics). Rotation of the superior vertebra will be contralateral to the direction of lateral flexion if the inferior vertebra rotates further to the right (in space). Considering the anatomy of the costovertebral joint, it is likely that the head of the rib would prevent end-range segmental ipsilateral coupling in lateral flexion.

Vertebrochondral region: The orientation and shape of the costotransverse joints in this region result in the right transverse process gliding in an ALI direction and the left gliding in a PMS direction during right lateral flexion (Fig. 2.17). Segmental coupling for rotation is variable.

Palpation of the thoracic costal osteokinematics and arthrokinematics

Vertebromanubrial and vertebrosternal regions: Palpate the rib just lateral to the tubercle and medial to the angle with your thumb. With your other thumb, palpate the transverse process of the same number as the rib. Ask the patient to side-bend their neck and thorax ipsilaterally to the level being palpated. Optimally, the thumb on the transverse process should move inferiorly relative to the thumb on the rib (Fig. 2.20A & B). On the contralateral side the transverse process should move superiorly relative to the thumb on the rib (Fig. 2.20C & D).

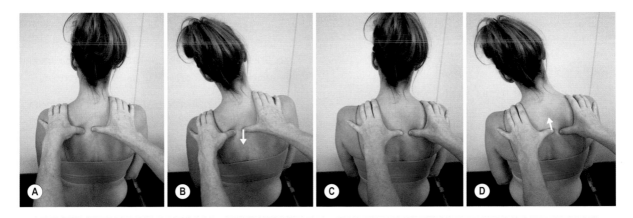

Figure 2.20

Vertebromanubrial and vertebrosternal regions: During left side bending of the neck and thorax the left transverse process should move inferiorly (arrow) relative to the left rib at the end of the available range of motion (A & B). The right transverse process should move superior (arrow) relative to the right rib (C & D).

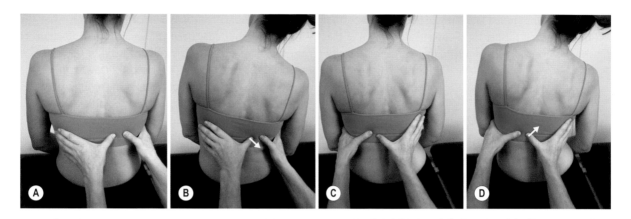

Figure 2.21

Vertebrochondral region: During right side bending of the thorax the right transverse process should move in an anterolateral inferior direction (arrow) relative to the right rib (A & B) and the left transverse process should move in a posteromedial superior direction (arrow) relative to the left rib (C & D).

Vertebrochondral region: Palpate the rib just lateral to the tubercle with your thumb and the body of the rib with the middle finger of the same hand. With your other thumb, palpate the transverse process of the same number as the rib. Ask the patient to side-bend their thorax ipsilateral to the level being palpated. Optimally, the transverse process should move in an ALI direction relative to the thumb on the rib (Fig. 2.21A & B). On the contralateral side the transverse process should move in a PMS direction relative to the thumb on the rib (Fig. 2.21C & D).

Axial rotation of the trunk

Axial rotation of the thorax is a component of many functional tasks and thus often an essential movement to assess. Overall, a gentle even concave curve on the same side of the rotation should occur (Fig. 2.22). When the thoracic ring rotates during right axial rotation of the trunk, the following biomechanics are proposed to be optimal (Fig. 2.23).

Thoracic spine osteokinematics

The superior vertebra rotates to the right in the VM, VS, and VC regions. If the superior vertebra is free to follow the orientation of the zygapophyseal joints then right lateral flexion also occurs. There is also a slight contralateral translation in the transverse plane of the superior vertebra

relative to the inferior (in this example the translation is to the left).

Thoracic spine arthrokinematics

During right axial rotation, the right inferior articular process of the superior vertebra glides inferiorly (and slightly posteriorly) and the left glides superiorly (and slightly anteriorly). The anteroposterior translation that couples with the glide likely depends on the amplitude, direction, and symmetry of inclination of the facets in the coronal plane. There is a slight left lateral translation of both the left and right inferior articular process of the superior vertebra.

Palpation of the thoracic spinal osteokinematics and arthrokinematics

All regions of the thorax: With the index fingers and thumbs, palpate the four transverse processes of the thoracic ring (Fig. 2.4). Ask the patient to rotate the head and/or thorax to the level being palpated. Optimally, the index finger should move toward the thumb on the ipsilateral side and away from the thumb on the contralateral side as the superior vertebra rotates and laterally flexes and the inferior articular process of the superior vertebra glides inferiorly on the ipsilateral side and superiorly on the contralateral side (Fig. 2.24).

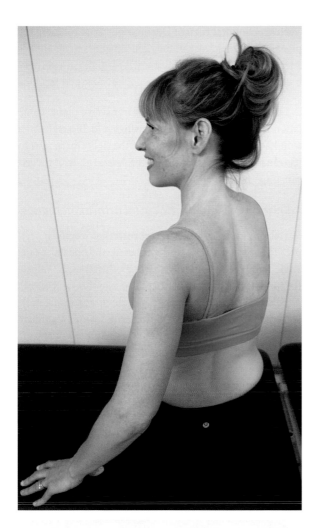

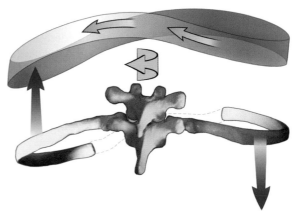

Figure 2.23

During right axial rotation of the neck and thorax the superior vertebra should rotate (yellow arrow) and side-bend to the right. The right rib should posteriorly rotate and the left rib should anteriorly rotate (red arrows). In addition, there is a small contralateral translation of both ribs and the superior vertebra relative to the inferior vertebra (green ribbon with yellow arrows). For example, at the 7th thoracic ring, the left and right 7th ribs together with T6, translate slightly to the left relative to T7.

Figure 2.22

Axial rotation of the trunk should produce a smooth even curve which is concave on the ipsilateral side. Note the lack of curvature in the vertebrosternal region during left thoracic rotation in this individual. This finding warrants further assessment of interthoracic ring mobility to determine where the impairment is.

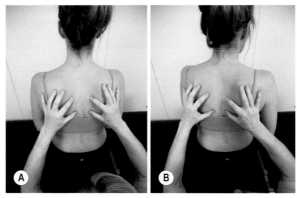

Figure 2.24 A & B

During right axial rotation of the thorax the index finger and thumb on the right should approximate while those on the left should move apart.

Costal osteokinematics

During right axial rotation, the right rib posteriorly rotates and the left rib anteriorly rotates both in space and relative to the vertebrae that comprise the thoracic ring. In addition, in the VS and VC regions (3rd to 10th thoracic rings) there is a slight contralateral transverse plane translation that occurs between the ribs and their relative transverse processes. A suitable metaphor for this motion is the linear translation that occurs when a screw is rotated into wood. This motion follows the noted contralateral transverse plane translation of the relevant thoracic vertebra. The 2nd thoracic ring is variable with respect to this transverse plane translation. The thoracic rings that are atypical (1, 11, 12) do not translate in the transverse plane during axial rotation. The only study to report on this motion is an in vitro one done on non-intact thoracic rings (Panjabi et al. 1976). The motion is small, yet palpable (Lee D G 1993, 2015; Lee D 1994, 2003; Lee L-J 2016).

Costal arthrokinematics

Vertebromanubrial and vertebrosternal regions: During right axial rotation, the convex articular surface of the right rib glides inferiorly and rolls posteriorly while the left rib glides superiorly and rolls anteriorly relative to the transverse process.

Vertebrochondral region: During right axial rotation, the planar articular surface of the right rib glides in an antero-lateral inferior direction while the left rib glides in a postero-medial superior direction relative to the transverse process.

The coupled contralateral (left) transverse plane translation that occurs from thoracic rings 3 to 10 results in a simultaneous anteromedial glide of the right rib (relative to its transverse process) and a posterolateral glide of the left (imagine the turning screw).

Palpation of the thoracic costal arthrokinematics

Vertebromanubrial and vertebrosternal regions: Palpate the rib just lateral to the tubercle and medial to the angle with your thumb. With your other thumb, palpate the transverse process of the same number as the rib. Ask the patient to rotate their head and thorax ipsilaterally to the level being palpated. Optimally, the thumb on the rib should move inferiorly relative to the thumb on the transverse process as the rib posteriorly rotates (Fig. 2.25A & B). On the contralateral side, the thumb on the rib should move superiorly to the thumb on the transverse process as the rib anteriorly rotates (Fig. 2.25C & D).

Vertebrochondral region: Palpate the rib just lateral to the tubercle with your thumb and the body of the rib with the

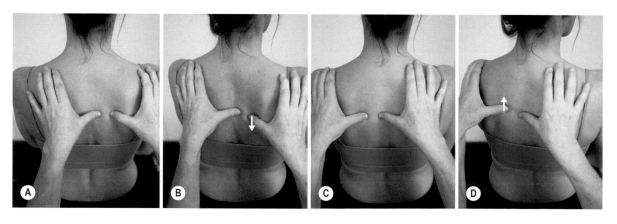

Figure 2.25 A–D

Vertebromanubrial and vertebrosternal regions: During right axial rotation of the neck and thorax the right rib should move inferiorly (arrow) relative to the right transverse process. The left rib should move superiorly (arrow) relative to the left transverse process. There is also a conjunct roll of both ribs that occurs with this motion but it is very difficult to discern in most patients.

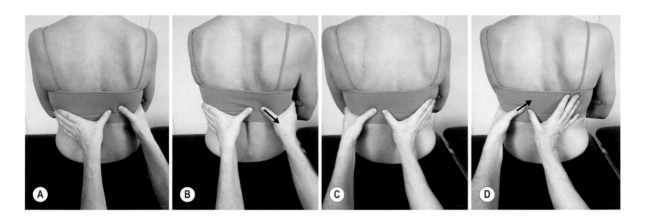

Figure 2.26 A–D

Vertebrochondral region. During right axial rotation of the thorax the right rib should move in an anterolateral and inferior direction (arrow) relative to the right transverse process. The left rib should move in a posteromedial and superior direction (arrow) relative to the left transverse process.

middle finger of the same hand. With your other thumb, palpate the transverse process of the same number as the rib. Ask the patient to rotate their thorax ipsilaterally to the level being palpated. Optimally, the rib should move in an anterolateral inferior direction relative to the thumb on the transverse process as the rib posteriorly rotates (Fig. 2.26A & B). On the contralateral side, the thumb on the rib should move in a posteromedial superior direction to the thumb on the transverse process as the rib anteriorly rotates (Fig. 2.26C & D).

Manubrium and clavicle osteokinematics

During right axial rotation of the head, neck and upper thorax the left clavicle anteriorly rotates, the right posteriorly rotates, and the manubrium rotates right and side-bends right (congruent with the upper two thoracic rings). The clavicular rotation occurs in the medial joint compartment of the sternoclavicular joint between the disc and manubrium (Pettman 2011).

Elevation of the arm

The thorax extends when both arms are elevated overhead (Edmondston et al. 2012), (Fig. 2.27A). During elevation of one arm, the upper and midthorax rotate and side-bend toward the side of the elevating arm (Fig. 2.27B). The variability of coupling noted by Theodoridis and Ruston (2002) is seen

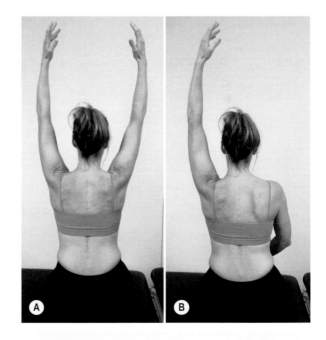

Figure 2.27

(A) When both arms are fully elevated the thorax should extend. (B) When one arm is fully elevated the upper thorax and midthorax rotate and side-bend to the side of the elevating arm.

clinically and often reflects variations in motor strategies for performance of this task.

Breathing

The following biomechanics are proposed to be optimal for each element of the thoracic ring during breathing.

Osteokinematics of inhalation

The ribs posteriorly rotate in the VM, VS, and VC regions. The number and location of ribs that posteriorly rotate depend on the depth of the inhalation and the posture and position of the rib cage.

Arthrokinematics of inhalation

Vertebromanubrial and vertebrosternal regions: During inhalation the rib glides inferiorly and rolls posteriorly relative to the transverse process at the costotransverse joint.

Vertebrochondral region: During inhalation the rib glides in an anterolateral inferior direction relative to the transverse process at the costotransverse joint.

Palpation of the thoracic costal osteokinematics and arthrokinematics

Osteokinematics: Palpate the left and right ribs of the same number just lateral to the tubercle and medial to the angle with your thumb. In the VC region, palpate the body of the rib with the middle finger of the hand palpating the rib. Ask the patient to inhale until the relative ribs are felt to move. Optimally, the thumbs should move inferiorly as the ribs posteriorly rotate (in an anterolateral inferior direction in the VC region). When the thoracic ring is in a neutral position, the amplitude of this motion should be symmetric. When the thoracic ring is translated and rotated, or the ribs are unable to fully anteriorly or posteriorly rotate, the starting position of the left and right ribs may be asymmetric and/or one phase of respiration (inhalation or exhalation) may be asymmetric (Fig. 2.28A–C).

Arthrokinematics: Palpate the rib and its related transverse process. Ask the patient to inhale until the relative costotransverse joint is felt to move. Optimally, the rib should move inferiorly or in an anterolateral inferior

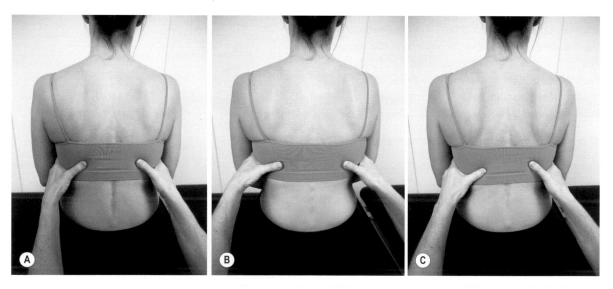

Figure 2.28

(A) This individual's 8th thoracic ring is translated right and rotated left in her neutral sitting position. Note the asymmetry of the therapist's hands. The right 8th rib is anteriorly rotated, the left 8th rib is posteriorly rotated. (B) During inhalation, the left and right rib alignment becomes symmetric and both ribs can fully posteriorly rotate. (C) During exhalation, the rib asymmetry is increased. The left rib cannot anteriorly rotate as far as the right and this restriction creates a rotation of the entire thoracic ring at the end of exhalation. Further assessment is required to determine the reason for this restricted mobility and its relevance to the clinical picture.

direction as the rib posteriorly rotates. The direction depends on the region (VM, VS or VC). When the thoracic ring is in a neutral position, the amplitude of this motion should be symmetric between sides unless there is a structural asymmetry in anatomy.

Osteokinematics of exhalation

The ribs potentially anteriorly rotate in the VM, VS, and VC regions. The number and location of ribs that anteriorly rotate depend on the depth of the exhalation and the posture or position of the rib cage.

Arthrokinematics of exhalation

Vertebromanubrial and vertebrosternal regions: During exhalation the rib glides superiorly and rolls anteriorly relative to the transverse process at the costotransverse joint.

Vertebrochondral region: During exhalation the rib glides in a posteromedial superior direction relative to the transverse process at the costotransverse joint.

Palpation of the thoracic costal osteokinematics and arthrokinematics

Osteokinematics: Palpate the left and right ribs of the same number just lateral to the tubercle and medial to the angle with your thumb. In the VC region, palpate the body of the rib with the middle finger of the hand palpating the rib. Ask the patient to exhale until the relative ribs are felt to move. Optimally, the thumbs should move superiorly as the ribs anteriorly rotate (in a posteromedial superior direction in the VC region). When the thoracic ring is in a neutral position, the amplitude of this motion should be symmetric.

Arthrokinematics: Palpate the rib and its related transverse process. Ask the patient to exhale until the relative costotransverse joint is felt to move. Optimally, the rib should move superiorly in a posteromedial direction as the rib anteriorly rotates. When the thoracic ring is in a neutral

position, the amplitude of this motion should be symmetric between sides.

Conclusion

When the proposed biomechanical model of the thorax is used in conjunction with a biopsychosocial, integrated approach, the relevant clinical findings can be determined. Since the thorax is integrated with the entire body, biomechanical impairments of alignment, movement, and control can impact body regions far removed from the thorax. Poor biomechanics of the thorax are often implicated in multiple conditions across a wide variety of populations and optimal thoracic function is paramount for good health.

In the opening keynote address of the 2012 IFOMPT conference in Quebec, Professor Gwen Jull said:'The future of physiotherapy continues with an informed clinically reasoned assessment approach to direct management of the individual patient.' Sackett et al. (2000) note that:

'External clinical evidence can inform, but can never replace individual clinical expertise, and it is this expertise that decides whether the external evidence applies to the patient at all, and if so, how it should be integrated into a clinical decision.'

In short, regardless of what you believe needs to be done, the individual with primary nociceptive pain often 'knows best' and when the appropriate change or changes in alignment, biomechanics and/or control is or are provided (to the thorax, pelvis, foot, hip, etc.) there is an immediate improvement in both performance and the experience of the meaningful task. This is not necessarily true for the patient whose nervous system is centrally sensitized. Clinical reasoning coupled with an informed understanding of the highly variable biomechanics of the thorax is the evidence-informed way forward for direct management of individual patients.

Assessment of the thorax and its relationship to the whole body

Introduction

Assessment and treatment of the whole person (body, mind and spirit) require an understanding of the relationship between, and the contribution of, various body regions, systems, thoughts, beliefs, and social behaviors or contexts that are ultimately manifesting as cognitive, emotional or sensorial dissonance or altered performance. In other words, a biopsychosocial approach is required. Collectively, this dissonance can be interpreted by the individual as threatening or dangerous and can manifest as pain anywhere in the body, fear of movement, anxiety, movement impairments, and a wide variety of system disorders. Patients with persistent pain have many of these features (comorbidities) and complex histories comprised of:

- Multiple past traumas to several areas of the body, caused by high load or accumulative low load or both, many of which are only partly resolved (suboptimal biology);

- Poor lifestyle habits, such as poor nutrition or hydration, alcohol or drug misuse, and lack of sleep (suboptimal biology);

- Beliefs and cognitions that present barriers to recovery (suboptimal psychology); and

- Lack of supportive relationships at home, at work, or in the community (suboptimal sociology).

Ultimately, conservative care should consider, and address, all relevant components (biology, psychology, sociology), which sounds difficult and yet is the challenge clinicians face daily.

Most individuals with persistent low back pain (LBP) believe their problem to be due to 'something physically defective' (degenerated discs, scoliosis, spondylolisthesis) and that once 'broken' it cannot be fixed, and they receive this information from health professionals (Setchell et al. 2017). Traditional physiotherapy training emphasizes the biological component of a biopsychosocial model, thus most feel more confident in offering postural, structural, movement training (motor control and movement strategies) for treatment to individuals with persistent LBP. For some individuals with persistent LBP, restoring their biomechanics (biology + mechanics) is what is required for full recovery. For others, it is not enough, nor relevant. Health care professionals are being asked to be evidence based in their clinical practice and to:

'shift [their] understandings of LBP beyond biological causes to consider psychosocial, cultural and institutional factors that constitute LBP. Our finding that patients believe they learnt their potentially harmful understandings from health professionals encourages further interventions to shift thinking within healthcare.' (Setchell et al. 2017)

However, 'shifting understanding' to include psychosocial and social factors does not mean letting go of the biological ones *if* they can be determined relevant to the clinical picture. All three components require consideration, individually and collectively.

The broad understanding of the whole person's experience, or the biopsychosocial components that collectively constitute their reality, can either overwhelm both the individual and the clinician, or highlight a path to change. The path is clearer when the patient's information is organized, prioritized, and the clinical relevance of each component and finding determined. This requires a theoretical framework, or model, for both assessment and treatment of the individual patient.

The neuromatrix or cortical body matrix approach

In 1990, Ronald Melzack proposed a neuromatrix model and suggested that the brain be considered as a mass of neural networks that produce 'outputs' in response to various 'inputs.' Each network of neurons was called a neurosignature.

Melzack's updated neuromatrix theory (Fig. 3.1) (2001) postulated that inputs to the neuromatrix from:

- cognitions – memories of past experience, attention, meaning, beliefs (psychology),

- sensations – cutaneous, visceral, visual, vestibular, musculoskeletal (biology), and

- emotions – fear, hypervigilance, anger, sadness, grief (biology and sociology)

lead to outputs that potentially produce:

- pain,

- involuntary and voluntary action patterns (increased neuromuscular activity in certain muscles, organs, vessels), and

- activation of the stress-regulatory system (cortisol, nor-epinephrine, and endorphin levels, immune system).

Moseley and Butler (2017) have expanded on Melzack's neuromatrix theory renaming it the 'cortical body matrix' theory (Moseley 2003, Moseley & Butler 2017, Moseley et al. 2012) and suggest there is a 'matrix of thalamocortical neural loops that subserve the protection and regulation of the body and the space around it, at both a physiological and perceptual level.' They coined the term 'neurotag' – of

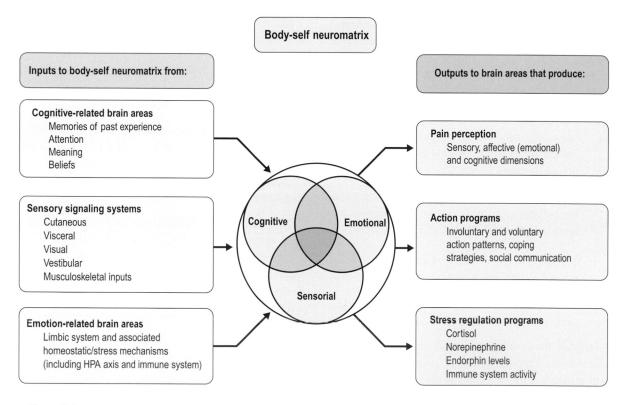

Figure 3.1

Melzack's body-self neuromatrix (2001) provides an introductory framework for understanding the possible cognitive, emotional and sensorial inputs to the embodied nervous system and how these inputs can collectively impact perceptions of pain, activate action programs (e.g., fight, flight, or freeze), change social behavior, suppress the immune system, and stimulate stress responses.

Redrawn with permission from Melzack R (2001) Pain and the neuromatrix in the brain. Journal of Dental Education 65(12) 1378–1382.

which there are two types, an action and a modulation neurotag – that expands on Melzack's original concept of a neurosignature. Moseley and Butler suggest the brain (and spinal cord) be considered as a mass of neurotags 'that are in a constant state of collaboration and competition, having influences over others and being influenced by others.'

The outputs from the cortical body matrix result from activation of the action neurotags and are related to threat, which is either real or perceived. Action neurotags exert influence beyond the brain (muscles, thoughts, feelings, etc.) whereas modulation neurotags exert influence only within the brain (visual data, odors, proprioceptive encoded data, etc.). The bigger the neurotag (high number of neurons) the greater potential influence it can have. The more often a neurotag is activated, the more efficient its synaptic connections become. The principles of neurotag size and efficiency are captured in Donald Hebb's 1949 phrase: 'Neurons that fire together, wire together' (Hebb 1949). 'Broadly speaking, this research speaks to the unity of the mind–body connection. What we mean by this mind–body unity is that we are one biological environment that is in constant state of change, correction and, well, *life*' (Moseley & Butler 2017).

What is the clinical significance of the cortical body matrix theory? It helps to explain why, and how, every individual with persistent pain will have a different experience or trigger in response to threat because the manifestation of pain (involuntary and voluntary action patterns, or activation of the stress-regulatory system) is influenced by what they do, what they think, and how they feel. Current evidence and clinical experience (Garner 2016, Hodges 2015, Hodges et al. 2013, Jones & Rivett 2004, Kent and Hartvigsen 2015, Moseley & Butler 2017, O'Sullivan et al. 2015, Sahrmann & van Dillen 2015) support an individual, clinically reasoned, biopsychosocial approach for complex patients that considers all inputs to, and outputs from, the cortical body matrix to promote adaptability and resilience for, well ... *life!*

Helping clinicians expedite their expertise in a biopsychosocial approach is a common goal of several postgraduate programs for physiotherapists (Table 3.1).

The Integrated Systems Model (ISM) (Lee D 2011, Lee L-J & Lee D 2011, Lee D G 2015) (Fig. 3.2) is an

Table 3.1
Postgraduate physiotherapy programs with a common goal of expediting clinical expertise as part of evidence-informed practice. This list is not complete and only contains those programs the author is familiar with.

PROGRAM	WEBSITE
Movement System Impairment Syndromes	https://pt.wustl.edu/education/movement-system-impairment-syndromes-courses/
Barral Institute	www.barralinstitute.com
Cognitive Functional Therapy	www.pain-ed.com
NOI Group	www.noigroup.com
Institute of Physical Art	www.instituteofphysicalart.com
Manual Concepts	www.manualconcepts.com
The North American Institute of Orthopaedic Manual Therapy (NAIOMT)	www.naiomt.com
Canadian Academy of Manipulative Physiotherapy	https://manippt.org/
The Integrated Systems Model	www.learnwithdianelee.com

evidence-informed, biopsychosocial approach, which aims to help therapists organize knowledge from multiple fields of science and clinical practice and is the approach that will be presented in this text. ISM is particularly useful for the individual whose major barrier to recovery is primarily due to tissue overload, inflammation, aberrant activation of primary nociceptors, or injury to nerves (Moseley & Butler 2017) whereby discrete or accumulative load demand (posture, suboptimal movement strategies) has exceeded the individual's tolerance (Hodges & Smeets 2015). While every individual will have psychological and social components to their story, the dominant barrier to recovery for the individual highly suited to ISM is a biological one, with secondary psychological or social contributors. A primary biomechanical or functional disturbance of body tissue, influenced by thoughts and feelings which are also biological events in the brain, collectively create threat to the cortical body matrix and modulate the individual's well-being: '... we are truly so interconnected, […] that we can't really think, feel or experience something

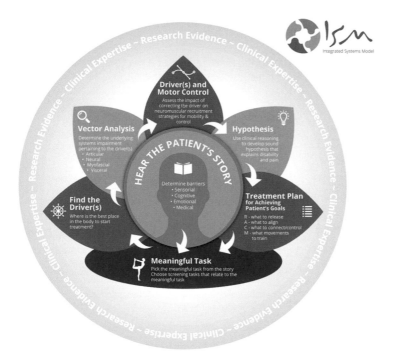

Figure 3.2

A graphic that represents key concepts of the Integrated Systems Model (ISM). ISM is a clinical reasoning framework for organizing knowledge and expediting clinical expertise.

without having additional bodily effects' (Moseley & Butler 2017).

Principles of the Integrated Systems Model approach

Hearing the story and identifying the meaningful complaint

An ISM assessment begins by hearing the autobiographical details of the patient's story. This reveals information about the patient's experience and how it changes over time and with load. Table 3.2 outlines specific questions that help to clarify the patient's sensorial experience, cognitive beliefs, lifestyle habits, and social contexts.

How the story is told (body language and words chosen) also provides information on the emotional contribution to this experience. Setchell et al. state: 'The language we use has a role in creating or constituting reality, rather than simply reflecting it' (Setchell et al. 2017).

Words that suggest catastrophizing thoughts and behaviors alert the therapist to potential cognitive and emotional barriers to recovery (e.g., negative beliefs, fear, depression, anger, anxiety). Specifically enquiring as to what the patient believes is 'going on' and 'why they haven't recovered' provides further information about their cognitive beliefs.

Each patient's experience has a varying degree of contribution from the sensory, cognitive, and emotional domains (Fig. 3.3) and each requires consideration for optimal recovery of function (Falla & Hodges 2017). The focus, and approach to care, will vary according to the percentage of each component in the individual's story.

The meaningful complaint is the primary reason the patient is motivated to seek help and is often the barometer they use to judge improvement. While everyone wants to be pain free, it is important that the patient understands the fundamentals of current evidence of persistent pain

Table 3.2

Hearing the story: Questions that provide information about the patient's experience and general health

QUESTIONS THAT PROVIDE INFORMATION ABOUT THE PATIENT'S SENSORIAL EXPERIENCE

- Was the onset of symptoms sudden or insidious?
- Was there an element of trauma? If so, was there a major traumatic event over a short period of time, such as a motor vehicle accident, or were there a series of minor traumatic events over a long period of time (postural or movement habit contributions).
- Is the patient presenting during the acute or chronic (persistent) stage of this event? Is this the first episode requiring treatment or is this a recurring problem?
- Where is the pain or dysesthesia? Is it localized or diffuse? Does it involve the whole body, one side of the body, or can it even be localized?
- Do the symptoms spread over time or with load? If so, where do they spread to and what words does the patient use to describe its quality (threatening versus safe language)?
- What activities, if any, aggravate the symptoms?
- How long does it take for this activity to produce symptoms (load tolerance)?
- Which activities (and how much activity) provide relief or cause irritability?
- Are the symptoms interfering with sleep?
  - What kind of bed is being slept in and what position is most frequently adopted?
  - Does rest provide relief?

QUESTIONS THAT PROVIDE INFORMATION ABOUT THE PATIENT'S COGNITIVE BELIEFS

- What do you think is going on?
- Why do you think this is happening?
- Why do you think your condition is not resolving?
- How do you think I can help you?

Is their language 'catastrophizing' suggesting they are very 'broken' and not 'fixable'? Are they still hunting for the right professional 'to find their problem,' or is their language more optimistic and are they looking for guidance toward improving their function and quality of life?

PERTINENT LIFESTYLE AND SOCIAL QUESTIONS

- Nutrition – any noted sensitivity to gluten, dairy, sugar (potentially inflammatory), hydration, drugs, alcohol?
- Social relationships (home, partner, work, extended family) – are the primary relationships supportive?

PERTINENT MEDICAL QUESTIONS

- How is the patient's general health?
- Is any medication being taken for this or any other condition?
- What are the results of any adjunctive diagnostic tests (X-rays, CT scan, MRI, laboratory tests)? What does the patient think about the relationship between these results and their current problem?

Sensorial dimension
Location and behavior of
primary complaint

Cognitive dimension
Beliefs and attitudes about their
experience

Emotional dimension
Feelings associated with experience;
anger, fear, anxiety, sadness

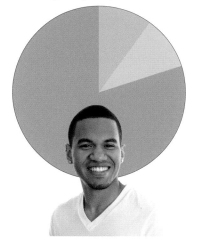
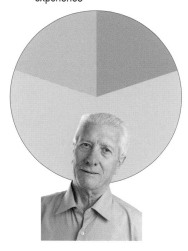
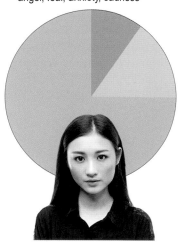

Figure 3.3

Every patient has a unique experience comprised of three components: sensorial, cognitive, and emotional. The first pie chart represents a patient in whom the dominant dimension is sensorial. They have some cognitive beliefs and emotional factors but none that are likely to be barriers to intervention that focuses on the musculoskeletal system. The second pie chart represents a patient in whom the dominant dimension is cognitive. There are biomechanical, sensorial, and emotional factors; however, priority for this session would be to address the patient's cognitive beliefs about their condition. The third pie chart represents a patient in whom the dominant dimension is emotional. The person's nervous system is under high threat and this must be addressed in conjunction with their beliefs. If biomechanical interventions (manual therapy and movement) help to change this patient's experience, the emotional dimension may reduce considerably. Consideration must be given to ensure safety is a priority.

and why pain should not be the only parameter used to measure improvement (Butler & Moseley 2003, Hodges & Smeets 2015, Moseley 2003, 2007, Moseley & Butler 2017, Smeets et al. 2006). Improvements in function (less effort to move, better range of motion, ease of breathing, improved quality of sleep, etc.) often precede pain reduction, and are better initial parameters for determining change. With reduced threat and improved function, pain often decreases. Threat can be reduced with knowledge (Butler & Moseley 2003, Moseley & Butler 2017) and by changing the patient's experience of their body, which is the goal of the ISM approach.

A positive, trusting, relationship between a therapist and patient is required for motivating change in behavior, whether cognitive (thoughts and feelings) or physical

(posture and movement). How the therapist hears a story (attentive versus distracted listening, eye contact, being present) is a critical first step toward establishing this relationship. Take time to be present and attentive and after the story is heard, repeat the key sensorial, cognitive, and emotional components for confirmation and ensure the patient knows that they have been heard. Confirm the meaningful complaint so that the patient understands what will be used to judge change in status during future sessions.

The next step of an ISM assessment is all about biomechanics (biology and mechanics) and consists of observing and palpating postures and movements that are relevant to the patient's functional goals and interpreting the findings through a biopsychosocial lens.

Determining the meaningful task

In the ISM approach, the movement tasks chosen for evaluation are not related to the location of pain but rather to activity or the functional goals, which come from the patient's story. If there are multiple activities that are problematic (e.g., sitting, walking, turning the head, lifting the arms overhead, leaking urine when sneezing, etc.), the patient is asked to choose which one has priority since different body regions can be responsible for impairing function in different tasks. This meaningful task then becomes the focus of the current assessment and treatment session. Meaningful tasks can be:

- Aggravating to the meaningful complaint;

- Difficult to perform yet desired (patient may be fearful or avoidant);

- Tasks that 'don't feel right';

- Tasks that create respiratory or urogynecological symptoms;

- Tasks that are not symptomatic and based on improving performance (e.g., improving a golf swing, becoming faster or more agile, or being able to perform a certain yoga pose).

The patient should be informed that any intervention pertaining to this meaningful task may not resolve their complaints during other tasks so that their attention to change is focused appropriately.

Screening tasks and finding the driver or drivers

Complex meaningful tasks are then broken down into component tasks, or screening tasks, that are easier to initially examine. Consider the following clinical scenarios. Two individuals present with persistent low back pain (LBP). One has chosen a meaningful task of sitting since they experience intensification of their LBP when they sit for more than 15 minutes. For this individual, it would be relevant to evaluate two screening tasks; the squat task and sitting posture. The other has chosen a meaningful task of walking since their LBP increases after

10 minutes of walking. For this individual, the squat task and sitting posture are irrelevant since these tasks do not relate to the meaningful task of walking. It is more relevant to evaluate the strategies they use for single leg standing, stepping forward and thoracic rotation, which are all component tasks for walking. It is not relevant to evaluate flexion or extension of the lumbar spine in either individual.

For each screening task, the entire body is assessed as the task is performed. The patient is asked to report on any sensations evoked during the performance of the screening task (production or reduction of symptoms, effort to perform, balance challenges, fear, or anything else they note). Pay attention to the words they use to describe their experience. This will provide information about their thoughts, beliefs, and sometimes fears relevant to this movement task.

Observe or palpate each region of the body as the task is performed and note any areas that demonstrate suboptimal alignment, biomechanics or control for that task. In this model, these regions are called sites of failed load transfer (FLT), in other words, areas of the body that are performing suboptimally and not transferring loads well. This requires an understanding of what optimal alignment, biomechanics, and control of each body region are for that task against which the patient's performance is compared. If you tend to tell your patient your findings as you find them, ensure that they do not leave feeling 'more broken.' Judge what information is empowering and safe, and what information will merely add more negative beliefs and threat about their condition. There are no rules here, be sure to ask them to repeat back to you what their understanding is of what you said. The words they use will tell you if you should have said anything, or not!

In Chapter 2, the optimal biomechanics of the thorax for forward, backward and side bending, axial rotation of the trunk, elevation of the arm and breathing were described. In this chapter, the requirements of the thorax for standing posture, squat, and head, neck, and thoracic rotation will be described as examples of how to assess thoracic function and find drivers in a whole-body task.

Optimal strategies for the transference of load through the entire body support multiple systems including the musculoskeletal, respiratory, and urogynecological systems. Suboptimal strategies produce sites that fail to transfer load and they often demonstrate suboptimal alignment, biomechanics or control, or are associated with:

- Excessive increases in pressure;

- Suboptimal breathing patterns (e.g., breath holding);

- Rigidity inappropriate for the task; and

- Impedance of blood flow (arterial supply and venous drainage).

Suboptimal strategies do not look, nor do they feel, good.

Subsequently, manual and verbal cues are given to change the strategy (alignment, biomechanics or control) used for one body region noted to be performing suboptimally, and the impact of this correction on the patient's experience, as well as any change in performance of other body regions, is noted. An enquiry is made as to the difference in the patient's experience when various body regions are corrected and controlled to not only confirm the hypothesis but to help the patient become aware of the differing experiences when sites distant from their pain are corrected and controlled. This step is critical. To understand the relevance of any suboptimal biomechanical finding, test it. The patient must report an improvement in their experience with the correction for the finding to be relevant. Some aspect of performance (range of motion, reduction in effort, more expansive breathing, etc.) must also occur.

In the ISM approach this is called 'finding the driver,' the region of the body or mind or both that when corrected results in the best improvement in the *experience and performance* of the task. Correction (manual or verbal) of the driver will result in the best correction of the other sites of failed load transfer (suboptimal alignment, biomechanics, control) for the chosen screening task. The low back, neck, and knee are often victims of suboptimal strategies for transferring load through the thorax, pelvis, hip or feet, particularly when pain is persistent, posture and movement patterns are habitually poor, and biology is the dominant component contributing to the cortical body matrix. The driver can change both within and between treatment sessions when the whole body is evaluated for each task. In the ISM approach, the driver merely informs the therapist of the next place to focus intervention. Sometimes, two areas of the body require equal intervention (co-drivers) and sometimes one area requires most treatment (primary driver) while another requires some attention for the best outcome (secondary driver).

Table 3.3 defines primary, secondary and co-drivers and provides clinical examples of how to use these terms appropriately.

Table 3.3
Definition of drivers in the Integrated Systems Model

TYPE OF DRIVER	DEFINITION	SITES OF FAILED LOAD TRANSFER AND MEANINGFUL TASK	CORRECTIONS
Primary driver (PD)	Correction of one body region results in complete correction of all other regions of FLT for the MT	**Task: Standing posture** • 4th thoracic ring translated left and rotated right • 7th thoracic ring translated right and rotated left • Pelvis: Left TPR and left IPT • Right femoral head anterior to left femoral head • Right foot pronated, left foot supinated • C7 translated left and rotated right • C2 translated right and rotated left	Correcting the 4th thoracic ring alignment improves all other sites of FLT completely *The thorax (4th thoracic ring) is the primary driver*

Table 3.3 *continued*

TYPE OF DRIVER	DEFINITION	SITES OF FAILED LOAD TRANSFER AND MEANINGFUL TASK	CORRECTIONS
Primary driver with secondary driver (PD with SD)	Correction of one body region (PD) results in complete correction of most regions of FLT and an improvement, but not full correction, in another area of FLT (SD) for the MT	**Task: Squat** *Starting alignment:* • 5th thoracic ring translated left and rotated right • 8th thoracic ring translated right and rotated left • Pelvis: Left TPR and right SIJ unlocked • Right femoral head anterior to the left femoral head • C7 translated left and rotated right • C2 translated right and rotated left • Right foot pronated, left foot supinated *Changes during the squat:* • Thoracic rings: No change • Pelvis and hips: No change • Hips and feet: No change	*Intra-regional:* • Thorax: Correcting the 5th thoracic ring results in complete correction of the 8th thoracic ring • Pelvis and hip: Correcting the pelvis (TPR and providing control to the right SIJ) results in complete correction of the right hip • Cervical spine: Correcting C7 results in complete correction of C2 *Inter-regional:* • Pelvis and thorax: Correcting the pelvis does not change the alignment, or the biomechanics, of the 5th or 8th thoracic rings • Thorax and pelvis: Correcting the 5th thoracic ring corrects the 8th thoracic ring and pelvic alignment in standing (TPR reverts to neutral in standing); however, the right SIJ still unlocks during the squat but later in the task • Thorax and cervical spine: Correcting the 5th thoracic ring results in complete correction of C7 and C2 *Best Correction:* • Correcting the 5th thoracic ring and pelvis during the squat completely corrects all other sites of FLT **The primary driver is the thorax (5th thoracic ring) and the secondary driver is the pelvis** • There can be multiple secondary drivers. If the C7 only partially corrected with the 5th thoracic ring correction, then the neck would also be considered a secondary driver

Continued

69

Table 3.3 *continued*

TYPE OF DRIVER	DEFINITION	SITES OF FAILED LOAD TRANSFER AND MEANINGFUL TASK	CORRECTIONS
Co-driver Type 1 (CD Type 1)	Correction of one body region results in worsening of ABCs for another body region for the MT; however, correction of *both* regions improves the task performance	**Task: Right head and neck rotation** *Starting alignment:* • 2nd thoracic ring translated left and rotated right • C5 translated right and rotated left *Changes during the HN rotation task:* • 2nd thoracic ring: No change • C5: No change	*Inter-regional:* • Correcting the 2nd thoracic ring worsens the alignment of C5 and does not improve the amplitude of right HN rotation • Correcting the C5 worsens alignment of the 2nd thoracic ring and does not improve the amplitude of right HN rotation • Correcting both the 2nd thoracic ring *and* C5 improves the amplitude, and the patient's experience, of right HN rotation ***The co-drivers are the thorax (2nd thoracic ring) and neck (C5)***
Co-driver Type 2 (CD Type 2)	Correction of one body region results in improvement of ABCs for another body region *and* correction of the other body region improves the ABCs of the first for the MT	**Task: Right single leg standing** *Starting alignment:* • 8th thoracic ring translated left and rotated right • 4th thoracic ring translated right and rotated left • C7 translated right and rotated left • C2 translated left and rotated right • Pelvis: Left TPR and left IPT • Right hip anterior to left • Right foot pronated, left foot supinated *Changes during right single leg standing* • Only notable change is that the right SIJ unlocks • All other findings remain the same	*Intra-regional* • Thorax: Correcting the 8th thoracic ring results in complete correction of the 4th thoracic ring • Pelvis and hip: Correcting the right hip corrects the pelvis alignment in standing and restores control of the right SIJ during the right single leg standing task • Cervical spine: Correcting C7 corrects C2, correcting C2 corrects C7 *Inter-regional* • Hip, pelvis and thorax: Correcting the right hip restores the alignment and biomechanics of the thorax and pelvis as well as the cervical segments and feet • Feet: Correcting the right foot corrects the right hip and thus the pelvis, thorax and neck ***The co-drivers are the right hip and right foot***

ABCs = alignment, biomechanics and control, CD = co-driver, FLT = failed load transfer, HN = head and neck, IPT = intrapelvic torsion, MT = meaningful task, PD = primary driver, SD = secondary driver, SIJ = sacroiliac joint, TPR = transverse plane rotation.

Understanding ideal alignment, biomechanics and control for task analysis is a recommended approach for the management of motor control disorders and the lumbar spine (Hodges et al. 2016).

'Although this proposed "ideal" postural alignment is unlikely to be ideal for all individuals ... It serves as a starting point for identification of features that can be evaluated for relevance to pain. In a way, it is the basic blueprint for postural alignment that acts as a starting point for assessment, but this needs to be molded by the specific presentation of the patient to identify the postural alignment that is ideal for their unique individual situation. If a feature of postural alignment is identified that deviates from ideal, it can be modified to assess the relationship to pain/muscle activation. If correction changes symptoms and/or reduces overactivity of muscle, then the feature is likely to be relevant to consider in planning of the [treatment program].' (Hodges et al. 2016)

Once the driver for a screening task is confirmed, the more complex meaningful task is repeated to:

- Confirm the hypothesis of the best place to begin treatment;

- Create patient confidence and understanding as to how the regions of the body relate and why

sometimes treatment should begin far distant from the site of their symptom or symptoms; and

- Give the patient a different experience of their body and thus begin to change the input to the cortical body matrix since changing a motor output begins by changing the sensory input.

If no correction in alignment, biomechanics or control of a body region changes the patient's experience during analysis of any task, and altered dural or perineural mobility is not suspected (see Dural and perineural mobility below), then their experience may not be dominated by a 'biology' component. Consider psychological components (extreme fear of moving, i.e., threatening beliefs) and sociological components (relationship contexts) (Moseley & Butler 2017).

Determining the system impairments related to the driver or drivers

If a driver is found, further tests, performed on the body region noted to improve the task experience best, will reveal the contribution of underlying system impairments (which could be articular, neural, myofascial or visceral) impacting the alignment, biomechanics and/or control of the driver (Table 3.4). The articular system includes

Table 3.4
Conditions associated with the various systems of the Clinical Puzzle.

Conditions associated with the various systems of the Clinical Puzzle	
SYSTEM	**ASSOCIATED CONDITION**

(A)	• Cognitive barriers (beliefs and memories from past experiences, thoughts 'attended to')
	• Emotional barriers (anger, fear, depression)
	• Physiological and medical considerations:
	  ○ Hormone health (neuroendocrine)
	  ○ Nutrition
	  ○ Hydration
	  ○ Disease (e.g., diabetes, cardiovascular disease)
	• Patient's values and goals (meaningful complaints and tasks)

Continued

Table 3.4 *continued*

SYSTEM	ASSOCIATED CONDITION
B	• Capsular sprain or tear • Ligament sprain or tear (Grades 1–3) • Labral or intra-articular meniscal tear • Intervertebral disc strain, tear, herniation, or prolapse • Fracture • Joint fixation or dislocation • Periosteal contusion • Stress fracture • Osteitis, periostitis, apophysitis • Osteochondral and chondral fractures, minor osteochondral injury • Chondropathy (e.g., softening, fibrillation, fissuring, chondromalacia) • Synovitis • Apophysitis • Fibrosis or osteophytosis of the zygapophyseal and intervertebral joints, sacroiliac joint, hip joint

C	• Intramuscular strain or tear (Grades 1–3)
	• Muscle contusion
	• Musculotendinous strain or tear
	• Complete or partial tendon rupture or tear
	• Fascial strain or tear
	• Tendon pathology – tendon rupture, partial tendon tears, tendinopathy (acute or chronic), paratendinopathy, pantendinopathy
	• Skin lacerations, abrasions, or puncture wounds
	• Bursa, bursitis
	• Muscular or fascial scarring or adhesions
	• Loss of fascial integrity of the anterior abdominal wall including:
	  ○ Diastasis rectus abdominis
	  ○ Sports hernia (tear of transversalis fascia)
	  ○ Hockey hernia (tear of the external oblique)
	  ○ Inguinal hernia
	• Loss of integrity of the vaginal wall leading to urethrocele, cystocele, enterocele or rectocele

D	• Peripheral nerve trunk or nerve injury (neurapraxia, neurotmesis, axonotmesis)
	• Central nervous system injury
	• Altered motor control:
	  ○ Absence of recruitment, inappropriate timing (early or late) of muscle recruitment
	  ○ Inappropriate amount (increased or decreased) of muscle activity (all relative to demands of task)
	  ○ Overactivity or underactivity of muscles at rest
	• Altered neurodynamics (dura or perineurium)
	• Sensitization of the peripheral or central nervous system
	• Altered central nervous system processing:
	  ○ Altered body schema or virtual body

Table 3.4 *continued*

SYSTEM	ASSOCIATED CONDITION
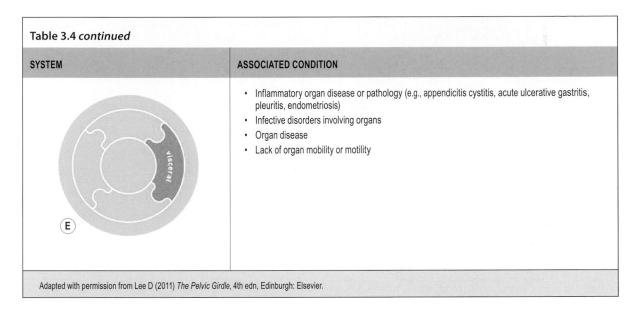	• Inflammatory organ disease or pathology (e.g., appendicitis cystitis, acute ulcerative gastritis, pleuritis, endometriosis) • Infective disorders involving organs • Organ disease • Lack of organ mobility or motility

Adapted with permission from Lee D (2011) *The Pelvic Girdle*, 4th edn, Edinburgh: Elsevier.

the bones, joints, ligaments and capsules. The myofascial system includes muscles, and their tendinous, fascial, and aponeurotic connections, as well as the regular dense and loose connective tissue. The neural system includes all components of the central and peripheral nervous systems. The visceral system includes all the viscera.

Note: Conditions can be combined; for example, it is possible to have a stiff joint and an overactive muscle further compressing the joint. The articular system impairment is not identifiable until the compression from the neural system impairment has been released.

Findings from the various system tests then determine the individualized treatment plan. These tests are specifically directed to the region of the driver or drivers. Once again, be careful with the words you choose to explain the biology of the patient's condition and ensure they understand that the treatment plan is *guidance from you* and *done primarily by them.* Avoid patient dependence or creating patient beliefs that 'only you can fix them,' 'you are special,' 'no one has ever found all these things wrong with me, you are the only one that understands how broken I am.' If you hear language like this from your patient, you have either created, or reinforced, a suboptimal neurotag (belief) that will not be helpful in the long run for empowering your patient toward maintaining their own health.

The Clinical Puzzle

The Clinical Puzzle (Lee D G et al. 2008, Lee L-J & Lee D 2011) (Fig. 3.4A & B) is a tool for reflection; it is not a charting tool. Reflecting on the patient's story and assessment findings helps to organize knowledge and determine the relevance of a finding. While not essential for every patient, for those with a complex story and multiple meaningful tasks, the Clinical Puzzle helps to keep knowledge organized and generate a sound hypothesis and plan for treatment. Furthermore, reflecting on a session often reveals things that were missed, which can then be included for subsequent investigation. Reflection is critical for developing clinical expertise (Butler 2000, Edwards & Jones 2007, Higgs & Jones 2000) and the Clinical Puzzle, while somewhat incomplete for all body systems, is useful for the systems relevant to musculoskeletal therapy.

Where to put the findings in the Clinical Puzzle?

Key features from the patient's story are noted in the center of the Clinical Puzzle (see Chapter 5 for examples) including:

- The meaningful complaint: The primary symptom, thought, emotion or feeling that has brought them for treatment (biology). What are they looking to change?

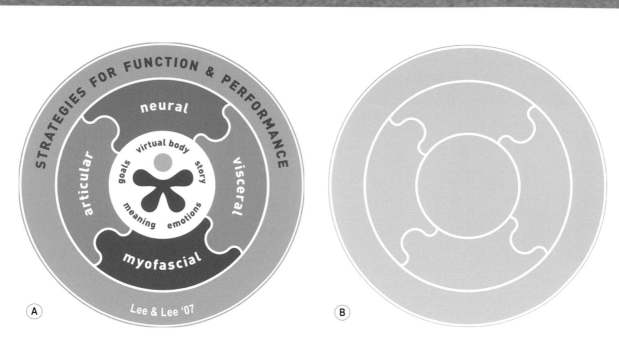

Figure 3.4

(A) The Clinical Puzzle is a reflection tool to help organize the assessment findings. The outer circle of the puzzle represents the strategies for function and performance that the patient currently uses for the screening tasks that relate to their meaningful task. The center circle of the puzzle represents several systems that relate to the person and the sensorial, cognitive, and emotional components of their current experience. It is the place where the meaningful complaint, and goals and barriers to recovery are noted. The four other pieces of the puzzle represent the various systems in which impairments are assessed and noted during the clinical examination. (B) The Clinical Puzzle template for reflection of findings.

- The current meaningful task or goal (biology): What are they looking to be able to do better?

- Any potential cognitive, emotional, or social factors that may be barriers to recovery (psychology, sociology).

- Any significant medical considerations.

The screening tasks (derived from the meaningful task) are entered on the outer circle of the Clinical Puzzle. The main sites of the body that demonstrate suboptimal alignment, biomechanics or control (FLT) are listed below each screening task. The driver or drivers for the screening task are identified as either a primary driver (PD), secondary driver (SD), or co-driver (CD).

The findings from further tests (articular, neural, myofascial, visceral – see details below for these tests) are noted in the relevant Clinical Puzzle pieces (middle ring of the puzzle). Reflection on the completed puzzle facilitates a sound hypothesis for treatment planning that is relevant to the underlying system impairments affecting the functioning of the body region or regions that have been determined to be the driver for the meaningful task.

Treatment planning

Each treatment session should include components of:

1. Release: Use education to 'release' suboptimal thoughts and beliefs. Use manual therapy or dry needling to release protective, maladaptive postures or movement patterns, stiff joints or myofascial or visceral impairments. Provide instructions for home exercises, meditation or breathwork practice to retain the release gained.

2. Alignment: Align the patient's knowledge, thoughts, and beliefs to the evidence and clinical picture

(e.g., Explain Pain [Butler & Moseley 2003, Moseley & Butler 2015, 2017]). Align the patient's posture and body to better receive and transfer the loads necessary to achieve their goals (running, swimming, sitting, etc.). Incorporate alignment awareness (release cues) in their movement tasks.

3. Connect and control: Teach or remind the patient of better recruitment strategies for neuromuscular support of the joints for both static loading and then through motion. Incorporate connect or control cues in their movement tasks (motor learning).

4. Move: Create a safe environment for a positive experience during functional movement training that ultimately pertains to the patient's meaningful task and goals. There are many ways to do this. The key principle is to create movement programs that feel safe, pain-free, and relevant. Pace the program according to perceived threat.

Summary

In closing her keynote presentation at the 2012 IFOMPT conference in Quebec, Professor Gwen Jull said: 'The advantage of a clinical reasoning approach is that it is responsive to new knowledge and evidence, is flexible and allows for change and growth.' The Integrated Systems Model is an evidence-informed, clinical reasoning approach. It is a framework – not a classification – that considers all three dimensions of the patient's experience and the barriers that each may present to the recovery process for both acute and persistent conditions and is thus a biopsychosocial approach.

In closing her presentation at the 9th Interdisciplinary World Congress on Low Back and Pelvic Pain in Singapore (November 2016), Dr. Julie Hides emphasized the importance of the clinical reasoning process and stated that: 'The Integrated Systems Model, which draws from several other approaches, may provide a very useful framework for therapists which could incorporate individual aspects of the evidence-based approaches presented [in her presentation]'. While several single case studies exist as part of ISM certification (see www.learnwithdianelee.com) and some in peer-reviewed chapter publications (Lee D 2016,

Lee D G & Jones [in press]), a Level 1 randomized clinical trial on the efficacy of the Integrated Systems Model has not been conducted yet. This approach does draw from the research evidence, as well as from clinical practice; however, it is acknowledged that with respect to levels of evidence it qualifies as Level 4 Grade 4, which, according to Moseley & Butler (2017), equates to: 'We have no idea whether or not a treatment is good, but it is worth doing a clinical trial to find out.' All in time, I hope.

Common screening tasks for assessment of function of the thorax

What follows is a description of how to analyze the biomechanics of three common screening tasks with a focus on the thorax that also considers its relationship to the whole body. The principles of the tasks described below can then be applied to other screening tasks. The corrections are described in detail in the first task – standing posture – and are not repeated in the other tasks. The entire process of finding drivers for the entire body in one screening task seems long and complicated when committing it to writing; however, once the skills are acquired to find findings quickly, the process only takes five to seven minutes per task. Rarely are more than three screening tasks evaluated per session.

This chapter will not cover the assessment of forward, backward or side bending as screening tasks for the thorax. If the meaningful task requires one of these as a screening task, assess the alignment and biomechanics as described in Chapter 2 and then apply the specific corrections that are described below to determine the driver or drivers. An analysis of standing posture, squat, and head, neck and thoracic rotation have been chosen for this chapter.

Standing posture

Many functional tasks begin from the standing position and this screening task is often part of the objective examination. Table 3.5 outlines the requirements for optimal standing posture.

It is not uncommon to find multiple body regions that are not optimally aligned in standing. The Integrated Systems Model helps to determine when the findings are

Table 3.5

Requirements for optimal standing posture

	SAGITTAL PLANE
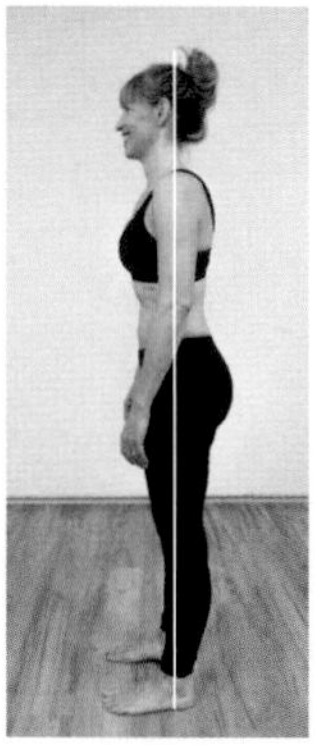	In the sagittal plane, a vertical line should pass through the external auditory meatus, the bodies of the cervical vertebrae, the glenohumeral joint, slightly anterior to the bodies of the thoracic vertebrae transecting the vertebrae at the thoracolumbar junction, the bodies of the lumbar vertebrae, the sacral promontory, slightly posterior to the hip joint, the center of the knee, and slightly anterior to the talocrural joint. The primary spinal curves should be maintained: Cervical lordosis, thoracic kyphosis, and lumbar lordosis. Very few individuals meet all the requirements for optimal standing posture. Figure 3.5 This individual's head and neck are slightly forward for optimal sagittal plane alignment and her knees are overextended.
	CORONAL PLANE
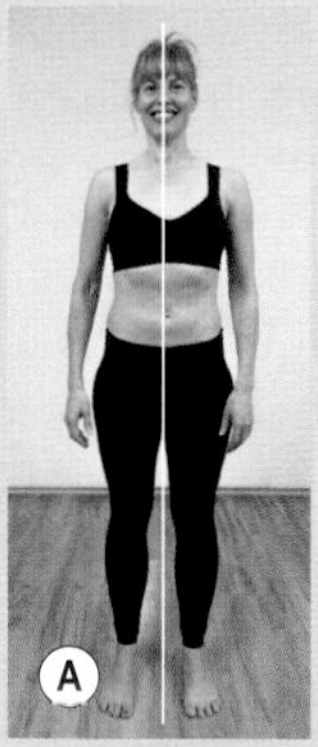	In the coronal plane, the eyes, ears and mouth should be level (i.e., the cranium should not be side-bent relative to the neck), the cervical vertebra should be aligned (i.e., no segment should be side-bent relative to the one above or below), the clavicles should be slightly elevated, and the manubrium and sternum should be vertical (not side-bent) and in the same plane as the pubic symphysis. The scapulae should be slightly elevated with the scapular spine at the level of the 3rd thoracic ring and the inferior angle and medial border approximated to the chest wall. Deviations in the coronal plane of the thoracic spinous processes are common and often insignificant. The thorax as a unit should be aligned over the pelvis, and the pelvis should be centered between the feet. The femoral heads should be centered such that the hip joints are neither abducted nor adducted, and the knees should be aligned (without any varus or valgus inclination). The calcaneus should be neutral such that the talus is well supported in the mortise and the Achilles tendon vertical. There should be a slight medial, lateral, and transverse arch in the foot with the toes aligned with the relative metatarsal. Figure 3.6 (A) This individual's thorax is slightly to the left of center and her head and neck are slightly side-bent to the right.

Table 3.5 *continued*	
	TRANSVERSE PLANE
	In the transverse plane, the cranium should be neutral with no rotation or intracranial torsion (ICT) (rotation between the temporal bones with or without a congruent or incongruent rotation of the sphenoid). The cervical vertebrae (C1–C7) should not be rotated in the transverse plane, and each thoracic ring should be in a neutral position with respect to the one above and below (no transverse plane rotation = no lateral translation). The lumbar vertebrae should be neutral as should the sacrum. The pelvis should not be rotated in the transverse plane without intrapelvic torsion. Both femoral heads should be centered in their respective acetabulum, and each other. The knee joints should be close to full extension and therefore the tibia externally rotated relative to the femur. The talus should be centered in the mortise (not tilted medially or laterally, nor anteriorly translated). The midfoot (navicular and cuboid) should be neutral such that the forefoot is neither internally, nor externally, rotated. All metatarsals and phalanges should be in neutral rotation. Figure 3.6 (B) From a posterior view, the thorax is slightly left of center.

relevant to the clinical picture and, which findings have priority (which corrections improve all other findings as well as the patient's experience).

It is important to find the driver or drivers for standing posture *if* standing is the meaningful task. Even if standing is not a meaningful task, standing posture is still an important screening task since it provides valuable information on the starting position of the body areas that are being assessed in the other screening tasks. In these instances, it is only important to note the starting position of the body regions that are not optimally aligned (without the need to determine the driver or drivers for standing) so that any change during the next screening task (for example, squat or step forward) can be determined.

To expedite the assessment, the body is divided into three functional units:

1. 3rd thoracic ring to the hip joints (T2–T3, left and right 3rd ribs to the hip joints).

2. 2nd thoracic ring to the cranium (the shoulder girdle and glenohumeral joint can be included in either the first or second functional unit depending on the story). The *cranial region* is part of the second functional unit and includes the cranium, C1 and C2.

3. Lower extremity (knee to foot) and upper extremity (elbow to wrist).

The driver or drivers are found first in each functional unit and then the relationship, or priority, is determined between the drivers of the units. This process determines the relevance of any finding to the clinical picture. Both the performance of the task and the patient's experience of the task should improve, if the finding is clinically relevant.

Third thoracic ring to the hips

Stand at the patient's side and note the sagittal plane relationship between the pelvis and the feet (anterior or posterior), the amount of extension of the knees and thus dorsiflexion or plantarflexion of the ankles, as well as the relationship between the thorax and the pelvis (whether the manubrium is anterior or posterior to the pubic symphysis). Additionally, note the degree of anterior or posterior tilt of the pelvis and the thorax (as a unit relative to the pelvis and then between the vertebrosternal (VS) and vertebrochondral (VC) regions) (Figs 3.7 and 3.8). Note the position of the cranium relative to the thorax in the sagittal plane (forward or vertical) and the degree of anterior or posterior tilt of the cranium (Fig. 3.9).

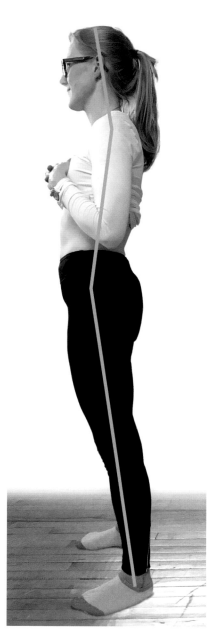

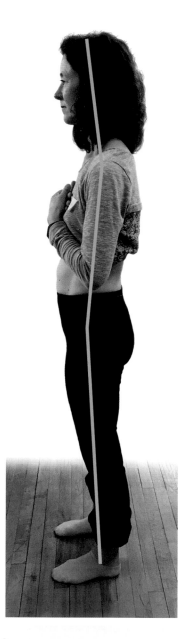

Figure 3.7

Sagittal plane relationship of the pelvis, lower extremity, and thorax. This woman stands with an anterior sway and posterior tilt of her pelvis and a posterior tilt of her thorax such that her manubriosternal symphysis is posterior to the pubic symphysis. Note the hyperextension of her knees.

Figure 3.8

Sagittal plane relationship of the pelvis, lower extremity, and thorax. This woman stands with her pelvis optimally aligned over her feet (compare this to Fig. 3.7); however, her thorax is posteriorly tilted in the sagittal plane and her cranium is anterior to the center of her thorax. The profile of her abdomen suggests she has a diastasis rectus abdominis.

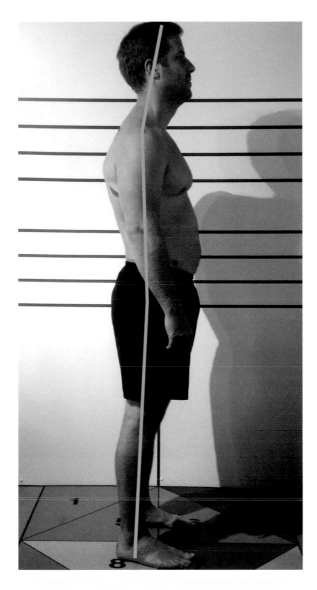

Figure 3.9

Sagittal plane relationship of the pelvis, lower extremity, thorax, and cranium. This man stands with his pelvis in an anterior pelvic sway and anterior tilt, his thorax in an anterior tilt, and his cranium anteriorly translated relative to his upper thorax and posteriorly tilted.

Reproduced courtesy of clinical anatomist, biomechanist, and ISM certified practitioner, Jo Abbott (https://joabbottmsc.com).

From the front or back, note the coronal plane relationship from head to toe (Figs 3.10–3.12). Then determine the transverse plane position of the pelvis as a unit (entire pelvic ring) by placing your hands such that the metacarpophalangeal joints rest over the left and right anterior superior iliac spines (ASIS) of the innominates (Fig. 3.13). This test requires the therapist to stand directly behind the patient in a neutral position and to set their scapulae such that their arm lengths are equal when flexed forward. Close your eyes and sense which arm is reaching further forward to access the same point on the patient's pelvis. If the right arm is reaching further forward, the pelvis is rotated in the transverse plane to the left; if the left arm is reaching further forward, the pelvis is rotated to the right.

Then move your hands to the anterior aspect of the VC region of the thorax (Fig. 3.14) and note the transverse plane rotation and whether the direction is congruent (in the same direction) or incongruent (in the opposite direction) to the pelvis rotation. When the lower thorax is rotated incongruent to the pelvis, the lumbar spine is under greater rotational load. Then determine which thoracic ring or rings is or are translated and rotated in the direction consistent with the rotation of the VC region. For example, if the VC region is rotated to the right, look for a thoracic ring that is translated to the left, relative to a thoracic ring above or below, since this translation is biomechanically coupled with right rotation (see Chapter 2 for the biomechanics of transverse plane rotation and Chapter 1 for how to landmark the position of the specific thoracic rings).

Next, determine the transverse plane rotation of the VS region by palpating the 3rd to 6th thoracic rings in the midaxillary line (see Chapter 1). Note if the VS region is rotated congruent with the VC region or is incongruent as this will determine the direction of the regional translation to look for. For example, if the VS region is left rotated relative to the VC region (which was right rotated in the example above), then look for a thoracic ring that is translated to the right (and therefore rotated to the left).

Finally, for this functional unit, determine the relative position of the head of the femur to its acetabulum as well

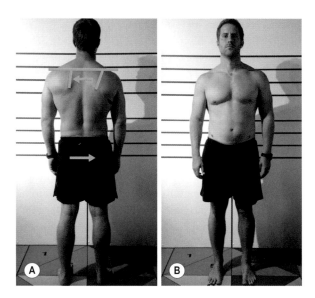

Figure 3.10

Coronal plane relationship of the pelvis, lower extremity, thorax, and cranium. (A) Posterior view. This man stands with his thorax to the left of his base of support. Specifically, more thoracic rings in the vertebrosternal region are translated left and rotated right than are translated right and rotated left. This results in 'net' right side bending of his thorax which has consequences for the alignment of his right scapula. Note the depression and downward rotation of the right scapula. (B) Anterior view. The depression of the right shoulder girdle is also evident from the anterior view of the coronal plane alignment. The center of mass of his cranium is translated to the right relative to the sternal notch and he has an intracranial torsion to the left with a congruent left rotation of his sphenoid (note the deep left orbit). The medial end of the left clavicle is elevated secondary to the right side bending of the manubrium that occurs in conjunction with the translation left and rotation right of the upper and middle thoracic rings.

Reproduced courtesy of clinical anatomist, biomechanist, and ISM certified practitioner, Jo Abbott (https://joabbottmsc.com).

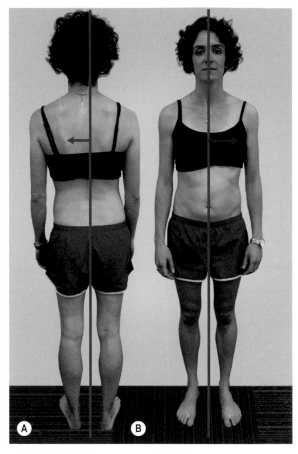

Figure 3.11

(A) Posterior view. This woman is standing with her pelvis rotated in the transverse plane to the left and the weight shift test for pelvic control revealed that in the standing position her left sacroiliac joint (SIJ) was unlocked. Her right hip was anterior compared to the left, which is congruent with the left transverse plane rotation of her pelvis. Her 3rd, 4th, and 5th thoracic rings were translated left and rotated right and this accounts for the apparent left lateral translation of her thorax in relationship to her pelvis. The 9th thoracic ring was translated right and rotated left. (B) Anterior view. The left translation of the middle thoracic rings is apparent from the anterior view as well. She appears to compensate for this lateral translation in her neck and cranium quite well.

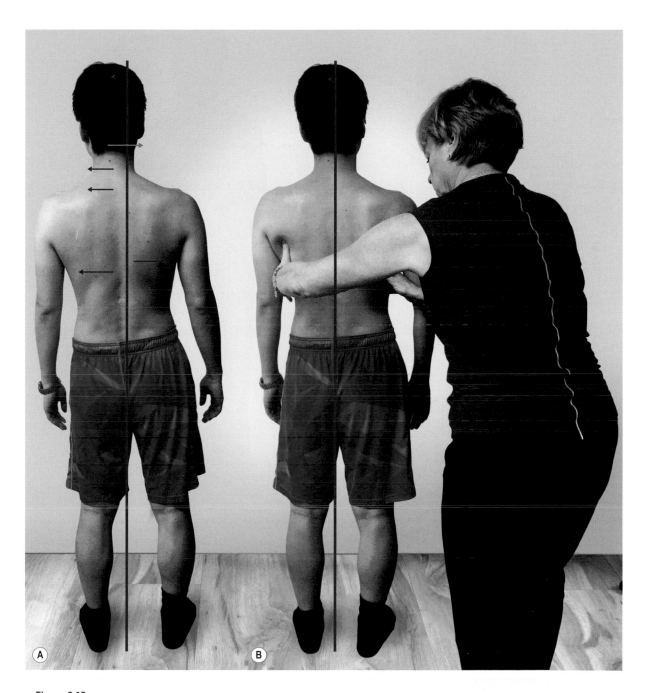

Figure 3.12

(A) Posterior view. This man is standing with his pelvis rotated in the transverse plane to the right, his 7th thoracic ring translated left and rotated right, 6th thoracic ring translated right and rotated left, 2nd thoracic ring translated left and rotated right, C7 translated left and rotated right, C2 translated right and rotated left, and he has a left intracranial torsion. B) Note the improvement in coronal plane alignment when the alignment of the driver (6th and 7th thoracic rings) is corrected.

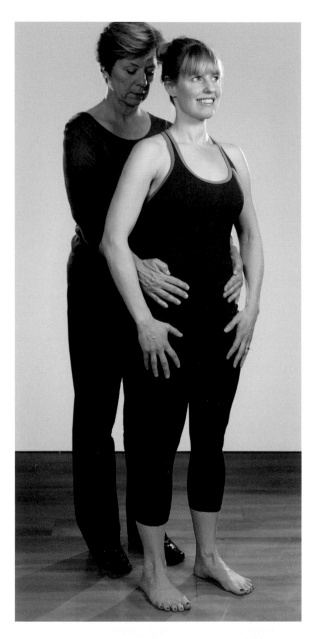

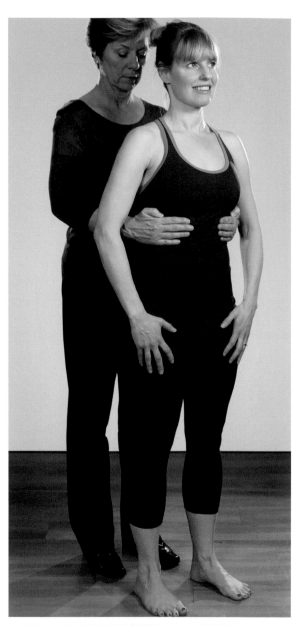

Figure 3.13

Hand placement for determining the transverse plane orientation of the pelvis as an entire ring. Kinesthetic sense is preferred to vision for reliability. Which arm must reach further forward to cover the anterior superior iliac spine? This informs the direction of rotation in the transverse plane.

Figure 3.14

Hand placement for determining the transverse plane orientation of the vertebrochondral region of the thorax. Kinesthetic sense is preferred to vision for reliability. Which arm must reach further forward to cover the anterior aspect of the lower thoracic rings? This informs the direction of rotation in the transverse plane.

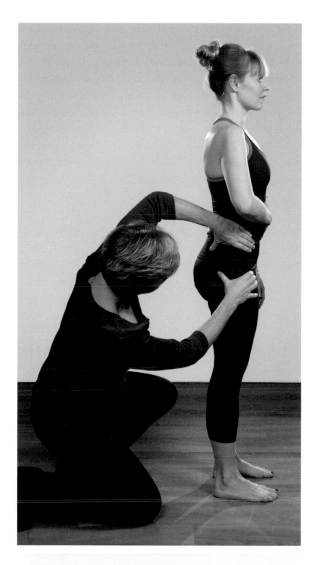

Figure 3.15

Hand placement for determining the position of the femoral head relative to the innominate and acetabulum. Returning to standing from a small squat is used to determine the resultant position of the femoral head relative to the acetabulum. It is easier to feel any loss of centering of the femoral head during motion than to determine static positional relationships.

as to the opposite femoral head. With one hand, palpate the innominate and with the other the femoral head (Fig. 3.15). Have the patient squat slightly and then return to standing. As they reach the standing position note any loss of centering of the femoral head, i.e., does it translate anteriorly or rotate internally or externally? Using movement to determine femoral head position appears more reliable than landmarking the hip in static tasks such as standing. Note if the position of the femoral head is congruent with the transverse plane rotation of the pelvic ring. If the pelvis is rotated to the left, the right femoral head should be more anterior than the left if the findings are congruent. If the left femoral head is anterior to the right and the pelvis is rotated to the left, these findings are incongruent with one producing the other.

So, let's assume that the pelvis is rotated in the transverse plane to the left, the VC region is rotated to the right (incongruent to the pelvis), with an associated translated left and rotated right 8th thoracic ring, and the VS region is rotated to the left (incongruent to the VC region) with an associated translated right and rotated left 4th thoracic ring. In addition, the right femoral head is anterior to the left (congruent with the pelvis). The next step is to determine the clinical relevance (determine the driver) of these findings before moving to the next functional unit. This requires manually and verbally correcting the alignment of one region and noting the impact of this correction on the alignment of the others.

Pelvic ring correction

Stand behind the patient, place your hands around the pelvic ring and correct its position in all three planes. Release the correction without releasing contact with the pelvis and feel the pelvis return to its original starting position. This test should confirm the prior visual and manual findings. The rotation between the left and right innominate that occurs with the transverse plane rotation can also be felt. When the pelvis is rotated to the left in the transverse plane there should be an associated left intrapelvic torsion (IPT) (Fig. 3.16) in which the right innominate anteriorly rotates relative to the left innominate and the sacrum rotates to the left (Lee D 2011). A right IPT would be incongruent with a left transverse plane rotation of the pelvic ring.

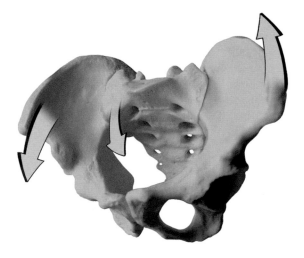

Figure 3.16

The relative position of the three pelvic bones in a left intrapelvic torsion. The right innominate is anteriorly rotated relative to the left innominate. The sacrum is nutated relative to both innominates, more so on the right such that the sacrum is rotated in space to the left (side of the posteriorly rotated innominate).

Once the pelvis is corrected in all three planes, maintain this correction and have the patient lift and replace each foot on the ground to reset the alignment of the feet in response to this correction. Maintain the pelvic correction and then note any change in the alignment of the lower (VC) and middle (VS) thorax and the femoral heads. If the pelvis is a primary driver, the alignment of all three regions (VC, VS and hips) will completely correct when the pelvis is manually corrected. Any other correction will worsen the alignment of the pelvis (Fig. 3.17A–C).

Hip correction

To understand the impact of a noncentered femoral head on pelvic and thoracic alignment, a hip correction is required. Stand to the side of the hip of interest and have the patient slightly squat. Decompress the hip joint by lifting the ischial tuberosity superiorly and slightly anteriorly with the heel of one hand. With the other hand, guide the femoral head posteriorly and laterally (Fig. 3.18). Maintain this correction and ask the patient to return to standing. Have them reset the position of their feet (lift and replace). Note the impact of this correction on the alignment of the pelvis, lower and middle thorax. If the hip is the driver, both will improve.

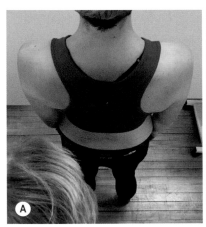
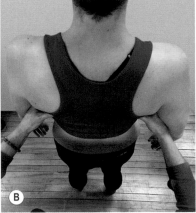
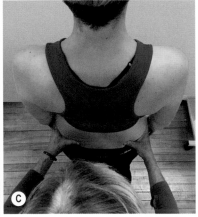

Figure 3.17

Pelvic correction and standing posture. (A) This woman is standing with her pelvis rotated in the transverse plane to the right (associated with a congruent right intrapelvic torsion) and her lower thorax is rotated to the left (associated with right translation of the 7th thoracic ring). (B) Correcting the alignment of the 7th thoracic ring causes the pelvis to rotate to the left; the alignment is not improved. (C) Correcting the alignment of the pelvis corrects the alignment of the lower thorax and the 7th thoracic ring. For this task, the pelvis is the driver.

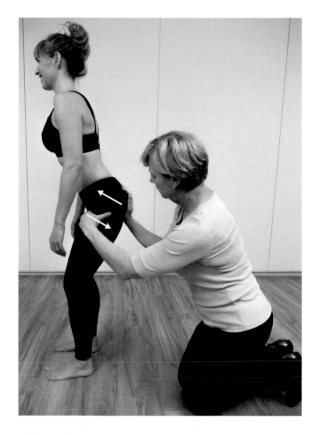

Figure 3.18

Left hip correction. The goal is to decompress the hip joint and reposition the femoral head in relationship to the acetabulum. Starting in a semisquat facilitates this correction regardless of the screening task.

Thoracic ring correction

Acknowledgment: The concept of a thoracic ring correction was developed by Linda-Joy Lee (2003a, 2016). The following technique is a modification of her original technique.

Let's continue with the scenario described above. The 8th thoracic ring of the VC region is translated to the left, which is coupled with rotation to the right (incongruent to the rotation of the pelvis). Palpate the left and right 8th ribs (see Chapter 1 for how to accurately landmark each rib of the thoracic ring for this test). When the 8th thoracic ring is translated left and rotated right, the left 8th rib is anteriorly rotated relative to the right 8th rib. Standing behind the

patient, the correction begins by gently lifting both 8th ribs (decompress the intercostal spaces between the 8th and 9th ribs to create space) (Fig. 3.19A). Wait, you are initially working in the nervous system. As the sensory input from this correction is interpreted by the cortical body matrix a change in the motor output may occur. This will be felt as a subtle softening of the resistance to further correction of the left 8th rib. Next, gently posteriorly rotate the left 8th rib by lifting the anterior aspect of the rib ever so slightly (Fig. 3.19B).

Wait. Wait. Wait. This is so important, it cannot be emphasized enough. Clinicians who struggle with learning this technique often have 'hard hands that are threatening to the patient,' squeeze, push or pull too hard or too fast, and do not wait long enough for a change to occur. In other words, they try to do something to the patient as opposed to 'offer an invitation to change' through the nervous system through their touch.

If it is possible for the thoracic ring to autocorrect (neural or visceral system impairment) the entire thoracic ring will automatically translate medially back to the neutral position and the ribs will derotate. No manual medial translation is required for this correction technique. When the thoracic ring autocorrects, the patient often spontaneously takes a deep, and local, breath and the thoracic ring feels like it is expanding. When this occurs be sure to ask the patient what they just felt. Note their words carefully and reinforce the positive, and possibility for change. If, however, there is an underlying articular or myofascial system impairment, the autocorrection may not occur since these impairments do not always respond to changing the sensory input. A myofascial system impairment may allow correction of the thoracic ring if more force is used, however the articular system impairment will not. Have the patient reset their feet by lifting one and then the other.

Hold the thoracic ring correction with your left hand (side of the previously anteriorly rotated rib) and note any change in alignment (translation) of the thoracic ring above (7th) or below (9th) (Fig. 3.20) on the opposite side of the thorax (right side in this case). Note any change in alignment of the previously noted translated right and rotated left 4th thoracic ring, the pelvis, and hips. If the 8th thoracic ring is the primary driver, the thoracic rings above

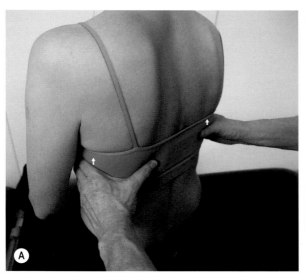
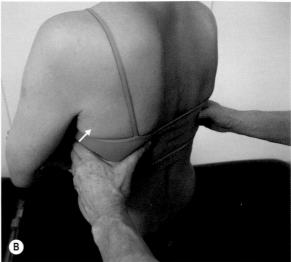

Figure 3.19

8th thoracic ring correction. This individual's 8th thoracic ring is translated left and rotated right. (A) The correction begins with gentle distraction of the 8th from the 9th thoracic ring. Wait for the nervous system to respond to this change in sensory input; a decrease in resistance to further correction of the left 8th rib should occur. (B) Next, gently posteriorly rotate the left 8th rib by lifting the anterior aspect of the rib slightly. If it is possible for the thoracic ring to autocorrect (neural or visceral system impairment), the entire thoracic ring will automatically translate medially back to the neutral position, the ribs will derotate, and the patient will spontaneously take a deep breath. Wait for the breath. The original concept of a thoracic ring correction was developed by Linda-Joy Lee (2003a, 2016).

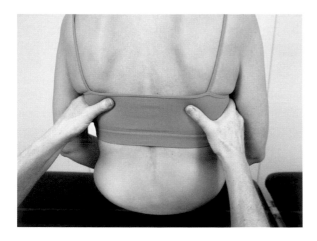

Figure 3.20

The left hand is holding the 8th thoracic ring correction and the right hand is noting any change (improvement or worsening) in the alignment of the 9th thoracic ring on the right with this correction.

and below will align, the 4th thoracic ring will completely correct as will the pelvis and hips. If it is difficult to determine the impact of this correction on the alignment of the pelvis or hip, note the change when the thoracic ring correction is released. If the alignment of the pelvis or hip worsens on release of the thoracic ring correction, this implies the alignment improved with the correction. However, it is not uncommon to find co-drivers (two body regions that require correction for the best result), secondary drivers (a body region that improves but does not completely correct when the primary driver is corrected) or two thoracic rings that are 'glued.'

A 'glued' thoracic ring is a term coined by Linda-Joy Lee (2003a, 2016) and used when two adjacent rings are incapable of independent motion. In the example above, if the 8th thoracic ring was glued to the 9th, the correction of the 8th thoracic ring would worsen the alignment of the 9th (often in the opposite direction). Correction of the 9th thoracic ring would worsen the alignment of the 8th. Glued thoracic rings can be found in all regions of the thorax except the thoracolumbar region and are usually the result of short interthoracic ring vectors (neural, myofascial or articular).

A co-correction of each thoracic ring is required when two adjacent thoracic rings are glued to prevent excessive elongation of the intercostal nerves and sympathetic ganglion (Fig. 1.50). When co-correcting two adjacent glued thoracic rings, one thoracic ring is partially corrected (through the anteriorly rotated rib) only until the adjacent one (above or below) is felt to worsen. The adjacent thoracic ring is then partially corrected (through its anteriorly rotated rib) until the first is felt to worsen. The corrections are alternated with plenty of time between each to allow for the motor output to respond to the changing sensory input. The co-correction is complete when the breath is felt to return to this region of the thorax, which then expands between your hands. If there are two adjacent thoracic rings translated in opposite directions and one automatically corrects with correction of the other, then these thoracic rings are not glued; one is compensating for the alignment of the other.

Multiple combinations of thoracic ring translations and rotations are found in the various regions of the thorax. Common findings include:

- Correction of one VS thoracic ring results in autocorrection of a contralaterally translated and rotated VC thoracic ring. For example, in the scenario above, correcting the 4th thoracic ring results in complete correction of the 8th. In this case, the 8th thoracic ring can be ignored since treating the 4th will result in autocorrection of the 8th.

- Correction of one VS thoracic ring results in worsening of a contralaterally translated and rotated VC thoracic ring. This is not the driver. The impact of correcting the VC thoracic ring on the alignment of the VS thoracic ring is then noted. If the VS thoracic ring autocorrects then it can be ignored and focus placed on the VC ring.

- Correction of one VS thoracic ring results in only a partial correction of a contralaterally translated and rotated VC ring. The VS thoracic ring may be primary but the 8th thoracic ring also requires attention.

Correct both thoracic rings and assess the impact of this correction on the alignment of the pelvis and hips, as well as the meaningful task. If correcting both the VS and VC thoracic ring results in complete correction of all other body regions, then the thorax is a primary driver, despite two thoracic rings requiring attention. Drivers pertain to body regions, not individual thoracic rings.

- Correction of two thoracic rings in two different regions of the thorax is required for improvement of whole body alignment and the meaningful task. Correcting each thoracic ring individually worsens the alignment of the other, as well as the performance of the task. Correcting both thoracic rings simultaneously improves the task performance. The thorax can still be considered a primary driver; however, two thoracic ring corrections are required for the best outcome in task performance and patient experience. If no other body region requires correction, the thorax is still the primary driver.

- Correction of one thoracic ring in two different regions of the thorax results in improvement of whole body alignment and the meaningful task. Correcting each thoracic ring individually improves the alignment of the other, as well as the performance of the task. If no other body region outside of the thorax required correction, then the thorax is still considered a primary driver; however only one thoracic ring (either one) requires treatment.

When the thorax is excessively compressed, and poorly controlled, three adjacent thoracic rings may translate and rotate in contralateral directions (e.g., the 4th thoracic ring translated right and rotated left, the 5th thoracic ring translated left and rotated right, the 6th thoracic ring translated right and rotated left). In this situation, the 4th and 6th thoracic rings are often compressed (side-bent) such that the right 5th rib is difficult to feel in the midaxillary line. The right scapula is often depressed and downward rotated on this side. Alternately, two thoracic rings may translate and rotate to the same side and the one above or below to the opposite side. The net effect is rotation and side bending of the thorax, which also results in depression and downward rotation of the scapula (Fig. 3.21). When the thorax is the driver, correcting the shoulder girdle does not change the alignment of the thoracic rings in either situation. When the shoulder girdle is the primary driver, the alignment of the thoracic rings is completely restored. If only a partial correction of the thorax occurs, the thorax may be a secondary driver. When correcting either the shoulder girdle

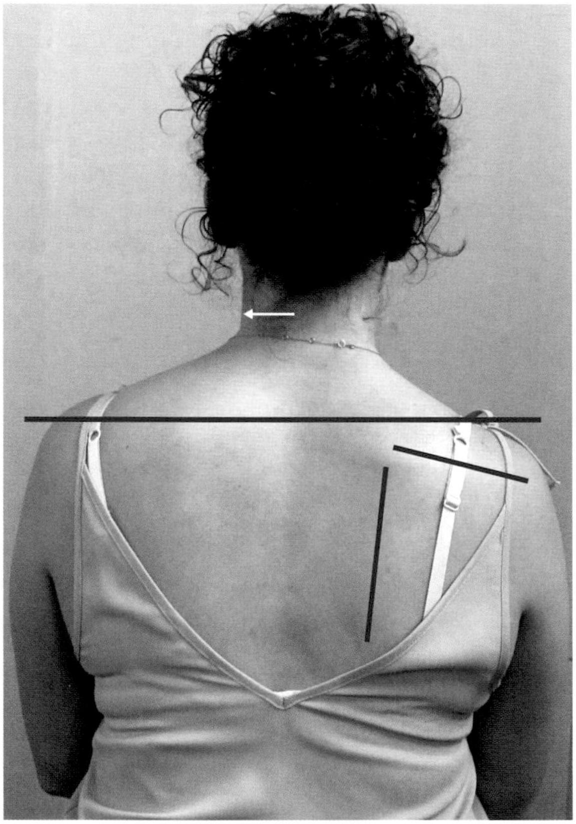

Figure 3.21

This woman's C7 is translated left (arrow) and rotated right, the 2nd and 3rd thoracic rings are translated left and rotated right, and the 4th thoracic ring is translated right and rotated left. Note the resultant depression and downward rotation of the right scapula. Correcting the position of the scapula did not change the alignment of C7 or the thoracic rings. Correcting the 2nd, 3rd, and 4th thoracic rings resulted in a positional correction of C7 and the right scapula. Her meaningful task was left head and neck rotation which also improved in both the range and experience with the thorax correction.

or the relative thoracic rings results in complete correction of the other, or if correction of both is required for the best improvement in standing posture, then they are co-drivers.

The correction of three alternating translated and rotated thoracic rings begins by creating space (distraction) between the two thoracic rings that are translated and rotated to the same side (4th and 6th in this scenario). Wait. Then the left 5th rib of the middle thoracic ring (5th) is gently posteriorly rotated and held. Wait for the medial translation and autoalignment of all three thoracic rings to occur and the regional breath to be restored. Note the impact of this correction on sites of suboptimal alignment in other body regions (head to toe eventually).

At this point, the best corrections between the 3rd thoracic ring and the hips for standing posture should be determined. The next step is to find the best correction (driver) in the second functional unit (2nd thoracic ring to the cranium) and then determine which of the two has precedence before moving onto the 3rd functional region.

Second thoracic ring to cranium

Note the position of the manubrium in the vertebro-manubrial (VM) region in the coronal and transverse planes (Fig. 3.22). Then note the relative position of the left and right 2nd ribs to determine the position of the 2nd thoracic ring (see Chapter 1 for how to landmark the 2nd thoracic ring) (Fig. 3.23A). If the right 2nd rib is more anterior than the left, then the 2nd thoracic ring is rotated to the left. It will also be slightly translated to the right; however, this is difficult to feel in the axilla in most individuals. Landmarking the 2nd thoracic ring can also be done from the anterior aspect of the chest (Fig. 3.23B & C). If congruent, the manubrium should also be rotated to the left and slightly side-bent left (ipsilateral side bending of the thoracic ring occurs with rotation; see Chapter 2). The position of the 3rd thoracic ring in relationship to the 2nd can also be noted from the anterior aspect of the thorax (see Chapter 1 for how to landmark the 2nd and 3rd thoracic rings from the front). It is not uncommon to find either congruent or incongruent rotations between these two thoracic rings.

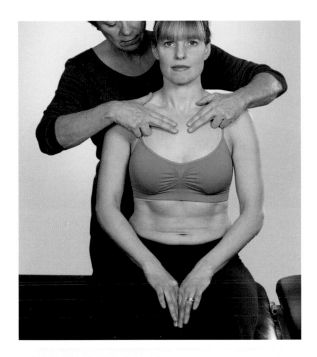

Figure 3.22

Positional testing of the manubrium. Note which side of the manubrium is more anterior. This determines the direction of rotation of the manubrium in the transverse plane.

Note the general alignment of the cervical spine and the coronal plane position of the cranium with respect to the neck (Fig. 3.24A–D).

Note the coronal plane position of the left and right clavicle (elevation or depression) and any rotation of one to the other (anterior or posterior rotation). Elevation of the clavicle should couple with anterior rotation, depression with posterior rotation (Pettman 1981, 1984). If the 2nd thoracic ring is rotated to the left, and the left and right shoulder girdle remain neutral (i.e., there is independent motion between the thorax and shoulder girdles), the right clavicle should be slightly depressed (lateral end horizontal with, or lower than, the medial end) and posteriorly rotated relative to the left clavicle, which is slightly elevated and anteriorly rotated (Fig. 3.25A–C). This is primarily due to the side bending of the manubrium (Fig. 3.26A–E). If the shoulder girdles follow the rotation of the 2nd thoracic ring (i.e., are incapable of independent motion from the upper thorax), the right clavicle will protract and anteriorly rotate relative to the left clavicle, which will retract and posteriorly rotate.

Palpate the transverse processes and laminae on the left and right sides of the cervical spine from C7 to C2 and note

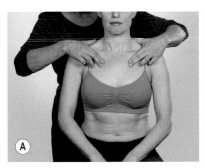
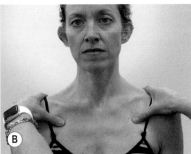
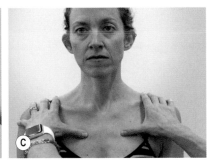

Figure 3.23

Positional testing of the 2nd thoracic ring. (A) Note which 2nd rib is further anterior. This determines the direction of rotation of the 2nd thoracic ring in the transverse plane. (B) It is important to be on the 2nd ribs and not the costocartilage when landmarking the position of the 2nd thoracic ring. This woman has a right rotated 2nd thoracic ring as indicated by the left and right 2nd ribs and the left rib is anterior in the transverse plane. (C) There is marked compression of the 2nd thoracic ring that is causing a 'buckling' of the costocartilage on the right. If the landmarking is done by palpating the patient's left and right costocartilages, the 2nd ring appears to be rotated to the left. There is marked tenderness over the right costochondral joint, which had been noted previously.

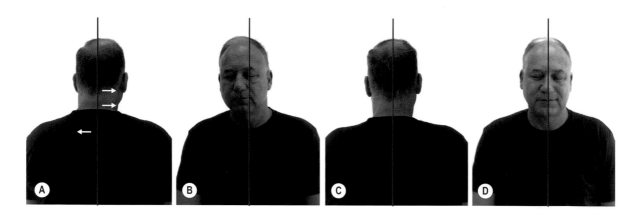

Figure 3.24

This man was struck by a cast iron grill on the top of his head and rendered unconscious for four seconds. His meaningful complaint was short-term memory loss, fogginess, headaches (pressure on the occiput), and increasing neck stiffness. (A, B) Seated posture analysis revealed translation of his entire head to the right of center associated with right rotation. The 2nd thoracic ring was translated left and rotated right, C7 was translated right and rotated left, C2 was translated left and rotated right, and his cranium was in an intracranial torsion to the right with an associated congruent right rotation of his sphenoid. The cranial region was his primary driver and the 2nd thoracic ring was a secondary driver. Vector analysis revealed increased tension in the posterior part of the left cerebellar tentorium and a right thoracic visceral vector was noted on correction and release of the 2nd thoracic ring. (C, D) Note the improvement in the patient's head-and-neck alignment after restoring venous drainage of the cerebellar tentorium and jugular vein. His pressure symptoms were immediately relieved and the range of motion of his head and neck improved.

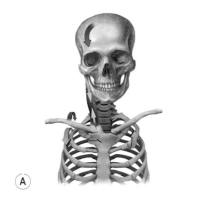
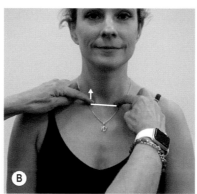
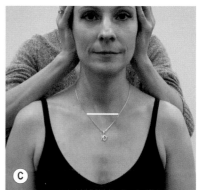

Figure 3.25

(A) This is a common postural pattern in the upper quadrant. The manubrium is rotated and side-bent to the left. The 2nd thoracic ring is congruent with the manubrial rotation and rotated in the transverse plane to the left (right 2nd rib is anteriorly rotated and the left is posteriorly rotated). The side bending of the manubrium impacts elevation of the left and right clavicle such that the right is more depressed and this induces a conjunct posterior rotation of the right clavicle and an anterior rotation of the left. The yellow arrows on the right sternocleidomastoid indicate that overactivation of this muscle is creating this postural pattern. This muscular vector results in side bending of the cranium and neck to the right. (B) This woman has a right intracranial torsion with a congruent right rotation of the sphenoid. Her 2nd thoracic ring is rotated to the left; the right clavicle is depressed and the medial end of the right clavicle is higher than the medial end of the left clavicle. (C) Her cranial region is the driver and correcting the alignment of the temporal bones, occiput, and sphenoid restores the alignment of her eyes, 2nd thoracic ring, manubrium, and clavicles.

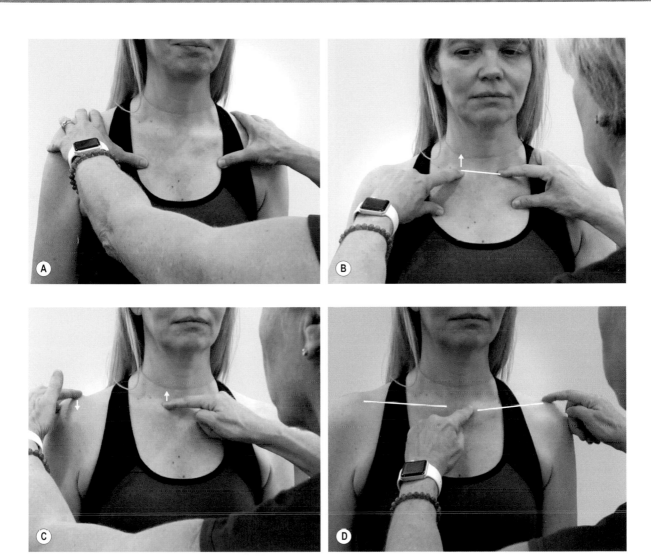

Figure 3.26

Impact of the 2nd thoracic ring on alignment and biomechanics of the clavicle and sternoclavicular joint (SCJ). (A) This woman's 2nd thoracic ring is rotated to the left. The right 2nd rib is anteriorly rotated and the left is posteriorly rotated. The manubrium is also rotated to the left and side-bent to the left. (B) The left side bending of the manubrium elevates the medial end of the right clavicle and this motion occurs in the medial part of the SCJ between the manubrium and the disc. (C) Elevation of the medial end of the right clavicle results in depression of the lateral end and osteokinematic posterior rotation of the right clavicle. (D) Compare the degree of elevation of the left and right clavicles. The left is more elevated. *Continued*

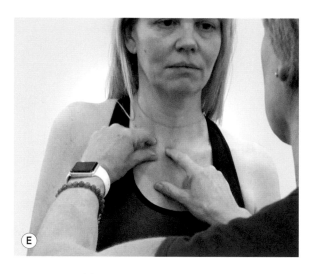

(E)

Figure 3.26 *continued*

(E) The alignment of the manubrium and 2nd thoracic ring prevents anterior rotation of the medial end of the right clavicle and disc relative to the manubrium during elevation of the clavicle and this has implications for tension in the deep and superficial fascia of the neck. Correction of the 2nd thoracic ring restored both the biomechanics of the SCJ and the alignment of the left and right clavicle.

any segmental lateral translation and rotation (Fig. 3.27). If C7 is translated to the right, it is also rotated and sidebent to the left and this would be congruent with a right translated and left rotated 2nd thoracic ring (Fig. 3.28). If C2 is translated to the left, it is also rotated to the right and this would be incongruent to both C7 and the 2nd thoracic ring. The atlas derotates the right rotation of C2 at the atlantoaxial joints.

The last thing to note is the presence of any intracranial torsion (ICT) (position of the temporal bones and occiput) and whether the position of the sphenoid is congruent or incongruent with the direction of rotation of the occiput. The temporal bones rotate about an axis through the petrous portion of the bone (Fig. 3.29). Like the ribs, clavicles and innominates, this motion in the ISM approach is called anterior and posterior rotation; whereas in osteopathic cranial therapy this motion is called external and internal rotation. When the right temporal bone rotates posteriorly, its mastoid process moves anteriorly and laterally. In a right ICT, this motion is associated with an anterior rotation of the left temporal bone during which the left mastoid process moves posteriorly and medially. When the temporal bones rotate relative to one another, the occiput follows the direction of the posteriorly rotating temporal bone (like the sacrum in the pelvis). The direction of the ICT is named according to the direction of rotation of the occiput. A right ICT is defined as a posteriorly rotated right temporal bone, anteriorly rotated left

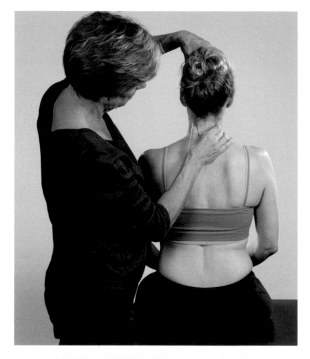

Figure 3.27

Positional testing of the cervical segments. Stabilize the cranium and gently palpate the left and right transverse processes and laminae of C7. Note any segmental lateral translation and rotation. Repeat for each cervical segment up to C1. The direction of translation informs the direction of rotation; a right translated C7 is also left rotated and side-bent.

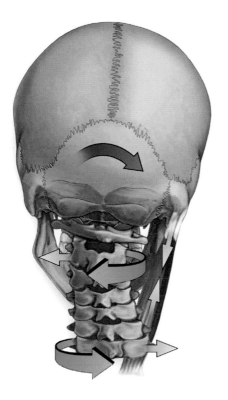

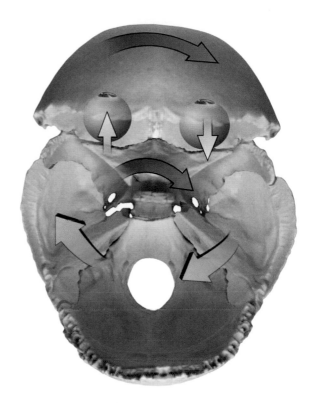

Figure 3.28

Potential impact of overactivation of the right sternocleidomastoid on the cervical segments. C7 is translated right and rotated left and C2 is translated left and rotated right.

temporal bone, and a right rotated occiput. The sphenoid should follow the direction of the posteriorly rotated temporal bone and right rotate with a right ICT (congruent). This motion deepens the right orbit and the eye appears deeper on this side (Fig. 3.30A & B). If the sphenoid is rotated incongruent with the ICT, then the opposite orbit will be deeper (Fig. 3.31A & B).

Let's continue with the scenario presented previously in the first functional unit. First functional unit findings:

- Pelvis: Left transverse plane rotation (TPR) and left intrapelvic torsion (IPT);

- Hips: Right femoral head anterior compared to the left;

Figure 3.29

Position of the temporal bones, occiput, sphenoid, and frontal bone in a congruent right intracranial torsion. The right temporal bone is posteriorly rotated (osteopaths call this internal rotation) about an axis through the petrous portion of the temporal bone and the left temporal bone is anteriorly rotated (osteopaths call this external rotation). The sphenoid follows the anteroposterior motion of the squamous portion of the temporal bone and rotates to the right. This motion deepens the right orbit. The frontal bone follows the sphenoid (right rotates) while the occiput follows the posteriorly rotated temporal bone and right rotates.

- Lower thorax: Right transverse plane rotation associated with a translated left and rotated right 8th thoracic ring;

- Middle thorax: Left transverse plane rotation associated with a translated right and rotated left 4th thoracic ring.

93

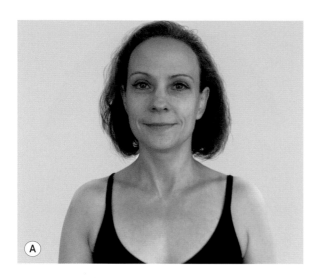

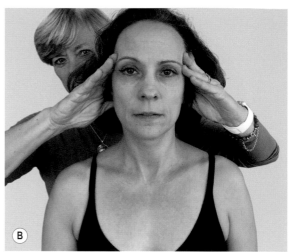

Figure 3.30

(A) This woman has an intracranial torsion to the left with a congruent left rotation of the sphenoid. Note the deepening of the left orbit. (B) Note the change in the depth of the left orbit and alignment of the head and neck when the intracranial torsion is corrected manually.

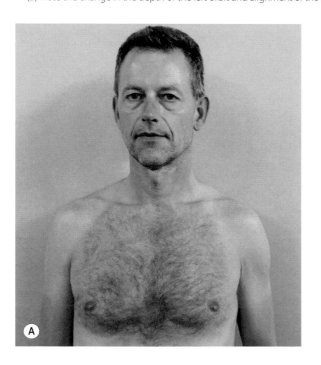

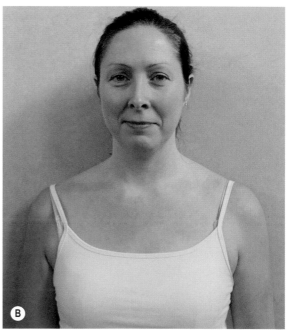

Figure 3.31

Incongruent intracranial torsion and sphenoid. (A) This cyclist suffered a head trauma when hit on his bike by a car. He has a right intracranial torsion (note the deviation of his mandible to the right of midline) and his sphenoid is rotated to the left (note the deeper left orbit). (B) This woman suffered head trauma as a driver in a motor vehicle accident. She also has a right intracranial torsion and a left rotated sphenoid (deeper left orbit).

Multiple possible combinations of drivers were presented for this scenario.

Let's assume further that:

- Upper thorax: Left transverse plane rotation associated with a left rotated 2nd thoracic ring;

- Clavicles: Right clavicle depressed and posteriorly rotated with left clavicle elevated and anteriorly rotated;

- Cervical: C7 translated right and rotated left with C2 translated left and rotated right;

- Cranial region: Right ICT with congruent sphenoid.

The next step is to determine the clinical relevance (determine the driver) of these findings, and then to compare the impact of correcting this driver on the ones found in the first functional unit.

Upper thoracic ring correction

It is easiest to correct the 2nd thoracic ring standing in front of the patient; however, the impact of this correction on the alignment of the cervical segments and cranium is more difficult to determine from this position. Stand beside the patient, and correct the upper thoracic rings (2nd and 3rd and sometimes 4th) with the fingers of one hand (Fig. 3.32A). Remember to wait with each part of this correction for the sensory input into the cortical body

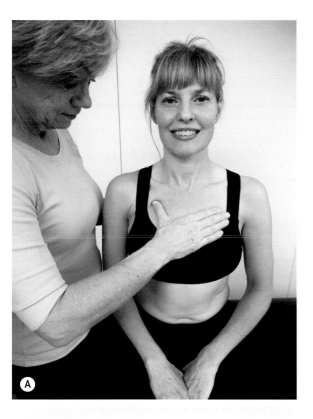 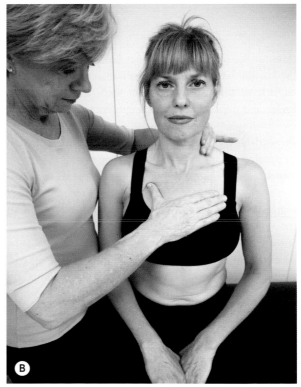

Figure 3.32

Impact of an upper thoracic ring correction on alignment of the cervical segments. This individual has a left rotated 2nd thoracic ring and a translated left and rotated right C7 (incongruent). (A) The 2nd thoracic ring is corrected by gently lifting the right rib (posterior rotation of the right 2nd rib) and pushing it slightly posterior rotating the thoracic ring to the right. Wait for the nervous system to respond to this change in sensory input. (B) The impact of this 2nd thoracic ring correction on the alignment of C7 is noted by palpating any change in position of C7 both during the correction and release. No change occurred.

matrix to evoke a motor output change. Lift the anteriorly rotated rib of the thoracic ring (right 2nd rib in this case) and wait. Then, gently derotate the 2nd thoracic ring ensuring it is capable of independent motion from the 3rd. If not, do a partial correction of the 2nd, followed by a partial correction of the 3rd, then a further correction of the 2nd then the 3rd, etc. until a complete correction of both thoracic rings is achieved. Note the impact of this correction of the upper thorax on the alignment of the cervical segments (C7 and C2 in this case) (Fig. 3.32B). If the cervical segments autocorrected, releasing the correction of the upper thorax will worsen their alignment. If the alignment of the cervical segments (one or more) worsened with correction of the upper thorax, the next step is to correct the cervical segment or segments and assess the impact of this correction on the alignment of the upper thorax.

Cervical segmental correction

Monitor the upper thoracic rings (2nd in this case) with the anterior hand and palpate the transverse processes and laminae of the cervical segment with the thumb, index finger and middle finger of the posterior hand (e.g., C7). Gently lift (distract) C7 and wait. Then, derotate the cervical segment and wait for the automatic medial translation to occur, if it can. Articular and strong myofascial system impairments will not allow the cervical segment to autocorrect whereas neural and visceral ones will. Once the cervical segment is aligned, note the impact of this correction on the alignment of the upper thorax (Fig. 3.33) and then on any other cervical segment that was previously noted to be suboptimally aligned (C2 in our scenario). Release the correction (C7) and note the response in the upper thorax and other cervical segments. It is often easier to feel the suboptimal alignment of the upper thorax or C2 return on release of the C7 correction than it is to feel the upper thorax or C2 autocorrect. Repeat the process for correcting C2.

Multiple combinations of correction effects are possible between the cervical segments and the upper thorax including:

- Correction of the upper thorax results in autocorrection of all cervical segments. The upper thorax is the primary driver.

- Correction of the upper thorax worsens the alignment of the cervical segments. The upper thorax is not the primary driver.

- Correction of the upper thorax results in a partial correction of the cervical segments. The upper thorax may be a primary driver with a secondary driver in another region (cranial or cervical spine).

- Correction of a lower cervical segment results in autocorrection of an upper cervical segment with either complete or partial improvement of the upper thorax.

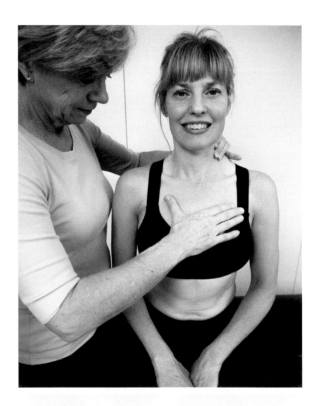

Figure 3.33

Impact of a segmental cervical correction on alignment of the upper thoracic rings. This same individual as in Figure 3.32 has a left rotated 2nd thoracic ring and a translated left and rotated right C7. Correcting the alignment of the 2nd thoracic ring did not impact the alignment of C7 (see Fig. 3.32B). Correcting the alignment of C7 immediately restored the alignment of her 2nd thoracic ring.

The lower cervical segment is a primary driver when complete correction occurs and either a co-driver or secondary driver to the thorax when only a partial correction occurs. A co-correction of both the lower cervical segment with the upper thorax then determines the relationship between these two regions and often a vector is found between the two.

- Correction of an upper cervical segment results in autocorrection of the lower cervical segment and upper thorax; however, the cranium does not correct (remains side-bent relative to the neck). If the cranial region is the driver and there is an ICT, the atlas will be rotated to follow the rotation of the occiput and C2 will rotate beneath the atlas (atlantoaxial joints) to compensate.

Cranial correction

A cranial correction (cranium, C1 and C2) requires both hands; therefore, the patient is often used as a 'second therapist' to witness any change in alignment of the upper thorax and later in the middle and lower thorax, pelvis, hips, and lower extremities. Teach the patient how to monitor the 2nd thoracic ring and C7 vertebra (Fig. 3.34).

If the sphenoid is rotated congruent with the ICT, then the cranial correction is focused on the temporal bones and no specific co-correction of the sphenoid is required. With the fingers of both hands pointing toward the ceiling and the thumbs abducted, place the entire thumb along the occipitomastoid sutures medial to the mastoid processes on the left and right sides of the cranium (Fig. 3.35A & B). Distract this suture by gently pulling the mastoid processes laterally. Wait. Derotate the ICT by pushing the mastoid process that is posterior and medial (this temporal bone is anteriorly rotated) anteriorly and laterally. Wait. Wait. Wait. Wait for a sensation of expansion to arrive between your hands. This feels like the posterior cranial fossa is filling with air. Then center the cranium as a unit over the atlas (C1) and axis (C2). Ask the patient if they noticed any motion or change in the alignment of the 2nd thoracic ring and C7. Release the cranial correction and assess if the suboptimal alignment of the upper thorax and C7 returns.

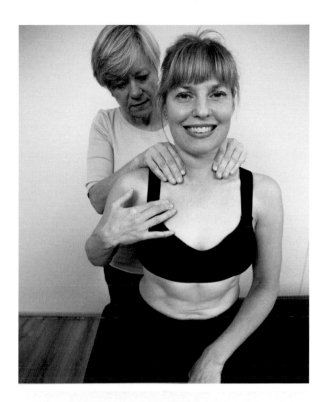

Figure 3.34

The patient is monitoring the alignment of the 2nd thoracic ring through the right 2nd rib as the therapist corrects C7.

If the sphenoid is rotated incongruent with the ICT, then the correction of the temporal bones is preceded by distraction of the sphenosquamous suture on the side that the sphenoid is rotated toward. With the fingers of both hands pointing toward the ceiling and the thumbs abducted, place the entire thumb along the occipitomastoid sutures medial to the mastoid processes on the left and right sides of the cranium. Now palpate the lateral aspect of the greater wing of the sphenoid with whatever finger can reach (Fig. 3.36A & B). Distract the sphenosquamous suture by gently pushing the greater wing of the sphenoid forward (toward the eyes), then distract the occipitomastoid sutures with the thumbs, wait, then derotate the temporal bones. To complete the cranial correction, center the cranium over the atlas and axis.

97

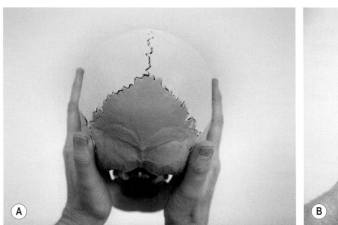

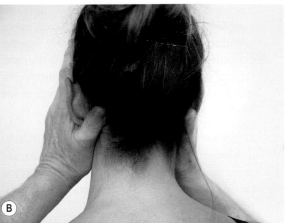

Figure 3.35

Hand placement for correction of an intracranial torsion associated with a congruently rotated sphenoid. (A) The thumbs are placed medial to the mastoid processes and along the occiptomastoid sutures. (B) The fingers rest gently on the rest of the cranium.

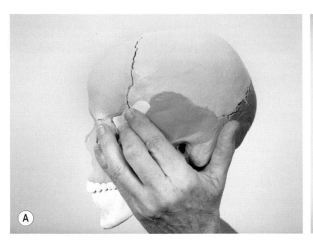

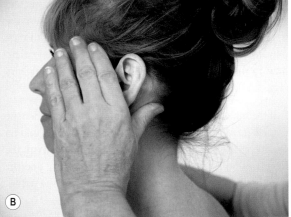

Figure 3.36

Hand placement for correction of an intracranial torsion associated with an incongruently rotated sphenoid. (A) The index or middle finger palpates the greater wing of the sphenoid on the side that it is rotated towards. (B) Decompress the sphenosquamous suture by gently pushing the greater wing of the sphenoid anteriorly toward the eye before decompressing the occipitomastoid sutures.

Clavicle and scapula correction

The clavicle is corrected by decompressing the sternoclavicular joint (distracting the clavicle laterally) and then repositioning the bone into slight elevation and neutral rotation. This is often done in conjunction with a correction of the scapula (Watson et al. 2009). The fingers of the anterior hand distract and rotate the clavicle (Fig. 3.37A) while the thumb of this hand supports the inferior aspect of the glenoid fossa. The posterior hand then corrects the

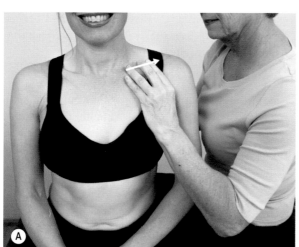
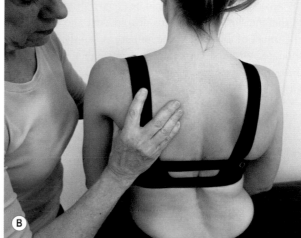

Figure 3.37

Shoulder girdle correction. (A) The thumb of the anterior hand supports the inferior glenoid of the scapula while the fingers distract the sternoclavicular joint and correct the rotation of the clavicle (arrow). (B) The posterior hand corrects the elevation, tilt, and rotation of the scapula.

scapular rotation (medially, laterally, upward), and the tilt (usually posteriorly), and both hands position the shoulder girdle in the appropriate amount of elevation (Fig. 3.37B). The spine of the scapula should be at the level of the 3rd rib with the clavicle slightly elevated. The impact of this correction on the upper, middle, and lower thoracic regions (VM, VS, VC), the pelvis or hip, the cervical segments and cranium is noted to determine the relationship between the cranial, cervical, and thoracic suboptimal alignments and the shoulder girdle position. When the thorax is the driver, correcting the clavicle and scapula does not improve the alignment of the thoracic rings. When the shoulder girdle is the driver, correcting the alignment of the clavicle and scapula corrects the thoracic rings. It is not uncommon to find vectors between the shoulder girdle and the VS and VM thoracic rings such that correcting one region results in correction of the other (co-drivers).

Correcting the position of the thorax and shoulder girdle can impact the position of the humerus relative to the scapula. Note the resting position of the head of the humerus relative to the scapula (Fig. 3.38). No more than a third of the head of the humerus should be anterior to

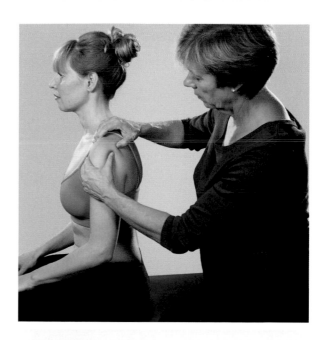

Figure 3.38

Positional testing of the head of the humerus. No more than a third of the humeral head should be anterior to the acromion.

the acromion and there should be equal resting activation of the anterior and posterior deltoid. Note the change in alignment of the head of the humerus when the thorax or shoulder girdle is corrected; they often, but not always, drive the positional changes noted at the glenohumeral joint.

Once the driver or drivers have been determined in the second functional unit, assess the impact of this correction on the driver(s) noted in the first functional unit. Does one correct the other? If so, it takes precedence for treatment. If not, then both require treatment.

Lower extremity

Note the coronal plane relationship of the femur, tibia, talus, and calcaneus (Fig. 3.39A–D). In standing, the tibia should be externally rotated relative to the femur (normal screw-home mechanism biomechanics for knee extension) (Fig. 3.40A & B).

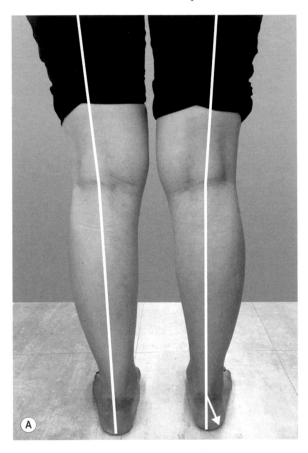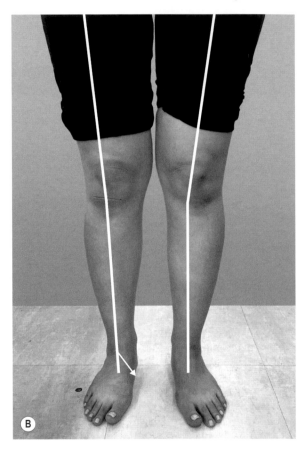

Figure 3.39
Coronal plane relationship of the lower leg and foot. (A) Posterior view. Note the increased abduction or valgus between the left tibia and femur. The left femur is also internally rotated in the transverse plane. The left foot has compensated for this change in coronal plane orientation and the hindfoot is well placed beneath the tibia. While the right femur and tibia have a more vertical orientation than the left (i.e., less valgus), the right hindfoot is not well positioned beneath the tibia. The calcaneus is excessively everted. (B) Anterior view. The displacement of the center of mass is clearly seen on the right talocrural joint. The talus is plantarflexed and adducted, the metatarsals are abducted (relative to the body midline), and the first toe is adducted (relative to the first metatarsal and 2nd metatarsal). The metatarsals are also somewhat abducted on the left foot.

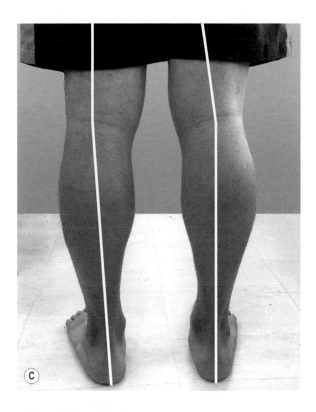
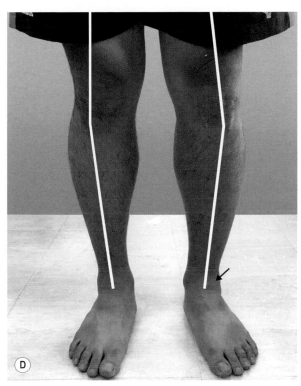

Figure 3.39 *continued*

(C) Posterior view of another subject. The coronal plane relationship of the left femur and tibia and calcaneus is optimal on the left. The right talus is excessively plantarflexed and adducted and the calcaneus therefore everted. (D) Anterior view. Note the crease in the anterolateral aspect of the left talocrural joint (arrow). This finding suggests that the left talus is also tilted in association with the plantarflexion and adduction.

Note the position of the patella: drop a visual plumb line from the infrapatellar tendon toward the ankle and it should bisect the talus. Note any tilting (medially or laterally) of the talus in the mortise joint and any excessive eversion of the calcaneus beneath the talus. An excessively everted calcaneus is often associated with a plantarflexed and adducted talus and a loss of the medial arch of the foot. Note the symmetry in length between the medial and lateral sides of the foot. Is one side apparently shortened indicating sickle- or C-shaped foot? Note any deviations of the toes in relationship to the relative metatarsals and any loss of the transverse metatarsal arch.

For the purposes of this text and understanding the relationship between the thorax and the whole body including the foot, it is only relevant to assess the impact of a hindfoot correction on the knee, hip, pelvis, thorax, etc. Once the foot is determined to be the driver, then a complete foot assessment, which is outside the scope of this text, is indicated. Alternately, assessing the impact of a distant correction on the hindfoot alignment (talus and calcaneus) is sufficient to determine which body region requires intervention first.

Hindfoot correction

Kneel beside the foot to be corrected. Have the patient shift their weight to the opposite foot and then plantarflex the ankle on the side of the foot being corrected such that they

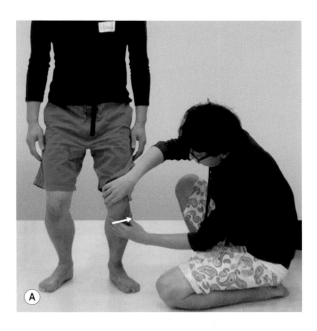
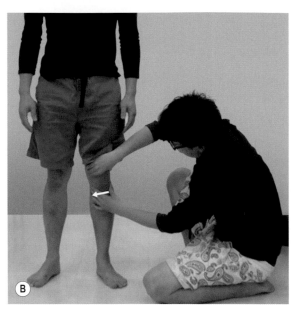

Figure 3.40

The knee joint in standing. The tibia should be relatively externally rotated to the femur when the knee is extended in standing. The tibia should immediately internally rotate during initiation of knee flexion. (A) To determine the conjunct rotation that occurs in weight-bearing knee flexion and extension and thus the position of the knee in standing, have the patient squat slightly and note the direction of rotation of the tibia during the initial stages of knee flexion. This subject has incongruent conjunct rotation in that his tibia externally rotates in the initial stages of knee flexion. (B) When he returns to the standing position, the tibia internally rotates as it extends. In Japan, this has been called the 'reverse screw-home movement' and is suboptimal alignment and biomechanics for this task. Ishii and Yamamoto (2008) reported on this finding in 20 per cent of healthy subjects between the ages of 20 and 65 during open kinetic chain knee extension. Many different drivers can immediately change the direction of this conjunct rotation.

are weight-bearing on the metatarsal heads (Fig. 3.41A). With both hands, center the talus in the mortise such that it is neither medially nor laterally tilted. Maintain this position with one hand and grasp the calcaneus with the other. Distract the calcaneus from the talus and evert or invert the subtalar joint to neutral (Fig. 3.41B). Then have the patient slowly lower their heel to the floor while maintaining the hindfoot correction. Note the impact of this correction on the position of the knee, patella, and the other regional drivers. Try to retain this foot alignment and correct the other hindfoot. If correcting the hindfoot (regardless of what happens to the midfoot and forefoot) is the best correction for the standing posture of the entire body, then treatment should be focused on improving

function (alignment, biomechanics and control) of the feet. Feet are often secondary drivers and become primary as treatment progresses. Correct the drivers of the other two functional units and note the impact on the position of the hindfoot. This will confirm the drivers and where it is best to start treatment. Remember, drivers should change as treatment progresses.

Squat

The squat is commonly assessed since it is a screening task for many meaningful tasks. The optimal biomechanics for a simple squat without arm motion, or eye tracking, are in Table 3.6. Analysis of the squat begins by noting key sites of suboptimal alignment in all three

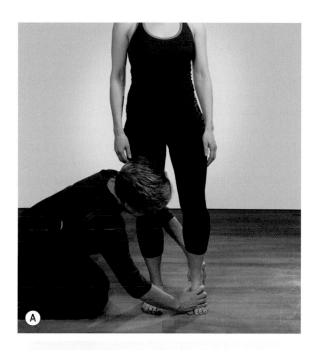
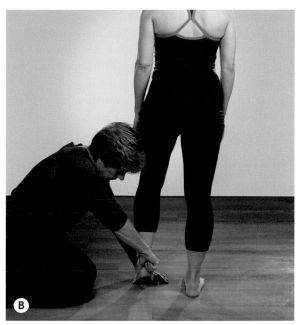

Figure 3.41

Hindfoot correction. (A) With the foot in partial weight-bearing, neutralize the talar tilt in the mortise. (B) Hold the talus, and neutralize the inversion or eversion of the calcaneus. Maintain the position of the talus and calcaneus as the patient returns the foot to the floor.

Table 3.6 Optimal biomechanics for a squat	
Pelvis	Should remain neutral in the transverse and coronal planes and anteriorly tilt in the sagittal plane. If the pelvis starts rotated or tilted, both should correct in the initial stage of the squat. The sacroiliac joint should not lose control. The innominate should remain posteriorly rotated relative to the sacrum on both sides.
Hips	Should flex. If the femoral head starts anteriorly translated relative to the acetabulum, it should center in the initial stage of the squat and remain centered throughout.
Knees	Should flex. The tibia should internally rotate relative to the femur in the initial stage of the squat as the knee comes out of full extension.
Hindfoot	The talocrural joint should dorsiflex relative to the mortise and plantarflex and adduct relative to the calcaneus as the calcaneus everts beneath it as part of pronation of the foot. The foot should lengthen as the midfoot and forefoot rotate (fan) around the 2nd metatarsal. The toes should remain extended and in line with their relative metatarsal.
Thorax	All regions should remain neutral in the transverse and coronal planes. The thorax as a unit should follow the anterior tilt of the pelvis but not anteriorly, nor posteriorly, tilt further. The manubriosternal symphysis should remain over the pubic symphysis.
Cranial region	The head should remain centered over the neck and thorax in all planes unless the eyes are fixed on a target and not the floor. The craniovertebral region will then extend or follow the target as may the cervical segments.
Shoulder girdle	Should remain congruent with the upper and middle thorax with the clavicle slightly elevated, scapula slightly upwardly rotated with the spine of the scapula at the level of the 3rd thoracic ring.

functional units in standing and their behavior (i.e., how they change) during the squat. The sites of suboptimal alignment in standing that improve (i.e., perform optimally during the squat) are ignored while those that remain suboptimally aligned for this task, or worsen during the task, are noted. Poor pelvic control is commonly seen during a squat and the thorax is often the driver of this impairment.

Pelvic control test in a squat

In standing, palpate the inferior lateral angle of the sacrum with one thumb. With the other hand palpate the iliac crest with the tips of the fingers allowing the hand to rest on the buttock (Fig. 3.42). The thumb of this hand may palpate the posterior superior iliac spine but the focus should not be only on the thumb. Have the patient shift their weight to the opposite side – the one not being palpated – and then shift back to the side being assessed for control. The innominate should remain posteriorly rotated relative to the sacrum and nothing should be felt between your hands (Hungerford et al. 2004, 2007). This is a controlled sacroiliac joint (SIJ). If there is control of the pelvis, ask the patient to squat (Fig. 3.43). The pelvis may posteriorly tilt as the squat deepens; however, the SIJ should never lose control. The innominate should always remain posteriorly rotated relative to the sacrum. Repeat the test on the opposite side.

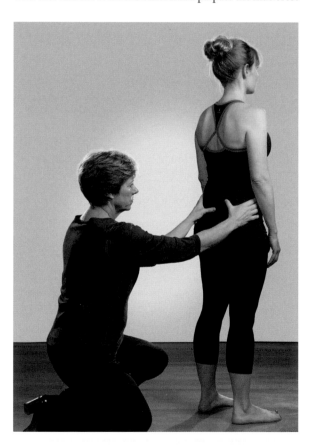

Figure 3.42

Hand placement for assessing control of the SIJ. The thumb palpates the inferior lateral angle of the sacrum while the fingers and thumb of the other hand palpate the ipsilateral iliac crest. The palm of this hand rests on the buttock.

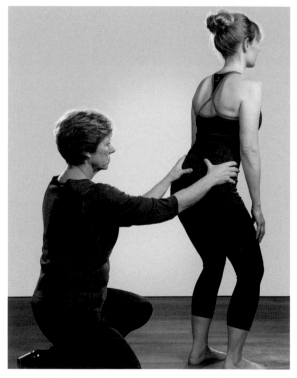

Figure 3.43

The SIJ should not move during a squat task. The pelvis should anteriorly tilt initially (hips flex), the sacrum should remain nutated between the left and right innominates, and no intrapelvic torsion or transverse plane rotation of the pelvis should occur throughout the task.

Impact of the thorax on pelvic control in a squat

The alignment findings will have already been noted in standing, but drivers may not have been determined if standing is not the meaningful task. Palpate the most significant translated and rotated thoracic ring found in standing and note the behavior (improvement or worsening of alignment) as the patient squats (Fig. 3.44). All translated and rotated thoracic rings that correct in a squat can be ignored. Those thoracic rings where the alignment remains suboptimal or worsens require correction, and the impact of this correction on pelvic control is noted. Remember to always determine if two adjacent translated and rotated thoracic rings are glued. The thoracic ring correction is held with one hand while the other hand palpates the SIJ (inferior lateral angle with the thumb and iliac crest with the fingers of the same hand, or just the innominate). If the thorax is the primary driver, pelvic control will be completely restored with correction of the thorax (Fig. 3.45). If the

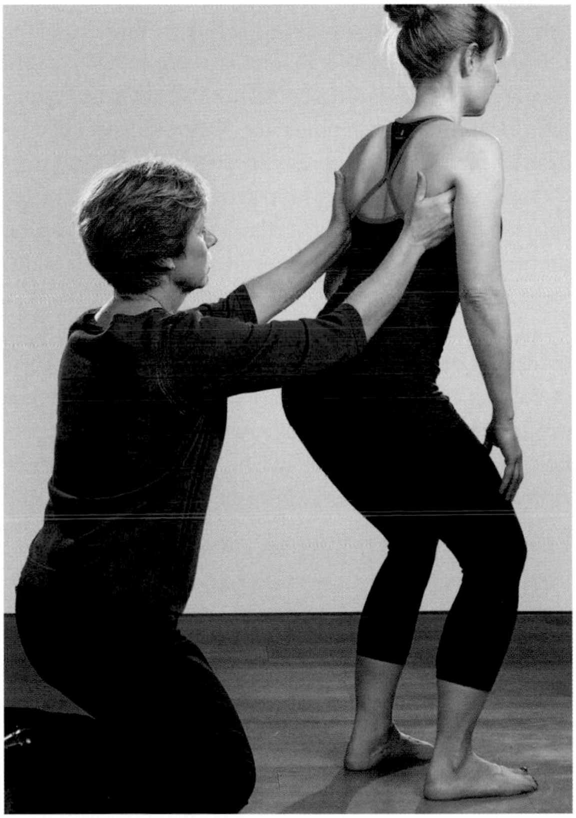

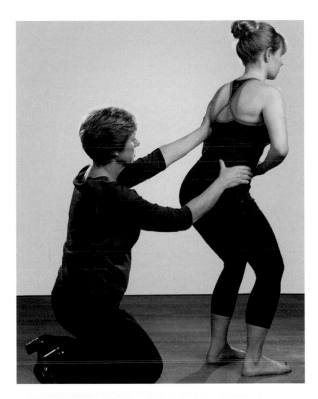

Figure 3.45

Assessing the impact of a single thoracic ring correction (vertebrosternal region translated left and rotated right in this subject) on control of the right SIJ during a squat task. The therapist previously determined that the right innominate anteriorly rotated relative to the sacrum in this task (i.e., lost control); therefore, if the innominate continues to anteriorly rotate relative to the sacrum when the thoracic ring is corrected, the SIJ is still losing control. If, however, there is no movement of the innominate relative to the sacrum during the squat with correction of the thoracic ring (the pelvis should anteriorly tilt relative to the femurs), then this correction has resulted in a change in the motor control strategy and SIJ control has been restored.

Figure 3.44

All the thoracic rings should remain aligned over the pelvis during a squat task. The thoracic rings should neither anteroposteriorly tilt nor translate and rotate during a simple unloaded squat task.

pelvis is a secondary or co-driver, loss of pelvic control will occur later in the squat task. Remember: with every correction ask the patient if their experience is better or worse or if there is no change. If the task feels better, ask them in what way. Help the patient to build new neurotags and to remember the sensations they will be asked to recreate with their movement training practice at home. Massed practice of better strategies for this task will reinforce the synaptic efficiency and mass of the new neurotag for this task (Moseley & Butler 2017).

Impact of pelvic control on alignment of the thorax

The pelvis can be manually controlled by compressing the SIJs and pubic symphysis with a belt, tape, or the patient's hands. Ensure that the SIJ is well controlled prior to assessing impact of this correction on the alignment of the thoracic rings. If restoring pelvic control improves the alignment of the thoracic rings noted to worsen during the squat, then the pelvis is the driver. If the thoracic rings continue to translate and rotate even when control is provided to the pelvis, then the pelvis is not a primary driver.

Once the driver is found within the first functional unit (3rd thoracic ring to the hip joints) for the squat task, the correction process is repeated for the second and third functional units to determine the best place to intervene to improve whole body function for the squat task.

Seated head, neck, and thoracic rotation

Seated, or standing, rotation of the head, neck, and thorax is another common screening task for many meaningful tasks. Table 3.7 outlines the optimal biomechanics for left rotation of the head, neck, and thorax. Note the amplitude of mobility for rotation of the head, neck, and thorax that is possible when the head and thorax are maintained aligned over the sacrum. This is the limit of functional rotation even if the patient can rotate further (Fig. 3.46A & B). Observe the ability of the cranium to rotate purely in the transverse plane (no anteroposterior tilting or side bending) as well as the quality of the formed C-curve in the cervical and thoracic spines. Compare the amplitude of movement from side to side. Note any areas of flattening, or kinking, of the spinal curve (Fig. 3.47A & B). This is where an incongruent rotation to the task is often occurring. Palpate those regions where the curve is suboptimal for any incongruent biomechanics for this task. List any incongruent thoracic ring, cervical segment, clavicle, or intracranial motion. Correct each incongruent site and note the impact of this correction on the patient's experience, mobility, and ability to maintain the head and thorax centered over the sacrum as they rotate (Fig. 3.48A & B). The driver (primary, secondary, or co-driver) will produce the most improvement in all aspects of the task experience. On occasion, a thoracic ring will be excessively translated and rotated *congruent* with the direction of rotation and will be driving the suboptimal strategy for rotation. This is an active motion control problem.

Table 3.7	
Optimal biomechanics for seated left rotation of the head, neck, and thorax	
Cranial region	Should rotate to the left maintaining the eyes, ears, and mouth in a level transverse plane (no side bending). This rotation should produce a left ICT with a congruent left rotation of the sphenoid.
Cervical segments	C1–C7 should translate right and rotate left. C2–C7 should also left side-bend. The occipitoatlantal and atlantoaxial joints right side-bend in conjunction with the left rotation. The zygapophyseal joints from C2–C3 to C7–T1 should glide inferomedially and posteriorly on the left and superoanteriorly and laterally on the right. The uncovertebral joints should glide inferiorly on the left and superiorly on the right.
Thoracic rings	Except for the 1st thoracic ring, all others should translate right and rotate left. The 1st thoracic ring rotates left but does not translate. The specific osteokinematics and arthrokinematics for each region are described in Chapter 2.
Clavicles	The left clavicle should posteriorly rotate and the right clavicle should anteriorly rotate. Neither clavicle should translate medially and compress the medial sternoclavicular joint as they rotate. If the medial sternoclavicular joint is compressed, clavicular rotation becomes limited.

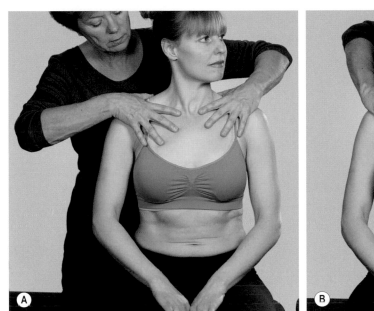
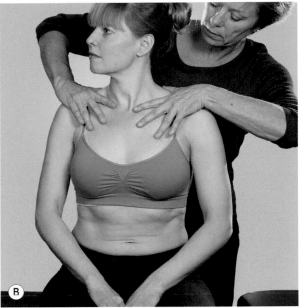

Figure 3.46

Left rotation (A) and right rotation (B) of the head, neck, and upper thorax while monitoring the biomechanics of the clavicles and upper thoracic rings. Note the limitation of left rotation.

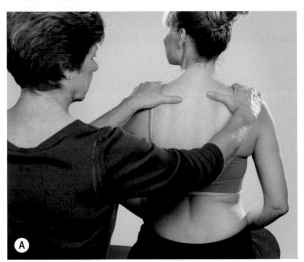
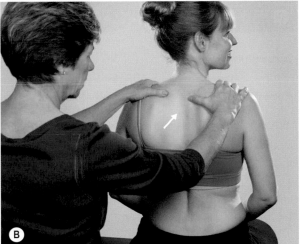

Figure 3.47

Left rotation (A) and right rotation (B) of the head, neck, and upper thorax. Note the lack of side bending in the vertebrosternal region (straight spine) during left rotation and the kink in the curve (arrow) during right rotation. These two findings suggest suboptimal biomechanics are occurring in this region during both left and right rotation of the head, neck, and upper thorax.

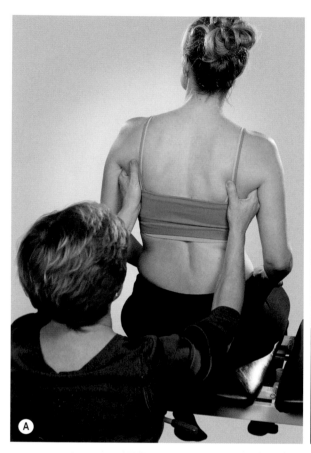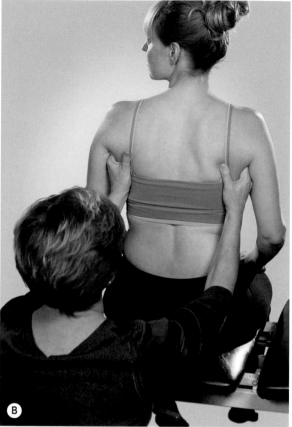

Figure 3.48

(A) The 4th thoracic ring is translated left and rotated right incongruent with the required biomechanics for left rotation of the head, neck, and upper thorax. Note the amplitude of possible motion and the persistent right side bending curve in the vertebrosternal region. (B) Note the change in the spinal curve as well as the increased range of motion when the alignment and biomechanics of the 4th thoracic ring are corrected.

The thoracic ring is translating and rotating in the correct direction; however, it is going too far. Correcting this thoracic ring during rotation requires preventing it from translating and rotating excessively.

This task can also be done in standing to determine the influence of the feet on thoracic function (Fig. 3.49A–C). Feet that are not adaptable, and cannot pronate and supinate, restrict the body's ability to twist. This loss of function must be compensated for by the hips and thorax. Test a full body twist in standing with, and without, a hindfoot

correction to assess the impact of immobile, nonresponsive feet on function of the thorax.

Summary

Understanding biomechanics is fundamental for assessment of the biological component (posture and movement) of the patient's biopsychosocial presentation. Furthermore, a knowledge of biomechanics is essential for knowing what, when, and how to correct various body regions to determine the best place to begin

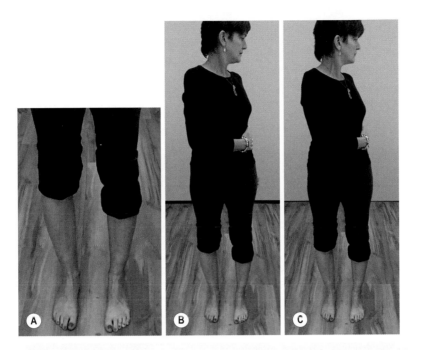

Figure 3.49

This woman's meaningful complaint is thoracic pain aggravated with left rotation tasks in standing. Standing posture: Pelvis: Right TPR and IPT, left hip anterior, 6th thoracic ring translated left and rotated right, 5th thoracic ring translated right and rotated left with (A) left hindfoot inverted, navicular externally rotated, and medial cuneiform internally rotated. (B) During a body twist to the left, her 6th thoracic ring translated further left and rotated further right and she tried to get more left rotation by 'torquing her thorax.' The left foot fails to supinate as it should in this task. Correcting the 5th and 6th thoracic rings did not improve the biomechanics of her pelvis, hips or feet in this task, nor her experience. (C) Correcting her left hindfoot and left midtarsal biomechanics improved her ability to left rotate her pelvis and corrected the biomechanics of both her hips and the two thoracic rings during the left body twist. She immediately noticed an improvement in the quantity of motion and a reduction in her midthoracic pain with this correction. This is a foot-driven thorax.

treatment regardless of pain or symptom location. Pain that is responsive to peripheral mechanical stimuli tends to change location or intensity when a biological driver or drivers are found. Further tests then help to determine the underlying system impairments, which then direct the individual treatment plan. Pain that is less influenced by biological and biomechanical factors tends not to respond to only changing the sensory input to the cortical body matrix through regional corrections of alignment, biomechanics, and control. This finding alone helps to direct treatment (see Chapter 4) without further testing of the musculoskeletal system.

Tests to determine the underlying system impairment of the driver or drivers

Let's assume that a body region has been located that when corrected results in an improvement in both performance and experience of the screening task. The next step is to determine what is causing the suboptimal alignment, biomechanics or control for that body region, or driver. Our ability to do this relies entirely on our ability to accurately perceive kinesthetic information during active mobility, passive mobility, and control tests. Treatment will depend on the interpretation of this information (clinical reasoning and hypothesis development).

Further tests – vector analysis

Active and passive mobility tests (physiological or accessory tests) provide information about more than the joint, although historically the findings from these tests have been interpreted through the lens of the articular system. Overactive muscles can increase compression across the joint's surfaces, effectively reducing mobility. Underactive muscles can reduce compression and thus increase mobility. Vectors of pull on the skeleton from visceral attachments can also produce joint compression and alter mobility. Changes in fascial integrity, tension or mobility can also change joint mobility and control. Therefore, when testing active or passive joint mobility, consideration must be given to more than the amplitude of motion or end feel to accurately determine which system is impacting function.

Vector analysis (Lee D & Lee L-J 2011b) differs from joint mobility testing in that focus is not placed on one system during assessment. As the driver is corrected, attention is paid to the location, direction and quality of vectors that limit or resist the correction, or that pull the driver out of alignment when the correction is released. If it is *not* possible to completely correct the alignment of the driver, then consideration should be given to the articular and myofascial systems since fibrosis can limit the required mobility for complete correction. If it *is* possible to correct the alignment, then an articular or myofascial system impairment is less likely and consideration is then given to the neural or visceral systems or both. So, the first test that determines the system for further analysis is done in conjunction with finding the driver. Once the driver is found, the correction is repeated with focus on learning more about the vectors.

'Active and passive listening' techniques are used during analysis of alignment, biomechanics and control, correction and release, to understand more about the vectors that are impacting the function of the driver. According to Dr. Gail Wetzler, physiotherapist and director of the Barral Institute of Advanced Manual Therapy, the term 'listening' was coined by osteopath Dr. Rollin Becker (2000). Dr. Jean-Pierre Barral (2007) introduced the concept of Becker's listening protocol to manual therapy through his novel ideas for assessing and treating the visceral system.

In this approach, both general listening of the entire body, and local listening of a specific structure within the body, are done passively; the patient is not asked to do anything actively. Dr. Gail Wetzler developed the 'Listening Courses' for the Barral Institute and introduced the concept of 'active and passive' listening. We had the opportunity in 2015 to discuss and integrate the visceral listening protocols to those of the Integrated Systems Model and came to the following agreement for use of the terms 'active and passive listening' (Wetzler & Lee 2015):

- Active listening occurs when manually analyzing the biomechanics and control of a body region as the patient is moving.

- There are two forms of passive listening:

  ○ Firstly, when correcting alignment or facilitating the biomechanics of a body region during a screening task, attention is paid to the location (left or right, front or back, inside or outside, etc.), length (long or short) and strength (strong, moderate, or weak) of the first vector resisting correction.

  ○ Secondly, as the correction is released, the hands remain in contact with the body region and attention is focused to determine:

    ▪ Which bone moved first? If two drivers (body regions) are being palpated at the same time, and both regions move simultaneously, then there is often a vector between the two drivers.

    ▪ What direction did the vector pull the bone to and did the force come from inside the thorax, abdomen, pelvis or cranium (visceral system), or from outside (neural, myofascial or articular systems)?

    ▪ How long and strong is the vector? Is it long, short, strong or weak?

Further palpation tests then attempt to confirm the specific structure and identify the system impairment. Sometimes, two structures create a net vector, and it is not possible to 'name it' anatomically. Even if it cannot be named, there are treatment techniques for releasing combined vectors that are impacting alignment, biomechanics, and control of the driver (see Chapter 6).

Articular system – assessment principles

Assessment of the articular system is indicated if complete correction of the driver is not possible and a stiff joint or joints is or are suspected. The principles of joint mobility testing will be discussed before specific techniques for the joints of the thorax are described.

All joints have two zones of motion – a neutral and an elastic zone (Panjabi 1992) (Fig. 3.50). The neutral zone is the part of the joint's range that is not influenced by the capsule or the joint's ligaments. In Maitland's terminology, this range has been defined as 0–R1 (neutral to first resistance) (Maitland 1986). The amplitude of neutral zone motion varies between joints in the same body and between individuals

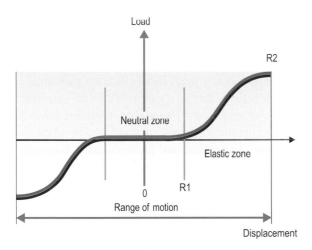

Figure 3.50

An adapted graphic representation of both Panjabi's (1992) neutral and elastic zone representation of joint motion and Maitland's (1986) joint movement diagram. Maitland's 0–R1 is equivalent to Panjabi's neutral zone and R1–R2 is equivalent to the elastic zone. Cyriax (1954) described several different qualities of R1 to R2 which he called 'end feel'.

comparing the same joint; however, the amplitude of both zones should be similar between the left and right sides in the same individual. The elastic zone is the range that is influenced by increasing tension in various parts of the joint's capsule and associated ligaments. Cyriax (1954) referred to the increasing tension at the end of a joint's range as 'end feel' and Maitland called this range R1 to R2 (from first resistance to the end of the joint's physiological range [R2]). It is important for the therapist to set their intention to feel the qualities of resistance throughout the entire range of motion (through both neutral and elastic zones).

Active physiological mobility tests

Active physiological mobility tests are incorporated into analysis of the screening task. For each task evaluated, the alignment, biomechanics, and control of the joints being assessed are compared against what is thought to be optimal. For example, during right rotation of the thorax the ribs on the right should posteriorly rotate, the ribs on the left should anteriorly rotate, the spinal vertebrae should right rotate and side-bend and the left and right ribs and the superior vertebra should translate slightly to the left relative to the inferior vertebra (Lee D G 1993, 2015) (Fig. 3.51). If the thoracic ring in question does something else during right rotation of the thorax (i.e., translates further to the right), then this is considered suboptimal performance. If the alignment and biomechanics of this thoracic ring cannot be manually corrected and facilitated during right thoracic rotation, then passive mobility tests are indicated to learn more about the potential mobility of the costal and zygapophyseal joints of the relevant thoracic ring.

Passive accessory mobility tests

It is critical to know the starting position of the thoracic ring, as well as the limitation of active physiological mobility, for interpretation of the findings from the passive accessory or arthrokinematic mobility tests. Consider a 5th thoracic ring that is translated left and rotated right (Fig. 3.51), with left thoracic rotation producing further left translation and right rotation of the 5th thoracic ring (suboptimal biomechanics for this task). In this example, complete correction and facilitation of optimal biomechanics is not possible.

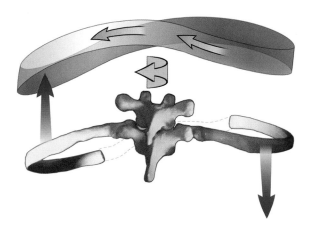

Figure 3.51

Osteokinematics and arthrokinematics of the 5th thoracic ring during right rotation of the thorax. Note the position of the zygapophyseal joints as well as the costotransverse joints in this position and clinically reason which joint glide restrictions could potentially limit left rotation.

The right T4–T5 zygapophyseal joint will be more extended (in inferior glide) and the left more flexed (in superior glide), the right 5th rib will be more inferiorly glided at the costotransverse joint (associated with a posterior roll) and the left will be more superiorly glided (associated with an anterior roll). If this impairment is due to an articular restriction, passive accessory or arthrokinematic mobility testing will reveal one or more of the following:

- Restriction of an inferior glide of the left zygapophyseal joint;

- Restriction of a superior glide of the right zygapophyeal joint;

- Restriction of a superior glide and anterior roll of the right costotransverse joint;

- Restriction of an inferior glide and posterior roll of the left costotransverse joint.

If the starting position of the thoracic ring is ignored, and this alignment is *not* due to an articular system impairment, asymmetry on passive mobility testing will be found when the two sides are compared (zygapophyseal and costotransverse joints) simply because the starting position for testing is different. This principle is true for any joint in the body.

Passive control tests

For every joint, there is a position called the close-packed position where there is maximum congruence of the articular surfaces and maximum tension of the major ligaments. In this position, the joint is under significant compression and the ability to resist shear or translation is enhanced by the tension of the passive structures and increased friction between the articular surfaces (form closure mechanism; Snijders et al. 1993a, 1993b, Vleeming et al. 1990). The close-packed position for all spinal zygapophyseal joints is end range extension (Bogduk 1997); for the SIJs it is full nutation of the sacrum, or posterior rotation of the innominate (van Wingerden et al. 1993, Vleeming et al. 1989a); for the hip joint it is extension combined with abduction and internal rotation (Hewitt et al. 2002); for the knee it is extension; and for the foot it is supination.

Passive control tests evaluate the form closure mechanism (Snijders et al. 1993a, 1993b): the ability of the passive components (capsule, ligaments) of the joint to resist shear forces. These tests are done in the joint's neutral and close-packed positions. A small amount of linear translation is possible between the thoracic rings in both the anteroposterior and mediolateral planes when in neutral; however, no anteroposterior translation should occur when the joints are close-packed, and no mediolateral translation should occur when one rib of the thoracic ring is prevented from translating relative to the transverse process of the same number. When there is a deficit in the form closure mechanism, motion will still be possible and palpable during these tests. If motion is well controlled, the articular system can be ruled out as being the cause of loss of joint control in loading tasks. If pain is provoked when the passive test moves beyond R1 (into the elastic zone) then primary nociception may be coming from the joint's capsule and ligaments.

Table 3.8 outlines the findings from active and passive mobility and control tests that identify and differentiate the various articular system impairments from the neural, myofascial or visceral impairments.

Table 3.8
Differentiating features of articular system impairments from the neural, myofascial and visceral system impairments

SYSTEM IMPAIRMENT	KEY FEATURES FROM THE STORY	ACTIVE OSTEOKINEMATIC MOBILITY	PASSIVE ARTHROKINEMATIC MOBILITY
Articular system: Acutely painful joint	Recent trauma or autoimmune, inflammatory disorder	Often too painful to test	Often too painful to test
Articular system: Stiff, fibrotic joint	Trauma that is not recent	Reduced	Reduced
Articular system: Fixated joint	Recent trauma or history of multiple acute episodes with intermittent relief with manipulation of the joint	Reduced	Reduced
Articular system: Lax joint	History of trauma (past or recent) with or without episodic joint fixation	Variable and may be reduced or not depending on neuromuscular compensation strategies	Excessive Form closure tests are positive for joint capsule or ligament laxity – this is the key differentiating feature
Neural system: Excessive force closure (compression) due to overactivation of muscles	Nothing in the story clearly differentiates this system impairment; usually nontraumatic	Inconsistent findings Mobility may be reduced, normal or excessive, and can vary with task and repetition of task Inconsistency of active mobility is a consistent finding	Often reduced, especially if the arthrokinematic mobility is tested with the driver in a non-neutral position
Neural system: Insufficient force closure due to under-activation of muscles	Tasks that increase loading of the driver are often aggravating	Inconsistent findings Mobility may be reduced, normal, or excessive, and can vary with task and repetition of task Inconsistency of active mobility is a consistent finding	Often normal or excessive mobility
Myofascial system: Diastasis rectus abdominis: Nonsurgical	Pregnancy-related or excessive intra-abdominal pressure secondary to a fatty omentum, or nonoptimal abdominal wall strategies in youth	Variable depending on compensatory strategy used to transfer loads through the lower thorax, lumbar spine, and pelvis	Variable
Myofascial system: Diastasis rectus abdominis: Surgical	Pregnancy-related or excessive intra-abdominal pressure secondary to fatty omentum	Variable depending on compensatory strategy used to transfer loads through the lower thorax, lumbar spine, and pelvis	Variable
Visceral system: Visceral vectors causing suboptimal alignment, biomechanics, and control of the thorax, abdomen, and pelvis	Nothing that differentiates	Often reduced	Vector analysis: The vector of pull comes from inside the thorax, abdomen or pelvis – this is the key differentiating feature of this system impairment
Visceral system: Inhibition of the abdominal wall secondary to visceral pain (pleura, mediastinum, pericardium, colon, bladder, uterus, etc.)	Certain foods or allergens (gluten, lactose, sugar, citrus or acidic foods, dust, pollen) often reported to irritate condition	Variable depending on compensatory strategy used to transfer loads through the lower thorax, lumbar spine, and pelvis	Often normal

Continued

Table 3.8 *continued*

SYSTEM IMPAIRMENT	TEST FOR WEIGHT-BEARING CONTROL	TESTS FOR PASSIVE CONTROL	INTERVENTION PRINCIPLES
Articular system: Acutely painful joint	Early loss of control Pain intensifies with any correction that compresses the painful joint – this is the key differentiating feature	If the passive structures of the joint are intact, the passive control tests will be painful but with a firm, solid end feel	Modalities for reducing intra-articular inflammation, gentle range of motion only, medical interventions
Articular system: Stiff, fibrotic joint	No loss of control when the joint is loaded	Normal	Vector-specific Grade 4 mobilization of restricted joints followed by reanalysis for mobility and control
Articular system: Fixated joint	No loss of control when the joint is fixated Loss of control after the joint is manipulated	No movement of the relative joint when there is a fixation. After the joint has been released, there is often an underlying loss of passive control	Specific distraction manipulation of impaired joint followed by taping for support, motor control training, and then movement training that includes strength and conditioning according to the meaningful task
Articular system: Lax joint	Loss of control early in task unless the force closure mechanism can compensate for the underlying articular system deficit	Loss of passive control in one or more directions	Motor control and movement training with or without prolotherapy to improve both the form and force closure mechanisms
Neural system: Excessive force closure (compression) due to overactivation of muscles	Loss of control at a variable time in the task, sometimes early, sometimes late – inconsistency is consistent finding	Normal	Release the overactive muscles and facilitate the underactive muscles (if necessary include motor control training for optimal synchronicity and synergy). This is followed by movement training that includes strength and conditioning for meaningful tasks
Neural system: Insufficient force closure due to underactivation of muscles	Inconsistent loss of control, varies with repetition and task	Often the passive control tests are falsely positive When these tests are repeated after four to six weeks of motor control training, the passive control tests are normal	Motor control training to restore optimal synchronicity and synergy followed by movement training that includes strength and conditioning for meaningful tasks
Myofascial system: Diastasis rectus abdominis: Nonsurgical	Loss of control with neural system deficits of insufficient force closure secondary to suboptimal motor control strategies	Normal	Motor control training to restore optimal synchronicity and synergy (brain training) then movement training that includes strength and conditioning for meaningful tasks. Goal is to restore tension in the linea alba and rectus sheaths for load transference across the abdomen and between the thorax and pelvis

Table 3.8 *continued*

SYSTEM IMPAIRMENT	TEST FOR WEIGHT-BEARING CONTROL	TESTS FOR PASSIVE CONTROL	INTERVENTION PRINCIPLES
Myofascial system: Diastasis rectus abdominis: Surgical	Loss of control with optimal neural system and motor control strategies that are unable to generate tension in the linea alba sufficient to force close and stabilize the joints of the lower thorax, lumbar spine or pelvis	Normal	Recti plication and abdominoplasty followed by motor control training, then movement training that includes strength and conditioning according to the meaningful task. If the diastasis rectus abdominis is secondary to obesity and visceral fat in the omentum then weight loss is required prior to surgery
Visceral system: Visceral vectors causing suboptimal alignment, biomechanics, and control of the thorax, abdomen, and pelvis	Often loss of control	Normal	Release the visceral vector specifically or with techniques that facilitate optimal alignment and use breathing or movement to generally release the visceral vectors. This is followed by motor control training of the driver, if necessary, and then movement training that includes strength and conditioning according to the meaningful task
Visceral system: Inhibition of the abdominal wall secondary to visceral pain (pleura, mediastinum, pericardium, colon, bladder, uterus, etc.)	Often loss of control due to inhibition of the abdominal wall		Treat the underlying visceral condition Gut and bowel: Nutrition Bladder: Avoid inflammatory foods

Articular system – specific tests

The following tests are done when the thoracic ring does not completely correct and an underlying articular system mobility impairment is suspected.

Active physiological mobility tests – costal joints

Palpate the left and right ribs of the thoracic ring of interest and note the starting position (neutral, translated left and rotated right, translated right and rotated left) (see the sections on landmarking in Chapter 1). Have the patient inhale fully and note the ability of the ribs to osteokinematically posteriorly rotate. Is the range of motion symmetric (Fig. 2.28B) or asymmetric? If one rib stops before the other, this rib may have an arthrokinematic restriction of inferior glide and posterior roll (VM or VS region) or anterolateroinferior glide (VC region) at the costotransverse joint.

Have the patient exhale fully and note the ability of the ribs to osteokinematically anteriorly rotate. Is the range of motion symmetric or asymmetric (Fig. 2.28C)? If one rib stops before the other, this rib may have an arthrokinematic restriction of superior glide and anterior roll (VM or VS region) or posteromediosuperior glide (VC region) at the costotransverse joint. There should be no difference in the amplitude of osteokinematic motion during an attempt to correct the thoracic ring if the system impairment is articular.

Active physiological mobility tests – thoracic zygapophyseal joints

Note the starting position of the thoracic ring of interest (neutral, translated left and rotated right, translated right and rotated left). With the index fingers and thumbs, palpate the four transverse processes of the two thoracic vertebrae related to the relevant thoracic ring (e.g., for the 4th thoracic ring, palpate the left and right transverse processes of T3 and T4) (Fig. 2.4A & B). If the thoracic ring is neutral, the left and right transverse processes should be equidistant apart. If the thoracic ring is translated left and rotated right T3–T4 should be slightly right rotated and side-bent and therefore the transverse processes should be closer together on the right. If the thoracic ring is translated right and rotated left T3–T4 should be slightly left rotated and side-bent and therefore the transverse processes should be closer together on the left. Have the patient forward bend with cues that specifically induce flexion of the thoracic spine and note the ability of the superior thoracic vertebra to flex relative to the one below; the fingers and thumbs should separate and end up equidistant apart (Fig. 2.5). Is the range of motion of each zygapophyseal joint symmetric or asymmetric? If one transverse process stops before the other there may be an arthrokinematic restriction of superior glide at the zygapophyseal joint.

Have the patient backward bend with cues that specifically induce extension of the thoracic spine and note the ability of the superior thoracic vertebra to extend relative to the one below; the fingers and thumbs should approximate and end up equidistant apart (Fig. 2.13). Is the range of motion of each zygapophyseal joint symmetric or asymmetric? If one transverse process stops before the other there may be an arthrokinematic restriction of inferior glide at the zygapophyseal joint. There should be no difference in the amplitude of arthrokinematic motion during an attempt to correct the thoracic ring if the system impairment is articular.

Passive accessory mobility tests – costal joints

Vertebromanubrial region

1st rib inferior glide test: This test is used to determine the ability of the right 1st rib to glide inferiorly relative to the transverse process of T1. This test is done when the 1st thoracic ring is held in left rotation and restricted in right rotation. The patient is supine with the head and neck comfortably supported on a pillow. With the lateral aspect of the metacarpophalangeal (MCP) joint of the index finger of the left hand, palpate, and stabilize, the superior aspect of the left transverse process of T1. With the lateral aspect

of the MCP of the index finger of the right hand, palpate the superior aspect of the right 1st rib just lateral to the costotransverse joint. Stabilize T1 with the left hand, distract the right 1st costotransverse joint slightly and then apply an inferior glide allowing the conjunct posterior roll to occur (Fig. 3.52A & B). Vary the direction of the glide to identify the specific direction that is limited. Be vector direction specific – feel for the sensation of a string (stiff vector) within a spring (more compliant direction). Compare the neutral and elastic zone behavior (amplitude, quality of first and second resistance, end feel) on both sides.

1st rib superior glide test: This test is used to determine the ability of the right 1st rib to glide superiorly relative to the transverse process of T1. This test is done when the 1st thoracic ring is held in right rotation and restricted in left rotation. The patient is supine with the head and neck comfortably supported on a pillow. Palpate the superior aspect of the right transverse process of T1 with the right thumb. Palpate the inferior aspect of the right 1st rib with the index and middle fingers of the right hand. Stabilize the 1st rib with the right index and middle fingers and glide the transverse process of T1 posteroinferiorly allowing the conjunct rotation to occur. This produces a relative superior glide of the 1st rib at the costotransverse joint (Fig. 3.53A & B). Vary the direction of the glide to identify the specific direction that is limited. Be vector direction specific – look for the string within a spring. Compare the neutral and elastic zone behavior (amplitude, quality of first and second resistance, end feel) on both sides.

Vertebrosternal region (including the 2nd thoracic ring)

4th rib inferior glide test: This test is used to determine the ability of the right 4th rib to glide inferiorly relative to the transverse process of T4. This test is done when the 4th thoracic ring is held in left rotation and restricted in right rotation; inhalation produces left rotation of the thoracic ring. The patient is prone with the head and neck in neutral rotation. With one thumb palpate the inferior aspect of the right transverse process of T4. Palpate the superior aspect of the right 4th rib just lateral to the tubercle with the other thumb. Fix T4 with one thumb, and with the other thumb distract the costotransverse joint slightly and glide the 4th rib inferiorly allowing the

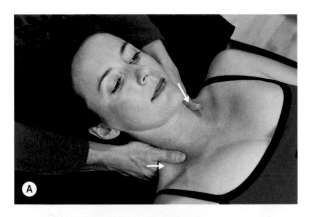

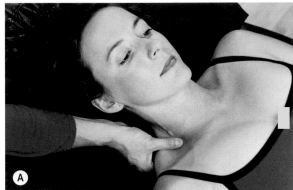

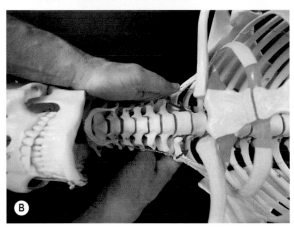

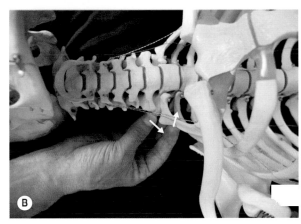

Figure 3.52

(A) This test is used to determine the ability of the right 1st rib to glide inferiorly relative to the transverse process of T1. (B) Distract the right 1st costotransverse joint by lifting the rib anteriorly with the MCP of the right index finger (arrows) prior to applying a posteroinferior glide to the rib.

Figure 3.53

(A) This test is used to determine the ability of the right 1st rib to glide superiorly relative to the transverse process of T1. (B) Distract the right 1st costotransverse joint by lifting the rib anteriorly with the right index and middle fingers prior to applying a posteroinferior glide to the transverse process of T1.

conjunct posterior roll to occur (Fig. 3.54A & B). Vary the direction of the glide to identify the specific direction that is limited. Be vector direction specific – look for a string within a spring. Compare the neutral and elastic zone behavior (amplitude, quality of first and second resistance, end feel) on both sides.

4th rib superior glide test: This test is used to determine the ability of the right 4th rib to glide superiorly relative to

the transverse process of T4. This test is done when the 4th thoracic ring is held in right rotation and restricted in left rotation; exhalation produces right rotation of the thoracic ring. The patient is prone with the head and neck in neutral rotation. Palpate the superior aspect of the transverse process of T4 with one thumb. Palpate the inferior aspect of the right 4th rib just lateral to the tubercle with the other thumb. Fix T4 and glide the 4th rib superiorly allowing the conjunct anterior roll to occur (Fig. 3.55A & B). Vary the

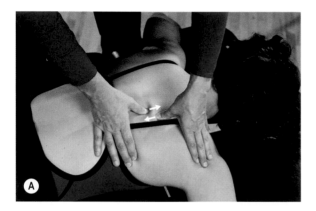

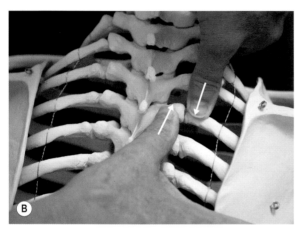

Figure 3.54 A & B

This test is used to determine the ability of the right 4th rib to glide inferiorly relative to the transverse process of T4.

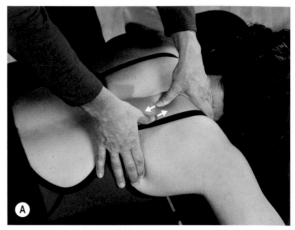

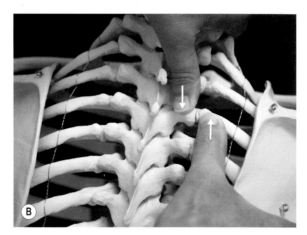

Figure 3.55 A & B

This test is used to determine the ability of the right 4th rib to glide superiorly relative to the transverse process of T4.

direction of the glide to identify the specific direction that is limited. Be vector direction specific – look for the string within a spring. Compare the neutral and elastic zone behavior (amplitude, quality of first and second resistance, end feel) on both sides.

Vertebrochondral region

9th rib anterolateral inferior glide test: This test is used to determine the ability of the right 9th rib to glide in an anterolateral and inferior direction relative to the transverse process of T9. This test is done when the 9th thoracic ring is held in left rotation and restricted in right rotation; inhalation produces left rotation of the thoracic ring.

The patient is prone with the head and neck in neutral rotation. With one thumb palpate the right transverse process of T9. With the other hand, palpate the 9th rib with the thumb just lateral to the transverse process of T9 and the index, or middle, finger along the body of the 9th rib. Fix T9 and glide the 9th rib in an anterolateral inferior direction (Fig. 3.56A & B). Vary the direction of the glide to identify the specific direction that is limited. Be vector direction specific – look for a string within a spring. Compare the neutral and elastic zone behavior (amplitude, quality of first and second resistance, end feel) on both sides.

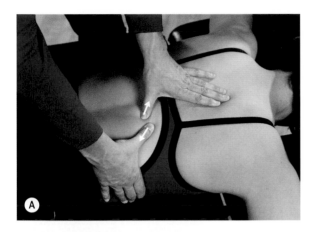

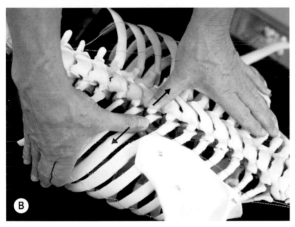

Figure 3.56 A & B

This test is used to determine the ability of the right 9th rib to glide anterolateroinferiorly relative to the transverse process of T9.

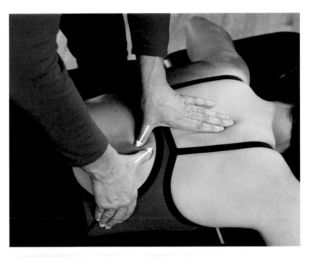

Figure 3.57

This test is used to determine the ability of the right 9th rib to glide posteromedially and superiorly relative to the transverse process of T9.

9th rib posteromedial superior glide test: This test is used to determine the ability of the right 9th rib to glide in a posteromedial superior direction relative to the transverse process of T9. This test is done when the 9th thoracic ring is held in right rotation and restricted in left rotation; exhalation produces right rotation of the thoracic ring. The patient is prone with the head and neck in neutral rotation. With one thumb palpate the right transverse process of T9. With the other hand, palpate the 9th rib with the thumb just lateral to the transverse process of T9 and the index or middle finger along the body of the 9th rib. Fix the

9th rib and glide the transverse process of T9 in an antero-lateral inferior direction (Fig. 3.57). This is a relative posteromediosuperior glide of the rib at the costotransverse joint. Vary the direction of the glide to identify the specific direction that is limited. Be vector direction specific – look for a string within a spring. Compare the neutral and elastic zone behavior (amplitude, quality of first and second resistance, end feel) on both sides.

Passive accessory mobility tests – thoracic zygapophyseal joints

These tests are used in the vertebromanubrial, vertebrosternal and vertebrochondral regions of the thorax.

T3 superior glide test: The following test is used to determine the ability of the right inferior articular process of T3 to glide superiorly relative to the superior articular process of T4. This test is done when T3 is held in extension with right side bending and restricted in flexion with left side bending. The patient is prone with the head and neck in neutral rotation. Palpate the inferior aspect of the left transverse process of T4 with one thumb. Palpate the inferior aspect of the right transverse process of T3 with the

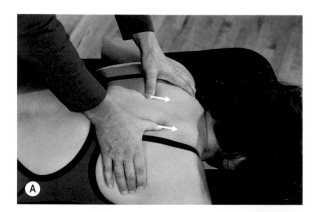

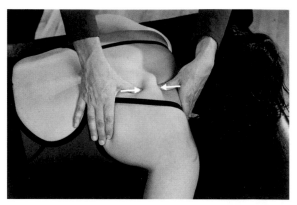

Figure 3.59

This test is used to determine the ability of the right inferior articular process of T3 to glide inferiorly relative to the superior articular process of T4.

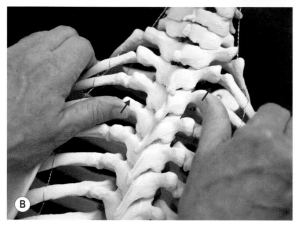

Figure 3.58 A & B

This test is used to determine the ability of the right inferior articular process of T3 to glide superiorly relative to the superior articular process of T4.

other thumb. Fix T4 and apply a superoanterior glide to T3 (Fig. 3.58A & B). Vary the direction of the glide to identify the specific direction that is limited. Be vector direction specific – look for a string within a spring. Compare the neutral and elastic zone behavior (amplitude, quality of first and second resistance, end feel) on both sides.

T3 inferior glide test: The following test is used to determine the ability of the right inferior articular process of T3 to glide inferiorly relative to the superior articular process of T4. This test is done when T3 is held in flexion with left side bending and restricted in extension with right side bending. The patient is prone with the head and neck in neutral.

Palpate the inferior aspect of the right transverse process of T4 with one thumb. Palpate the superior aspect of the right transverse process of T3 with the other thumb. Fix T4 and apply an inferior glide to T3 (Fig. 3.59). Vary the direction of the glide to identify the specific direction that is limited. Be vector direction specific – look for a string within a spring. Compare the neutral and elastic zone behavior (amplitude, quality of first and second resistance, end feel) on both sides.

Mediolateral translation – interthoracic ring mobility

The 2nd to 10th thoracic rings are capable of a small amount of mediolateral translation that occurs in conjunction with rotation (see Chapter 2). This test is used to determine interthoracic ring mediolateral mobility in the transverse plane. This motion is necessary for full rotation to occur. For full right rotation of the 6th thoracic ring, the left *6th* rib must be able to glide posterolaterally relative to the left transverse process of T6 and the right *6th* rib to glide anteromedially relative to the right transverse process of T6. T5 translates laterally relative to T6 when this motion occurs. This is left mediolateral translation of the 6th thoracic ring.

The patient is sitting with the arms crossed to opposite shoulders. The therapist is standing at the patient's left side. With a finger of the left hand, palpate the right 6th rib in the midaxillary line. With the index finger and thumb of the right hand, palpate the left *7th rib* in the midaxillary line (Fig. 3.60A). Stabilize T6 by approximating the left *7th rib* medially. With the left hand and arm translate the 6th ribs and T5 to the left in the transverse plane (Fig. 3.60B). The superior costovertebral joint of the left 7th rib prevents T6 from translating laterally with the 6th ribs. The motion is very small, but palpable and essential for optimal biomechanics of thoracic rotation. Compare the amplitude of motion to that of the thoracic rings above and below.

Passive control tests

These tests are used in the vertebromanubrial, vertebrosternal, and vertebrochondral regions of the thorax when the story and objective findings on analysis of the screening tasks suggests there may be a segmental interthoracic ring or intrathoracic ring form closure deficit. Several of the following tests were developed by Janet Lowcock (1990).

Anterior translation – thoracic spinal segment (intrathoracic ring)

The following test assesses the integrity of the anatomical structures that resist anterior translation between two thoracic vertebrae (intrathoracic ring). The patient is prone with the head and neck in neutral rotation. With the thumb and flexed proximal interphalangeal (PIP) joint of the index finger of the same hand, stabilize the transverse processes of the inferior vertebra of the thoracic ring

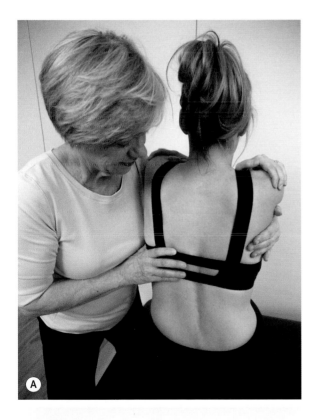
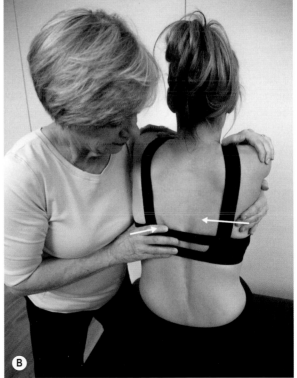

Figure 3.60

The 2nd to 10th thoracic rings are capable of a small amount of mediolateral translation that occurs in conjunction with rotation. This test is used to determine interthoracic ring mediolateral mobility in the transverse plane. (A, B) These figures illustrate a left mediolateral mobility test for the 6th thoracic ring.

of interest. With the opposite thumb and flexed PIP joint of the index finger of the same hand palpate the transverse processes of the superior vertebra. Stabilize the inferior vertebra and apply a straight posteroanterior force through the superior vertebra (Fig. 3.61). The orientation of the zygapophyseal joints in the thoracic spine limits anterior translation of the superior vertebra. There should be minimal palpable motion in this test. Excessive anterior translation suggests loss of osseous integrity (previous fracture).

Posterior translation – thoracic spinal segment (intrathoracic ring)

The following test assesses the integrity of the anatomical structures that resist posterior translation between two thoracic vertebrae. The patient is sitting with the arms crossed to opposite shoulders (3rd to 10th thoracic ring), or with hands behind the neck and fingers interlaced (1st and 2nd thoracic rings). The therapist is standing at the patient's side. With the thumb and flexed PIP of the index finger of the dorsal hand, stabilize the transverse processes of the inferior vertebra of the thoracic ring of interest. With the ventral arm and hand, position the segment such that the thoracic ring of interest is neither flexed nor extended (i.e., is in neutral). Apply an anteroposterior force to the superior vertebra through the thorax (through the patient's crossed arms or through their elbows) while fixing the inferior vertebra (Fig. 3.62). There may be a small amount of posterior translation with the segment in neutral flexion extension, but not excessive (compare this to the segments above and below). Then fully flex the thoracic spinal segment and retest the amplitude and end feel of anteroposterior translation. Then fully extend the thoracic spinal segment and retest the amplitude and end feel of anteroposterior translation. There should be no translation palpable in either full flexion or full extension if the articular system is intact. If the thoracic spinal segment stops translating posteriorly on one side and continues to translate posteriorly on the other, this suggests a loss of passive transverse plane rotational control.

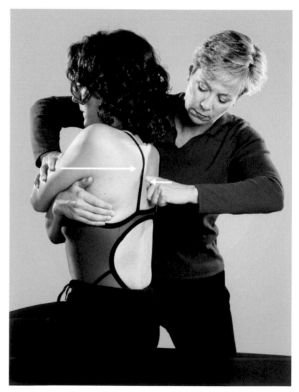

Figure 3.62

This test assesses the integrity of the anatomical structures that resist posterior translation between two thoracic vertebrae.

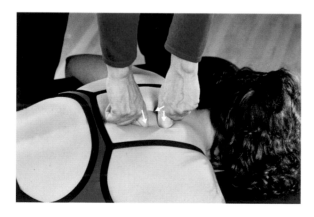

Figure 3.61

This test assesses the integrity of the anatomical structures that resist anterior translation between two thoracic vertebrae.

Anterior distraction – costotransverse joint (intrathoracic ring)

The following test assesses the integrity of the anatomical structures that resist distraction or separation of the posterior aspect of the rib (from the head to the tubercle) from the transverse process. Both the lateral costotransverse ligament and the ligament of the neck of the rib (costotransverse ligament) are part of the form closure mechanism for this test. The patient is prone with the head and neck in neutral rotation. With the thumb and flexed PIP of the index finger of the same hand, stabilize the contralateral transverse processes of the vertebrae to which the rib attaches (e.g., for the right 4th rib, stabilize the left transverse process of T4 and T3). With the pisiform or thumb of the other hand, palpate the rib just lateral to the tubercle. In the vertebromanubrial and vertebrosternal regions, stabilize the thoracic vertebrae and apply a posteroanterior force to the rib on the opposite

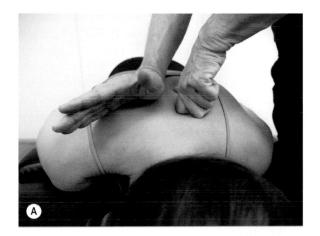

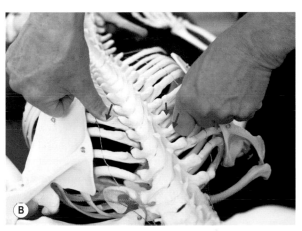

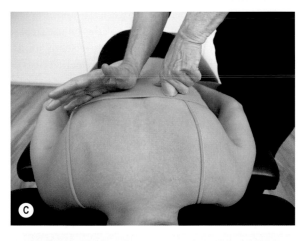

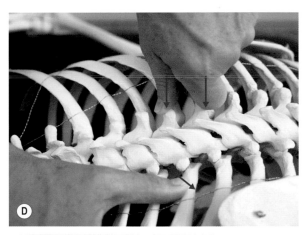

Figure 3.63

(A, B) Vertebromanubrial or vertebrosternal region: This test assesses the integrity of the anatomical structures that resist distraction, or separation, of the posterior aspect of the rib from the head to the tubercle from the transverse process. The vertebrae are stabilized on the contralateral side and the direction of force is primarily anterior to distract the costotransverse joint. (C, D) Vertebrochondral region: Note the difference in the direction of force required to distract the costotransverse joint in this region of the thorax.

side (Fig. 3.63A & B). In the vertebrochondral region the rib is on top of the transverse process; therefore, distraction requires the force to the rib to be superior, lateral, and anterior (Fig. 3.63C & D). Note any provocation of local symptoms, the amplitude of motion, and the end feel and compare to levels above, below and on the opposite side of the same thoracic ring.

Posterior translation – costochondral and sternocostal joints (intrathoracic ring)

The following test assesses the integrity of the anatomical structures that resist posterior translation of the rib relative to the costocartilage or the costocartilage relative to the sternum. When the articular integrity of the sternocostal or costochondral joints is compromised, a gap or step can be palpated at the relevant joint line. The patient is lying supine with head and neck in neutral. With one thumb, stabilize the anterior aspect of the sternum (sternocostal joint) or the costocartilage (costochondral joint). With the other thumb, palpate the anterior aspect of the costocartilage or the rib. Apply a straight anteroposterior force to the costocartilage or the rib (Fig. 3.64). There

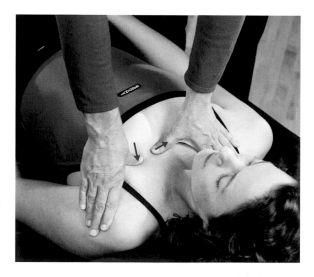

Figure 3.64

This test assesses the integrity of the anatomical structures that resist posterior translation of the rib relative to the costocartilage or the costocartilage relative to the sternum.

should be immediate resistance to this applied force and no provoked pain. Compare the amplitude of motion as well as the end feel and compare to levels above, below, and on the opposite side of the same thoracic ring.

Lateral translation (intrathoracic ring)

The following test assesses the integrity of the anatomical structures that resist excessive mediolateral translation between two adjacent vertebrae when the ribs between them are fixed. The primary structure being tested is hypothesized to be the intervertebral disc and the superior costovertebral joint (Lee D G 1996). To test left lateral translation control of the T6–T7 segment, the patient is sitting with the arms crossed to opposite shoulders and the therapist stands on the left side of the patient. Palpate the right 7th rib with the left hand. The therapist's left arm rests either over the patient's crossed arms or underneath the arms on the thorax. Palpate the left 7th rib with the right hand, and prevent this rib from translating laterally by compressing the head of the rib into the vertebral bodies of T7 and T6. Attempt to laterally translate T6 to the left by pulling the right 7th rib with the left hand toward you (Fig. 3.65). With the left 7th rib fixed there should be no palpable movement. If movement persists between T6 and T7, this suggests there is loss of integrity of the intervertebral disc and possibly the left and right costovertebral joints. This is an intrathoracic ring form closure deficit (loss of passive control).

Neural system – assessment principles

The neural system is extensive in that it includes all components of the central and peripheral nervous systems. There is an extensive body of research that suggests that motor control strategies (produced by the neural system) are individual and task specific (Hodges et al. 2013) and that changes are variable across patients with pain (van Dieën et al. 2017). The common link between individuals in pain is that the strategy used is suboptimal for the task; otherwise, everything can be different. When the motor control strategy is suboptimal for the task, various regions of the body will demonstrate altered alignment, biomechanics or control.

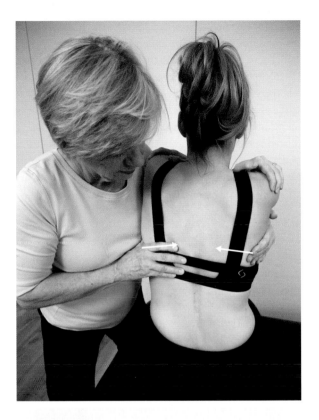

Figure 3.65

This test assesses the integrity of the anatomical structures that resist excessive mediolateral translation between two adjacent vertebrae (T6–T7) when the ribs between them are fixed.

Specific to low back and neck pain, the following is known (van Dieën et al. 2017, Falla & Hodges 2017):

- The deep muscles are often compromised; recruitment is absent, reduced or delayed (transversus abdominis, pelvic floor muscles, deep fibers of the multifidus, diaphragm). Superficial muscles are often augmented. Recruitment is dominant, excessive or early (erector spinae [iliocostalis, longissimus], superficial multifidus, sternocleidomastoid, anterior scalenes). Back pain patients have reduced variability of muscle recruitment patterns and tend to use strategies that generate rigidity as opposed to strategies that involve discrete activation of muscles

to 'fine-tune' intersegmental motion. These changes are accompanied by changes in brain organization.

- The specific pattern of altered recruitment strategies is generally unique to the individual patient, and within the individual they may be unique to the movement, posture or task that is assessed.

- There is not one strategy of muscle activation that is universally ideal for control of the spine and pelvis and not one strategy universally adopted by all patients in pain.

- Back and neck pain patients present with a redistribution of activity within and between muscles rather than inhibition or excitation of muscles in a stereotypical manner. The redistribution of activity leads to poorly controlled intervertebral motion and excessive compression.

- All the multisegmental muscles of the trunk contribute to movement and control.

- The current hypothesis is that spinal pain causes adaptive motor control changes through reinforcement learning.

- Motor control is influenced by thoughts, beliefs, emotions, and sensorial experiences that are both task and individual specific. The adaptive motor control changes may contribute to reorganization of the sensory and motor cortex.

- If the goal of rehabilitation (for example, using motor learning strategies) is to modify the adaptation (remove, modify or enhance), then this needs to be considered on an individual basis with respect to the unique solution adopted by the patient.

All the multisegmental muscles of the trunk contribute to movement and control and when their activity is redistributed they can produce specific vectors of force that contribute to suboptimal translation and rotation of the thoracic rings and rotation and torsion of the pelvis. Clinically, it is rare to find only one muscle that is overactive; therefore, it is impossible to predict exactly what one overactive muscle will do with respect to thoracic ring alignment, biomechanics, and control. Vector analysis facilitates the clinical reasoning process as to which muscle, tissue, or organ to release first (see Tests to determine which muscles to release below). Reassessment (vector analysis) following release of the primary vector then determines the second vector to release. The process is repeated until all vectors (from all systems) restricting mobility of the drivers are released. Reassessment of the screening task and meaningful task then determines if the distribution of muscular activity has improved or if further tests are necessary to determine which muscles are underactive (see Active control tests and Thorax Drivers and Motor Control Strategies below). There is a subgroup of individuals whose strategies for function immediately improve after release of the primary and secondary vectors (see Jennifer's story and Amanda's story in Chapter 5). This group does not require individual muscle motor control training although movement training is still critical for their home practice. There is another subgroup whose strategies for function do not improve sufficiently to control loads after release of the vectors (see Christine's story in Chapter 5). This group requires further tests to determine which muscles require specific motor control training along with movement training (see Active control tests and Thorax Drivers and Motor Control Strategies below).

Neural system – specific tests

Tests to determine which muscles to release

Active and passive listening techniques are used during motion analysis, specific body region correction and release to understand more about the vectors that are impacting function (alignment, biomechanics, control) (see Further tests – vector analysis). If the neural system impairment produces muscle dyssynergies, the alignment and biomechanics of the driver can be corrected with manual and verbal cuing; passive listening during correction provides some information about the primary vector. When the correction is released, passive listening also helps to determine the location (left or right, front or back, inside or outside the thorax, abdomen, or pelvis), length (long or short), and strength (strong, moderate, or weak) of the primary vector.

Correct the thoracic ring or rings previously determined to be the driver for the screening task. Slowly release the left

and right rib simultaneously and note which rib is pulled into anterior or posterior rotation first. Repeat the correction. Focus now on the 1st rib that moved and note whether the vector of pull came from the front, back, or side and whether the pull is from the inside or outside of the thorax. Is the vector long or short, strong or weak? If the vector is on the outside of the thorax, palpate the muscles and fascia related to the vector for excessive overactivity or tension and tightness to confirm the specific structure responsible for the suboptimal alignment and biomechanics. This structure should be released first in the treatment plan.

Sometimes, two muscles, or structures, create a net vector, and it may not be possible to identify the structure anatomically. As previously mentioned, even if it cannot be named, there are treatment techniques for releasing combined vectors that are impacting alignment, biomechanics, and control of the driver (see Chapter 6).

Redistributed muscle activity (Hodges & Smeets 2015) associated with overactivation of the superficial muscles creates vectors of force that can alter alignment and biomechanics of the physical body. These are classified as neural system impairments since the overactivation is a result of altered motor control strategies, and is influenced by the central and peripheral nervous systems. For example, overactivation of one fascicle of the right iliocostalis thoracis and iliocostalis lumborum can cause posterior rotation of the right rib and thus result in left translation and right rotation of the thoracic ring; the entire thoracic ring responds to this vector. The fascicle of the right external oblique attached to this ring may respond to the posterior rotation of the right rib and may also be overactive. Palpation of both the right iliocostalis thoracis and iliocostalis lumborum and the right external oblique may reveal tender trigger points. Knowing the biomechanics of the thorax combined with vector analysis facilitates the decision as to which muscle is the primary vector, and should be released first, and which muscle is reacting, and should be left alone (Fig. 6.24A). The case reports in Chapter 5 will provide further examples of the wide varieties of vectors that perturb the alignment, biomechanics, and control of the thoracic rings and how to clinically reason what requires release, when to specifically train an individual muscle, and how to prescribe movement training that is individual and meaningful.

Tests to determine when to release the nervous system

A mobility impairment of the dura is also classified as a neural system impairment since the dura is always in relationship with the nervous system. When a lack of dural or perineural mobility is the primary system impairment causing suboptimal alignment, biomechanics, and control of a body region, correcting that region often makes the patient's symptoms worse and reduces the performance of the meaningful task. No body region correction seems to improve the experience or performance of the task when there is a lack of dural or perineural mobility. The current hypothesis is that the body is 'changing shape' to reduce the tension on the dura or perineural tissue. If, on the other hand, a body region correction (thorax, pelvis, hip, neck, cranial region or foot) reduces neural symptoms (burning, tingling, numbness, etc.) and improves the performance of the screening task as well as the meaningful task, then the hypothesis is that the suboptimal alignment is the cause of the dural or perineural tension. In the first instance, specific release of the dura or a specific nerve is indicated (see the section on dural and perineural system impairments in Chapter 6). In the second instance, vector analysis to determine the primary vector impacting the alignment of the body region driver and subsequent treatment is indicated.

Active control tests

Active control tests evaluate the force closure mechanism provided by the chosen motor control strategy, which is known to be individual and task specific. These tests are incorporated into analysis of the screening task. For each task evaluated, the alignment, biomechanics and control of the joints being assessed are compared against what is thought to be optimal. For example, during right rotation of the thorax the thoracic rings should translate slightly to the left. If the thoracic ring in question translates too far to the left, then this is considered suboptimal performance and control tests are indicated. When resistance is applied to trunk rotation through bilateral flexed arms, the lumbar segments should remain still. During single leg standing, the innominate should not rotate anterior relative to the sacrum (Hungerford et al. 2004); this is referred to as

'unlocking or giving way' of the sacroiliac joint. During elevation of one arm, the cervical segments should not move until elevation has reached 120–130 degrees.

Passive control tests rule in or rule out a form closure deficit (see above). Active control tests assess the ability of the deep segmental muscles to control the excessive or undesirable motion or alignment regardless of whether the underlying system impairment is articular or neural. Verbal and manual cues are given, which aim to facilitate recruitment of the deep segmental muscles, and the screening task is repeated to determine the impact of a different motor control strategy on the performance of the body region being tested.

When the neuromuscular recruitment strategy is optimal, all motion should be controlled even when the joint is positioned in neutral. This does not mean that the joint should not move if movement is a requirement of the task, rather the joint's motion should be congruent with the optimal biomechanics. The amount of neuromuscular activation necessary to control translation or motion of a neutral joint varies according to the amplitude of the applied load.

Thorax – interthoracic ring control

These tests are used in the vertebromanubrial, vertebrosternal, and vertebrochondral regions of the thorax when the story and objective findings on analysis of the screening tasks suggest there may be a segmental interthoracic ring active control impairment with or without an underlying passive control impairment.

The deep segmental muscles responsible for thoracic interthoracic ring control include the deep fibers of the multifidus, the rotatores brevis and longus, the levator costarum, and the internal and external intercostal muscles. The deep and superficial muscles of the posterior thorax have been shown to have differential activity with respect to the direction of trunk rotation when induced by arm movement (Lee L-J et al. 2009). At T5, T8 and T11, both multifidus and rotatores and longissimus act as spinal extensors (i.e., are not activated differentially) when perturbed in the sagittal plane (Lee L-J et al. 2011). Conversely, with transverse plane perturbations, the multifidus, rotatores, and longissimus thoracis activate to control opposite directions of rotation. The longissimus thoracis is most active with contralateral arm movements, and is an ipsilateral rotator of the thorax, while the multifidus and rotatores are most active with ipsilateral arm movements, and are contralateral rotators of the thorax (Lee L-J et al. 2009) (Fig. 3.66). No studies have been done to investigate the impact of pain on motor control in the thorax. Clinically, it has been noted that atrophy or inhibition of the deep segmental muscles is often present when there is an active control impairment (Lee L-J 2003b); however, atrophy is not always present with thoracic pain. Interthoracic ring control tests are done after all vectors impeding alignment and biomechanics have been released. The thoracic ring merely drifts back into the translated and rotated position on release of the alignment correction. Alternately, the alignment of the thoracic ring may be restored but only for a few repetitions of loading.

In sitting or standing, palpate the deep and superficial muscles of the posterior thorax at the level of poor active thoracic ring control. Palpate the multifidus and rotatores bilaterally between the spinous and transverse processes. Press firmly but gently into the tissue and note the degree of tissue firmness (resting activation) and the size of the muscle. Compare the firmness and size to the contralateral side and to levels above and below (Fig. 3.67A). Ask the patient to lift one arm; the recruitment of the multifidus and rotatores should increase. Palpate the longissimus thoracis in the muscle belly just below its attachment to the transverse process and adjacent rib. Press firmly into the muscle and roll the tissue in the coronal plane (Fig. 3.67B). When there is increased activation in a specific fascicle of the longissimus thoracis this feels like a pepperoni stick in the middle of a salami. Repeat this palpation for the iliocostalis thoracis and iliocostalis lumborum.

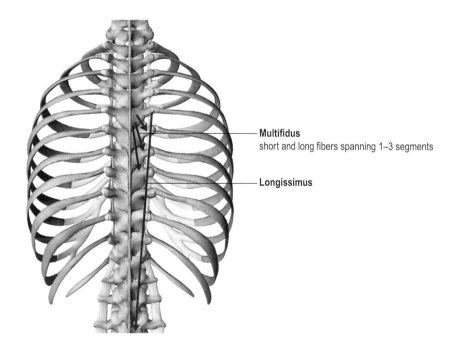

Multifidus
short and long fibers spanning 1–3 segments

Longissimus

Figure 3.66

Longissimus is an ipsilateral rotator of the thorax, while multifidus is a contralateral rotator; therefore, during rotary perturbations they are recruited differently (Lee L-J et al. 2009).

Reproduced from Essential Anatomy 5 3D4Medical with permission.

Both the iliocostalis thoracis, iliocostalis lumborum and longissimus thoracis can create a contralateral translation of a thoracic ring when overactive. Palpate the relevant thoracic ring and ask the patient to lift the right and then the left arm. Note the behavior of the thoracic ring and the recruitment response of the deep and superficial muscles of the posterior thorax. When there is an active control impairment the thoracic ring will translate and rotate further during a unilateral arm lift task (Lee L-J 2003b, 2016). When the patient can recruit the deep segmental muscles responsible for interthoracic ring alignment and control with a 'connect cue' (see Chapter 7), the thoracic ring will automatically correct as the motor control strategy changes. The superficial muscles will relax and the deep segmental muscles will activate (Fig. 3.67C & D).

The relationship between active control of a thoracic ring, pelvis and hip control is tested by finding the best 'connect cue' for interthoracic ring control (see Chapter 7) and then assessing whether this cue automatically aligns the thoracic ring and subsequently restores a strategy that provides better pelvic and hip alignment and control.

Lumbar spine – intersegmental control and thoracic ring drivers

This test is used to determine the active control of a lumbar segment and the impact of correcting a thoracic ring driver on lumbar segmental control. The patient is seated with the pelvis in neutral (with no transverse plane rotation or intrapelvic torsion and in a neutral anteroposterior tilt). Palpate the spinous processes of the lumbar segments of interest. Loss of active control would have previously been noted in a screening task and the segment of interest determined. Ask the patient to flex their arms and with their elbows extended, place the palms of their hands together.

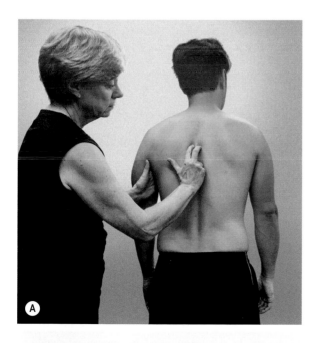
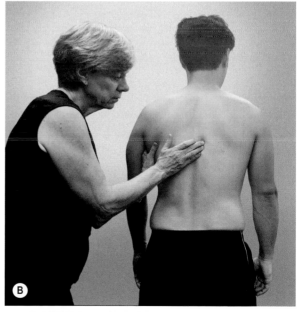

Figure 3.67

This man is standing with his 6th thoracic ring translated left and rotated right. (A) There is notable inhibition of the segmental multifidus and rotatores at T5–T6 and (B) over-activation of a fascicle of longissimus thoracis that inserts into the right transverse process of T6 and the right 6th rib. *Continued*

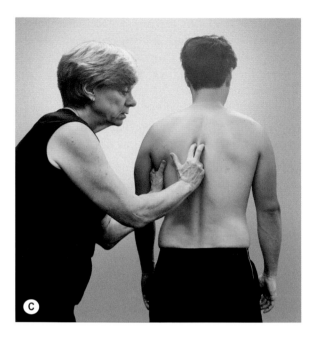

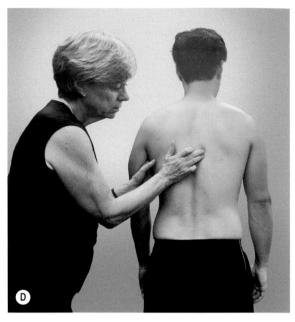

Figure 3.67 *continued*

(C) When the appropriate connect cue is given, the 6th thoracic ring is felt to automatically correct (therapist's left hand) as the recruitment of the segmental multifidus and rotatores increases. (D) Simultaneously, the overactivation of the right longissimus thoracis decreases.

Resist flexion, extension, and left and right rotation of the trunk through the arms and note the patient's ability to resist the force as well as any movement of the lumbar segment (Fig. 3.68A). Any loss of the neutral position in the lumbar segment indicates an active control impairment of this segment.

Correct the thoracic ring driver previously found for the screening task, hold the correction with one hand and repeat the test. Note any change in the patient's ability to resist the force and watch for any loss of neutral of the lumbar segment of interest (Fig. 3.68B, C). If there is no change in performance during this test, a specific evaluation of the deep segmental muscles responsible for control of the lumbar spine is indicated (Lee D & Lee L-J 2011b). If segmental lumbar control is automatically restored when the thoracic ring driver is corrected, a specific evaluation of these muscles is not indicated. Treatment should be directed to the thoracic ring driver.

Pelvis – sacroiliac joint control and thoracic ring drivers

The single-leg-standing test is a valid and reliable test of active control for the SIJ (Hungerford et al. 2004, 2007) (Fig. 3.69A–F). Palpate the inferior lateral angle of the sacrum with one thumb and the iliac crest of the ipsilateral innominate with the fingers of the opposite hand. Do not palpate the posterior superior iliac spine and S2 spinous process for this test; reliability has not been shown for this landmarking (Dreyfuss et al. 1994, Potter & Rothstein 1985, Carmichael 1987, Herzog et al. 1989, Meijne et al. 1999, Wurff et al. 2000). Ask the patient to shift their weight to the contralateral leg (i.e., unload the SIJ on the side being tested) and then take their full weight through the leg on the side being tested. No movement should be felt between your hands. The innominate should remain posteriorly rotated relative to the sacrum. If the innominate anteriorly rotates relative to the sacrum, then the SIJ has lost active control. If the SIJ remains controlled,

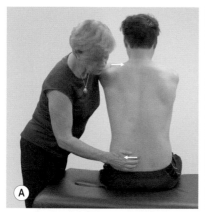 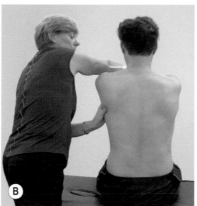 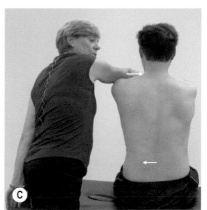

Figure 3.68

Lumbar spine: Intersegmental control and thoracic ring drivers. (A) This man has a longstanding history of low back pain. When either a flexion or right rotation load (right arrow) is applied to his trunk through his elevated arms, the L4–L5 loses neutral alignment and rotates to the right (left arrow). He finds it difficult to resist a right rotation force applied to his trunk. The 6th thoracic ring is translated left and rotated right and the overactivation of the right longissimus noted in standing (see Fig. 3.67B) persists in sitting. (B) When the alignment of the 6th thoracic ring is corrected, the longissimus relaxes and the deep fibers of multifidus at L4–L5 automatically contract and control L4–L5 during the resisted right rotation task. He can generate more force against a right rotation load. (C) When the 6th thoracic ring correction is released, the subject loses control at L4–L5 (left arrow) and immediately feels less able to resist a right rotation load. Note the increased activation of the right longissimus.

further load can be applied by having the patient single-leg-stand, squat or step forward. At no time should the innominate anteriorly rotate relative to the sacrum on the weight-bearing side.

Correct the thoracic ring driver previously found for the screening task, hold the correction with one hand and palpate the SIJ with the other. Repeat the single-leg-standing test and note any change in the performance of the SIJ when the thoracic ring driver is corrected. If the thoracic ring is a primary driver, full control will be restored to the SIJ. If the thorax is a primary driver and the pelvis a secondary driver, the loss of SIJ control will occur later in the task. If there is no change in performance of the SIJ during this test, the pelvis may be a co-driver.

Hip – control and thoracic ring drivers

This test is used to determine the active control of the hip and the impact of correcting a thoracic ring driver on alignment and control of the hip. With the patient standing, palpate the femoral head and greater trochanter of the femur with one hand and the innominate with the other. Note the starting position of the femoral head (see the section Standing posture, 3rd thoracic ring to the hips). Ask the patient to shift their weight to the contralateral and then the ipsilateral side and note any change in position of the femoral head relative to the acetabulum. It should remain centered. If the femoral head translates or rotates away from the centered position, there is a loss of active control.

Correct the thoracic ring driver previously found for the screening task, hold the correction with one hand and palpate the femoral head with the other. Repeat the weight shift and then the single-leg-standing test and note any change in the performance of the hip when the thoracic ring driver is corrected. If the thoracic ring is the primary driver, there should be complete restoration of alignment and control of the hip in the single-leg-standing task. If the hip is a secondary driver, an improvement (but not complete correction and control) will occur and a specific evaluation of the hip joint is indicated.

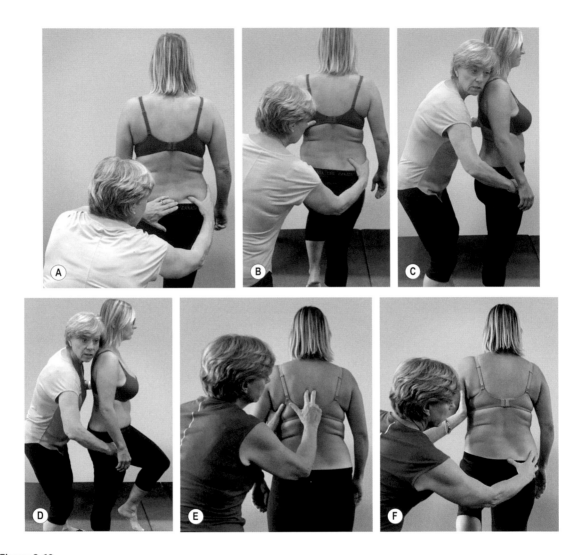

Figure 3.69

(A) Points of palpation for assessing control of the SIJ in vertical loading. Palpate the inferior lateral angle of the ipsilateral sacrum with one hand and the iliac crest (multiple points) with the other. Note any loss of control of the SIJ as weight is taken through the leg before testing any task that begins with load through the leg. This woman's meaningful task is running and the one-leg-standing task is used to screen her ability to maintain pelvic control during single-leg loading. During this weight-shift task to the right her right SIJ loses control (the right innominate anteriorly rotates relative to the right side of the sacrum). (B) Her 7th thoracic ring also translates further left and rotates further right during this task and when the 7th thoracic ring alignment is corrected and controlled, she can shift her weight to the right and flex her left hip without losing control of the right SIJ. (C) Her right hip is anteriorly translated relative to the left in standing and translates further anteriorly during the right weight-shift task. (D) This suboptimal alignment and control of the right hip is also corrected and controlled when her 7th thoracic ring is aligned and controlled during this task. The 7th thoracic ring is the primary driver for her loss of pelvic and right hip alignment and control for the right single-leg-loading task. (E) After releasing the relevant vectors, an appropriate cue for restoring the alignment and control of the 7th thoracic ring is found. (F) If the cue is effective, the right pelvis and hip alignment and control will be restored during the right single-leg-loading task. Subsequent motor control and movement training follows (see Chapter 7).

Cervical spine – intersegmental control and thoracic ring drivers

This test is used to determine the active control of a cervical segment and the impact of correcting a thoracic ring driver on cervical segmental control. With the patient either seated or standing, palpate the cervical segment previously noted to lose active control during a screening task. Ask the patient to elevate one arm to 90 degrees and note any loss of cervical segmental control (Fig. 3.70A). Further load can be applied to the neck by adding resistance in a variety of directions to the arm (Fig. 3.70B). The more robust the motor control strategy, the greater the load that can be managed.

Correct the thoracic ring driver previously found for the screening task, hold the correction with one hand and repeat the test. Note any change in the patient's ability to resist the force to the elevated arm and watch for any loss of neutral of the cervical segment of interest (Fig. 3.70C). If the thorax is the driver, there should be complete restoration of alignment and control of the cervical segment throughout the task (Fig. 3.70D). Partial improvement in alignment and control suggests the cervical segment may be a secondary driver and a specific evaluation of the deep segmental muscles responsible for control of the cervical spine is indicated.

Visceral system

Many intrathoracic visceral structures attach to the skeletal thorax and can impact alignment, biomechanics and control of individual, or multiple, thoracic rings. The visceral system is implicated when the passive listening response on release of the correction of the thoracic ring is felt to go inside the thorax. The Barral Institute

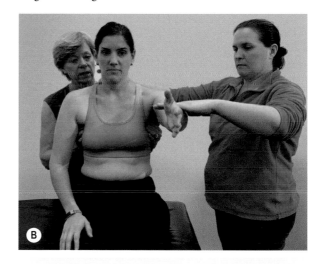

Figure 3.70

This test is used to determine the active control of a cervical segment and the impact of correcting a thoracic ring driver on cervical segmental control. (A) This woman's C7 is translated left and rotated right and there is no change in this position during elevation of the left arm. She notes that elevation of her left arm requires more effort than elevation of the right. (B) The 5th thoracic ring is translated left and rotated right and the 4th thoracic ring is translated right and rotated left. When an extension force is applied to the elevated left arm, the 4th thoracic ring translates further right and rotates further left and C7 translates further left and rotates further right. *Continued*

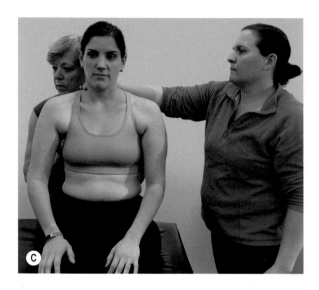

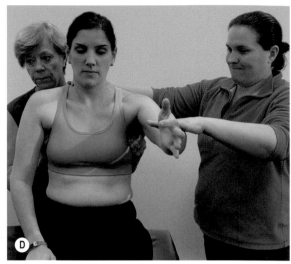

Figure 3.70 *continued*

(C) Correcting both the 4th and 5th thoracic rings resulted in complete correction of the alignment of C7. (D) Less effort was required to elevate the left arm and more load could be applied. C7 remained controlled when the 4th and 5th thoracic ring correction was maintained. This is a thorax-driven neck control problem for left arm elevation.

(http://www.barralinstitute.com) offers an extensive series of courses for therapists interested in learning how visceral system impairments impact function and readers are encouraged to explore this curriculum. The Barral Institute teaches a different way of listening to the body both globally and locally than presented in this text and the two methods integrate well (Wetzler & Lee 2015). One specific impairment that has significant impact on the alignment and biomechanics of the thorax will be described here.

Pericardial vectors and posture

The pericardium of the heart is firmly attached to the diaphragm (Fig. 1.32) as well as the posterior sternum and the anterior aspect of T4, T2 and C6 (Fig. 3.71A). When the central tendon of the diaphragm is persistently low in the thorax secondary to pregnancy, phrenic or vagal nerve facilitation, poor breathing habits, etc., vectors from the pericardial attachments to the spine create a classic posture (Fig. 3.71B). The vertebrochondral region remains flexed whereas the vertebrosternal region becomes extended. The vertebromanubrial region overly flexes and it not uncommon to see a segmental extension crease at the level of C6. Inversion of the trunk (as in downward facing dog pose or dolphin pose) often dramatically reverses these curves since in these postures the central tendon of the diaphragm ascends due to the influence of gravity and the vector is somewhat released (Fig. 3.71C). In these cases, treatment should then be directed to the diaphragm (see the section on hypopressive exercise and Low Pressure Fitness™ in Chapter 7).

Myofascial system

Myofascial system impairments of the thorax include surgical scars in any tissue that can impact the thoracic rings as well as loss of sliding mobility between the superficial and deep muscles of the thorax (loose connective tissue adhesions or loss of hydration). Whenever a scar is seen on the trunk (including the abdomen), its mobility should be assessed. Sometimes the passive listening when correcting

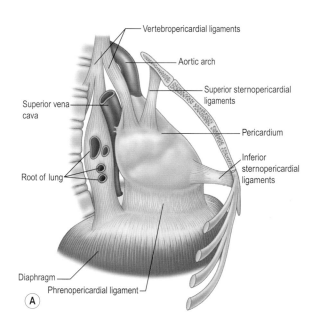

Vertebropericardial ligaments

Aortic arch

Superior sternopericardial ligaments

Superior vena cava

Pericardium

Inferior sternopericardial ligaments

Root of lung

Diaphragm

Phrenopericardial ligament

(A)

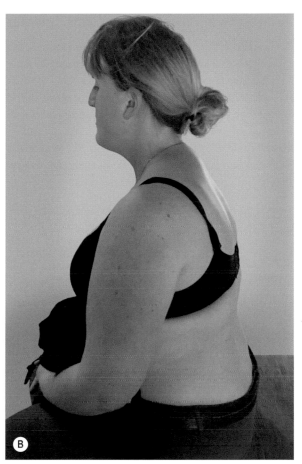

(B)

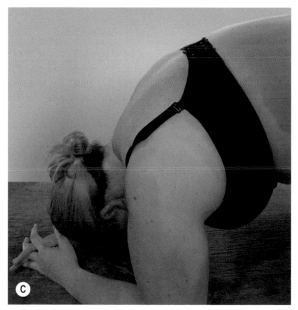

(C)

Figure 3.71

(A) The pericardium of the heart attaches to the sternum and the anterior aspect of the T6, T4 and C6 vertebra. (B) When the diaphragm is habitually low in the thorax this classic posture of midthoracic extension, cervicothoracic flexion, and excessive extension at C6 is seen. (C) When inverted as in the downward facing dog pose, the spinal curves reverse. This woman has also had thyroid surgery and there are myofascial restrictions around C6 that prevent her neck from elongating in this inverted position. Note the change in her midthorax in this position.

(A) Reproduced from *The Fasciae: Anatomy, Dysfunction and Treatment* (2006) by Serge Paoletti with permission of Eastland Press Inc.

and releasing a thoracic ring goes directly to a scar, which then needs to be released. When there is loss of mobility between the layers of muscles because of the adhesions from a scar, the alignment, biomechanics, and control of multiple thoracic rings can be impacted. Significant myofascial system impairments can prevent complete correction of the thoracic rings and require release before the impact of correcting alignment and biomechanics are understood.

Thorax drivers and motor control strategies

Redistribution of activity within and between muscles that control the spine and pelvis can be influenced, in some, by correcting the alignment and biomechanics of the drivers. The influence of suboptimal alignment of the thorax on recruitment patterns of the abdomen and back muscles was brought to my attention by Linda-Joy Lee. The following tests help to differentiate the patients that require specific muscle training for restoration of alignment, biomechanics, and control from those who do not.

Thoracic deep and superficial back muscle recruitment strategies

Palpate the segmental multifidus and rotatores (Fig. 3.67A), longissimus thoracis (Fig. 3.67B), iliocostalis thoracis and iliocostalis lumborum for resting activation at the level of the thoracic ring driver. If these superficial long back muscles are causing the thoracic ring to be translated and rotated, they should be overactive on the contralateral side of the thoracic ring translation. The right longissimus thoracis, iliocostalis thoracis and iliocostalis lumborum cause a left translation and right rotation of a thoracic ring (Fig. 3.72). If the thoracic ring is translated and rotated to the same side as the noted overactive superficial muscles, then these muscles are reacting to another vector.

Note the behavior of the thoracic ring and the recruitment response of the deep and superficial muscles of the posterior thorax when the patient is asked to lift one arm and then the other (Fig. 3.73A). Note which arm is heavier or harder to lift.

Correct the thoracic ring with both manual and verbal cues and have the patient repeat the arm lift. Note if the thoracic ring correction made the task easier. Hold the thoracic ring correction with one hand, palpate the multifidus and rotatores with the other and repeat the arm lift task. Note any difference in the recruitment strategy of the multifidus and rotatores. Repeat the task while maintaining the thoracic ring correction and palpate the recruitment strategy of the longissimus thoracis, iliocostalis thoracis and iliocostalis lumborum (Fig. 3.73B). It is not uncommon to find the recruitment strategy for both

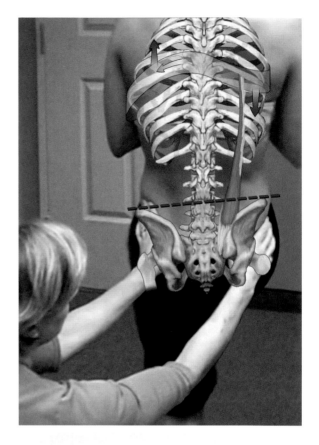

Figure 3.72

In this example, the fascicle of the right iliocostalis that inserts onto the right 7th rib is overactive. During the left single-leg-standing test, this overactivation prevents posterior rotation of the right innominate relative to the sacrum and causes the right 7th rib to posteriorly rotate more than the ribs above and below. This results in left translation and right rotation of the 7th thoracic ring during this task.

the deep and superficial back muscles normalize when the thoracic ring is corrected. This is a possible mechanism for why the effort to lift the arm decreases when the thoracic ring is corrected. When the effort to lift the arm does not change, and the recruitment strategy for this task remains suboptimal for either the deep or superficial back muscles, local treatment of the muscle or muscles is required.

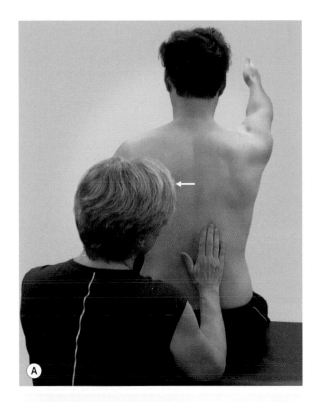 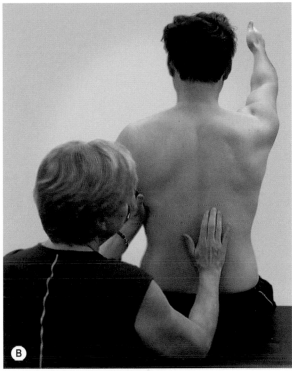

Figure 3.73

This is the same man as in Figures 3.67 and 3.68. In addition to persistent low back pain, he reports difficulty initiating elevation of the right arm. (A) The right longissimus thoracis is noted to overactivate during this task and the 6th thoracic ring translates further left and rotates further right. (B) Correction and control of the 6th thoracic ring changes the motor control strategy for the arm elevation task. The longissimus thoracis relaxes and the deep segmental muscles that control the 6th thoracic ring are activated. He notes that it is much easier to initiate elevation of the right arm.

Abdominal muscle recruitment strategies

The nerve supply to the abdominal muscles comes from the thorax and it is not uncommon to see a relationship between a translated and rotated thoracic ring and altered recruitment strategies of the abdominal muscles. Lee reports: 'In thoracic driven abdominal wall dysfunction, transversus abdominis muscle contraction occurs in response to a cue directed to control of the thoracic rings, not in response to abdominal wall cues' (Lee L-J 2016).

In this author's experience, in thorax driven abdominal wall dysfunction, a symmetric bilateral transversus abdominis (TrA) muscle contraction is often restored in response to both abdominal wall and pelvic floor cues when the thoracic ring driver is corrected (Fig. 3.74). A similar change in the abdominal wall recruitment response with a thoracic ring correction has also been noted during a short head and neck curl-up task (Fig. 3.75A & B) (Lee D 2017a).

Response to verbal cue – transversus abdominis and the pelvic floor

It is known that a 10–15 per cent contraction of the levator ani should induce a contraction of the middle fibers of the transversus abdominis that is isolated from the internal oblique (Hodges et al. 2003). Redistributed activity between

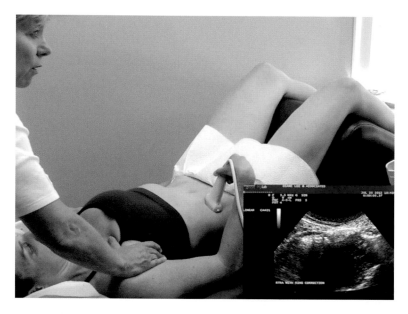

Figure 3.74

The behavior of the transversus abdominis muscle (in all three regions), in response to a cue to contract the pelvic floor, can be impacted when translated and rotated thoracic rings are manually corrected. This response does not occur in all patients; assessment is required to determine who requires specific motor control training in addition to treatment which improves alignment and biomechanics of the thorax and its relationship to the pelvis.

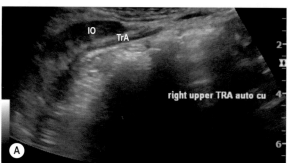

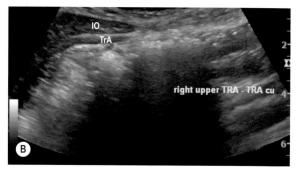

Figure 3.75

Ultrasound image of the right upper abdominal wall during a short head and neck curl-up task. (A) Automatic strategy. When there is a lower translated or rotated thoracic ring, it is common to see absent or delayed recruitment of the transversus abdominis during a short head and neck curl-up task. This is an image of the upper abdomen during a curl-up task. There is no response in the upper fibers of the right transversus abdominis. (B) Correcting, and maintaining, the alignment of the 8th thoracic ring during the task immediately changed the recruitment strategy of the lateral abdominals and resulted in co-activation of both the right transversus abdominis and internal oblique. auto = automatic, cu = curl-up, IO = internal oblique, TrA = transversus abdominis.

the left and right transversus abdominis (one or both delayed, absent, or asymmetric) or between the transversus abdominis and the internal or external oblique is commonly seen in patients with lumbopelvic pain, incontinence, pelvic organ prolapse, and diastasis rectus abdominis. What has not been investigated, yet is commonly observed clinically, is the impact of correcting the alignment of the thoracic ring driver on the recruitment strategy of the abdominal muscles in response to a verbal cue.

With the patient in supine lying, palpate the transversus abdominis at the level of loss of active control (Fig. 3.76A–C). Note the resting activation of the external oblique and internal oblique prior to reaching the layer of

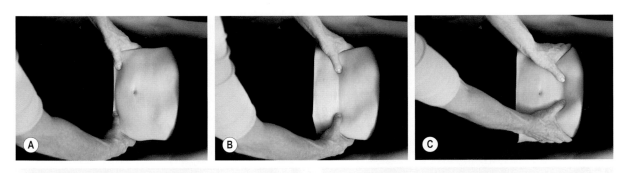

Figure 3.76

Points of palpation to assess the lower, middle, and upper fibers (A, B and C respectively) of the transversus abdominis and the intervening internal and external oblique.

the transversus abdominis (Lee D 2017a). Ask the patient to 'gently tighten the muscles around the anus and to then draw the anus up towards the pubic bone.' This is a cue specifically for the levator ani group of muscles (Peng et al. 2007) and a gentle contraction (10–15 per cent) should produce a bilateral, isolated contraction of transversus abdominis. Note any delay, absence or asymmetry in the recruitment strategy of the transversus abdominis.

Correct the thoracic ring driver for the screening task, have the patient maintain the correction, and note any difference in the recruitment strategy of the left and right transversus abdominis, internal oblique or external oblique (Fig. 3.77A & B). Ultrasound imaging is a useful tool for assessing the change in the recruitment strategy of the transversus abdominis with correction of a thoracic ring or any other driver (see Amanda's story in Chapter 5).

It is not uncommon to find the recruitment strategy for both the deep and superficial abdominal muscles normalize when the thoracic ring is corrected (Lee D 2017a, Lee L-J 2016). One mechanism is that the neural drive to the abdominal muscles changes when the thoracic ring position changes. When the recruitment strategy remains suboptimal for either the deep or superficial abdominal muscles, Stage 1 motor control training (see Chapter 7) of the muscle or muscles is required.

Short head and neck curl-up task

A short head and neck curl-up task requires co-activation of all abdominal muscles (Andersson et al. 1997). At rest, there

should be no distortion of the linea alba and tension should be maintained throughout the curl-up task (Lee D & Hodges 2016) (Fig. 3.78). The inter-recti distance should remain consistent between rest and the curl-up position, whether a cue is given to preactivate the transversus abdominis or not (Lee D & Hodges 2016). Dyssynergies of the abdominal muscles are common across multiple conditions, including those which create thoracic, lumbopelvic, and hip pain. In those with diastasis rectus abdominis (DRA), the linea alba is wider than normal and narrows during a short head and neck curl-up task (Lee D & Hodges 2016, Mota et al. 2015, Pascoal et al. 2014, Sancho et al. 2015), and this narrowing can be reduced with preactivation of the transversus abdominis (Lee D & Hodges 2016) (Fig. 3.79). When the inter-recti distance narrows during a curl-up task, the distortion of the linea alba often increases (Fig. 3.80). When the transversus abdominis contracts, the inter-recti distance is less narrow and less distorted. Forces can be transferred between sides of the abdomen when there is sufficient tension in the linea alba. In some individuals, the distance is too wide, and the distortion is too great for the lateral abdominals to effectively tense. These individuals demonstrate loss of active control at the level (thorax, lumbar spine, or pelvis) related to their DRA. A surgical recti plication may be required for these individuals to regain optimal function of their abdominal wall. A high DRA impacts active control of the lower thoracic rings, a DRA around the umbilicus impacts active control of the midlumbar region, and a low DRA impacts active control of the SIJs.

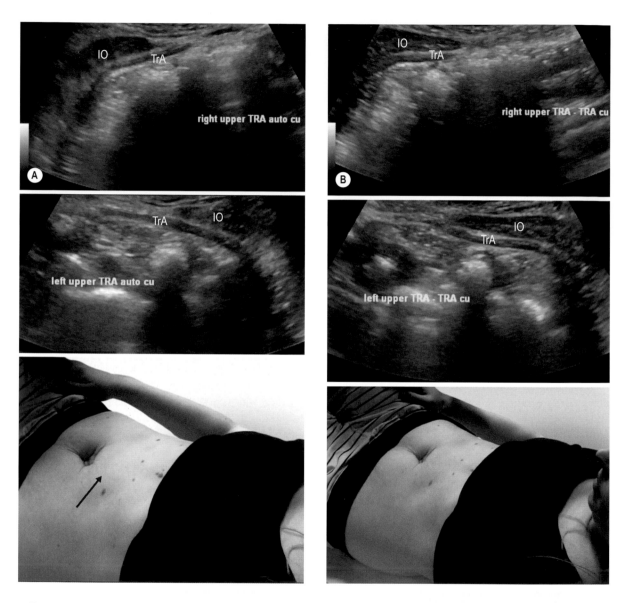

Figure 3.77

This patient's full story is presented in Chapter 5 (see Amanda's story). She has a diastasis rectus abdominis. (A) Upper abdominals during automatic curl-up. Note the lack of recruitment (i.e., lack of broadening and lateral slide) of the left and right upper fibers of the TrA during her automatic strategy for a curl-up task. Doming (distortion and lack of tension) of the linea alba (arrow) occurs. (B) Upper abdominals with correction of the 8th thoracic ring. Correcting the alignment of the 8th thoracic ring facilitated a better response from both the left and right upper fibers of the TrA and reduced the doming of the patient's linea alba. This suggests that the TrA could generate more tension in the linea alba. auto = automatic, cu = curl-up, IO = internal oblique, TrA = transversus abdominis.

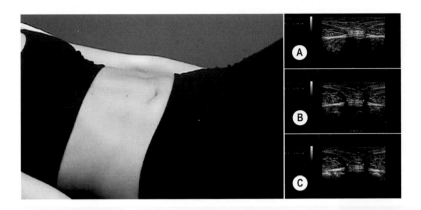

Figure 3.78

A short head and neck curl-up requires co-activation of all abdominal muscles. There should be no distortion of the linea alba and tension should be maintained throughout the curl-up task. The inter-recti distance should remain consistent between rest and the curl-up position, whether a cue is given to preactivate the transversus abdominis or not (Lee D & Hodges 2016). (A) Rectus abdominis and linea alba at rest. (B) Rectus abdominis and linea alba during an automatic strategy for a curl-up. (C) Rectus abdominis and linea alba during a curl-up with preactivation of the TrA muscle.

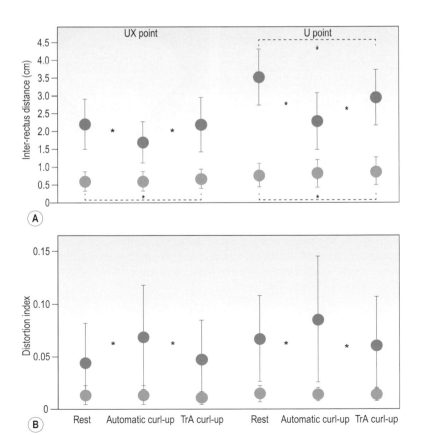

Figure 3.79

Inter-rectus distance (A) and distortion index (B) at rest and during the automatic curl-up and curl-up with preactivation of the TrA muscle. Mean standard deviation values of group data are shown for controls (blue circles) and participants with diastasis rectus abdominis (orange circles). *$P <.05$ for comparison between tasks. TrA = transversus abdominis, U point = just above the umbilicus, UX point = halfway between the U point and the xiphoid.

Reproduced with permission from Lee D and Hodges (2016) and the Journal of Orthopedics and Sports Therapy.

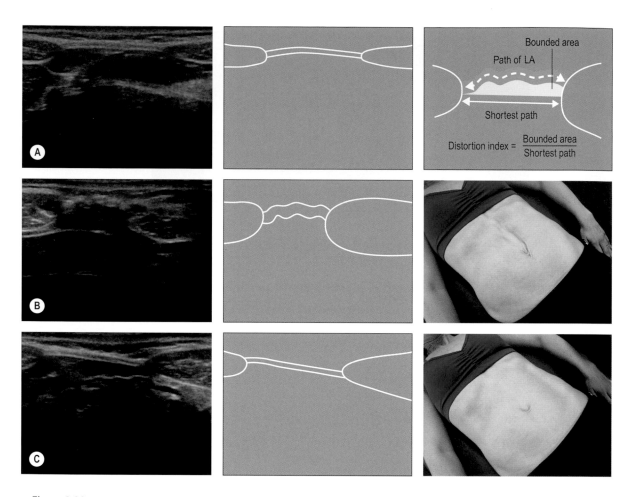

Figure 3.80

The distortion index and its interpretation. (A) Rectus abdominis and linea alba at rest and how the distortion index was determined.
(B) Automatic strategy for a curl-up with no co-activation of the transversus abdominis. The inter-rectus distance is reduced and distortion
is increased compared to rest. (C) Curl-up with voluntary TrA precontraction. There is no change in the inter-rectus distance and distortion is
not increased compared to rest. Left panel: Ultrasound images. Middle panel: Line drawings of ultrasound images; Right, bottom two images:
Photographs of the abdominal wall during the curl-up tasks. The inset at top right defines the calculation of the distortion index from the
area bounded by the path of the linea alba from the automatic curl-up task and the shortest distance between the linea alba attachments.
Note the distortion of the linea alba with the narrower inter-recti distance during the automatic curl-up and the wider inter-recti distance but
more direct path of the linea alba in the TrA curl-up (less distortion). LA = linea alba.

The following test evaluates the impact of a translated
and rotated thoracic ring, and its correction, on the recruitment strategy of the abdominal muscles during a short head
and neck curl-up task and the ability of the lateral abdominals to generate tension and reduce distortion in the linea
alba. Palpate the linea alba from the xyphoid to the pubic

symphysis and note any regions of excessive distortion or
laxity. The more distorted the linea alba, the further you can
sink your fingers into the abdomen. At the level of greatest
linea alba laxity, note if the left and right rectus abdominis
can be manually separated. With no specific transversus
abdominis cuing, ask the patient to slowly lift their head

towards their upper thorax and then flex their upper thorax to the level of the spine of the scapulae. Note any abdominal bulging (suggests absence of transversus abdominis recruitment) in the upper, middle or lower abdomen, or doming of the linea alba (suggesting lack of tension). Cue a bilateral contraction of the transversus abdominis. The patient must be able to recruit the left and right transversus abdominis and sustain this contraction throughout the short head and neck curl-up task to determine the impact of this recruitment strategy on the profile of the abdomen and tension of the linea alba. Note any change in the abdominal profile, such as bulging, and linea alba doming.

Ultrasound imaging is a useful tool for assessing the behavior of the linea alba in both the automatic curl-up task and the preactivation of the transversus abdominis curl-up task. If the patient cannot recruit or sustain the transversus abdominis, note the impact of correcting the thoracic ring driver (or any other noted driver) on their ability to do so. It is not uncommon to find a translated and rotated thoracic ring impacting the ability to recruit or sustain recruitment of the transversus abdominis and therefore impact the ability to generate tension in, and transfer forces across, the linea alba.

Pelvic floor muscle recruitment strategies

The pelvic floor forms the bottom of the abdominal canister and is integral for bowel, bladder, sexual, and musculoskeletal function. Overactivation of the pelvic floor muscles (three layers of 14 muscles) is common; however, these muscles are often reacting to other vectors or to increased intra-abdominal pressure. Knowing when to directly treat overactive pelvic floor muscles and when to treat other body regions to reduce their reaction is a key component of the Integrated Systems Model approach. It is outside the scope of this text to describe the complete external and internal examination of the three layers of muscles that comprise the pelvic floor. What is described below is how to determine the role the thorax is playing in the behavior of the pelvic floor muscles once examination techniques for the pelvic floor have been attained. Ultrasound images pertaining to the pelvic floor behavior in response to driver correction can be found in the case reports authored by Calvin Wong and Tamarah Nerreter in Chapter 5.

With the patient in supine lying, with hips and knees flexed, palpate the overactive pelvic floor muscle externally or internally. Not all muscles are accessible using one approach so both skills are necessary for a complete evaluation of the pelvic floor muscles. Note any tenderness on palpation, resting activation, ability to recruit, and ability to relax the muscle of interest. Teach the patient how to correct their driver, have them maintain the correction, and note any change in palpable tenderness, resting activation, ability to recruit, and ability to relax the muscles of the pelvic floor. When the pelvic floor muscle is reacting to other vectors, or to increased intra-abdominal pressure, its behavior will change when the driver is corrected. The driver may not be the thorax. If a cranial correction improved the performance of the screening task, then correct the cranial region and note the impact on the behavior of the pelvic floor. If a foot correction improved the performance of the screening task, then correct the foot and note the impact on the behavior of the pelvic floor. If no distal body region correction improves the behavior of the pelvic floor muscles, then local treatment is indicated. Once skill is attained to assess the pelvic floor in supine hook lying, the principles of this test can be applied in other positions that are more relevant to the meaningful task (standing, squat, lunge, etc.).

Dural and perineural mobility

Both the central and peripheral nervous systems, as well as their coverings, have some capacity to elongate to permit movement; however, once this capacity is exhausted symptoms often follow. The capacity for elongation can be reduced when nerves are required to adapt to increased pressure, which alters venous drainage and thus arterial supply to the nerve, or when the nerve and dura are subjected to traction forces due to suboptimal alignment of the body. In addition, intracranial dural tension (in the cerebral falx and cerebellar tentorium) can be influenced by impairments that impact drainage of the intracranial venous sinuses. The venous sinuses drain via the internal jugular veins, which merge with the subclavian veins to become the brachiocephalic veins, which merge into the superior vena cava. The intersection of the left and right brachiocephalic veins with the superior vena cava is posterior to the costocartilage of the right 2nd rib. Venous drainage can be compromised by suboptimal alignment of the cranium, neck, clavicle, manubrium or upper thoracic rings. The Integrated Systems Model helps to differentiate whether the suboptimal alignment is adaptive for an inability of the neural or dural tissue to elongate, or maladaptive and causing the inability of the tissue to elongate.

The following tests evaluate the mobility of the cerebellar tentorium, spinal dura, and the peripheral nervous system in both the upper and lower limbs. Clinical reasoning of the test findings differentiates whether the suboptimal alignment is responsible for loss of dural or perineural mobility or whether loss of dural or perineural mobility is responsible for the suboptimal alignment.

At this stage of the assessment, it would be known whether correcting the cranial region (correcting an ICT) improved or worsened the meaningful task. If correcting the cranium improved the task, and passive listening upon release of the correction revealed an intracranial vector, then an assessment of mobility of the cerebellar tentorium is indicated. If the passive listening revealed a vector outside of the cranium, then further assessment of that vector is indicated. If no correction of alignment of the skeletal body improved the patient's experience, nor the meaningful task, then mobility of the cranial and spinal dura, as well as the associated peripheral nervous system, is indicated.

With the patient sitting with a neutral pelvis, note the alignment of the cranium, cervical segments, thoracic rings, and position of the hindfoot. The full slump position with hip flexion, knee extension, ankle dorsiflexion, and hindfoot eversion requires full elongation of the cranial and spinal dura and posterior nerves of the lower extremity. Note any change in alignment in the complete slump position. Note the possible range of motion before the onset of symptoms.

Correct any site of suboptimal alignment and note the impact of this correction on the other noted sites of suboptimal alignment. When the dural and perineural system has exhausted its capacity to elongate, a correction in alignment of one body region will worsen the alignment in another (Fig. 3.81A–C). When the alignment of the body is the cause of the inability of the dural and perineural

system to elongate, correcting the alignment will improve the ability of the system to lengthen and more range of motion will be gained (Fig. 3.82A–F).

With the patient sitting with a neutral pelvis, note the alignment of the cranium, cervical segments, clavicle, and upper thoracic rings. Have the patient abduct the arm, pronate the forearm, bend the elbow and extend the wrist and note the range of possible motion before the onset of symptoms. This posture requires full elongation of the nerves of the upper extremity and when mobility is limited the alignment of the cranium, neck, upper thorax or clavicle is often impacted.

Correct any site of suboptimal alignment and note the impact of this correction on the mobility of the upper extremity in various positions that require lengthening of the nerves. When the dural and perineural system has exhausted its capacity to elongate, a correction in alignment of one body region will worsen the alignment in another as well as the performance of the task. When the alignment of the body is the cause for this inability to elongate, correcting the alignment will improve the ability of the dural and perineural system to lengthen and more range of motion will be gained (Fig. 3.83A–C).

When the driver for the task is somewhere in the skeleton, vector analysis of the driver subsequently determines the underlying system impairment and the required treatment intervention. When the system impairment is the dural and perineural system, then this system requires release (see the section on dural and perineural system impairments in Chapter 6) before suboptimal alignment, biomechanics, and control of the skeleton can be addressed.

Conclusion

The Integrated Systems Model is an evidence-informed, biopsychosocial approach for individual care. It is a framework, not a classification, that considers all three dimensions of the patient's experience (sensorial, cognitive, emotional) and the barriers that each may present to the recovery process for both acute and persistent conditions. When assessing the biological component (alignment, biomechanics, control) the body or person can no longer be considered as individual parts or problems in either

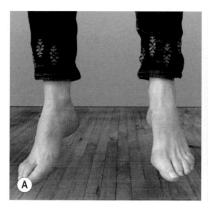
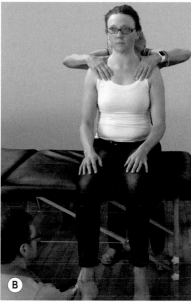
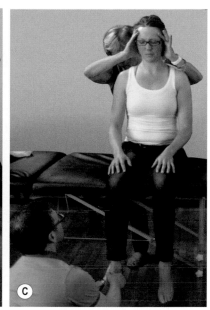

Figure 3.81

This woman has impaired mobility of the dural and perineural system from her cranium to her right foot. (A) Note the inversion of the right foot in sitting. This position decreases tension of the posterior tibial nerve at the medial malleolus. (B) She also has multiple translated and rotated thoracic rings (2nd translated left and rotated right, 3rd translated right and rotated left, 4th translated left and rotated right, 5th translated left and rotated right, 6th translated right and rotated left). This often occurs when the thorax is trying to shorten to reduce tension on the nervous system. (C) The subject also has a left intracranial torsion with a congruent left rotation of the sphenoid. All corrections of the thorax, cranial region, and foot worsen the alignment of another body region. Treatment should be directed to the dural and perineural system (see Chapter 6) prior to addressing any of the suboptimal alignments.

assessment or treatment. Most tasks involve the whole body; therefore, assessment must include an analysis of the relationship between the body regions and the impact and interplay of these regions.

Finding drivers requires the skill to not only interpret a finding but to find it reliably. For therapists, visual and kinesthetic perceptions are foundational tools for assessing the human form in function. Understanding our individual strengths, weaknesses, accuracies, and misperceptions enhances the reliability and skills that are necessary to find a finding. Jo Abbott is a biomechanist, clinical anatomist, clinician, and ISM Series graduate (https://joabbottmsc.com) who is currently doing her PhD, part of which is testing

ISM principles for the interpretation of manual positional assessment. Her preliminary findings suggest that manual palpation findings are 'better than random' for most clinicians and not 'better than random' for some. She is investigating what is different about the clinicians whose results are 'not better than random.' No inter-tester reliability study to date has considered why the interpretation of manual findings is different for some clinicians, or identified what is common amongst those who see or feel things differently from others. Once we can reliably identify and then eliminate the testers whose results are 'no better than random' from our studies, perhaps the evidence will increase for support of manual palpation assessment.

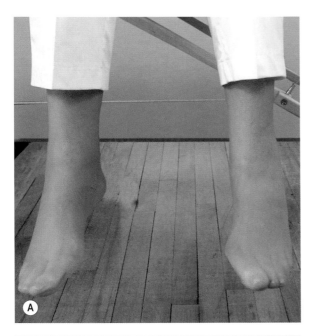

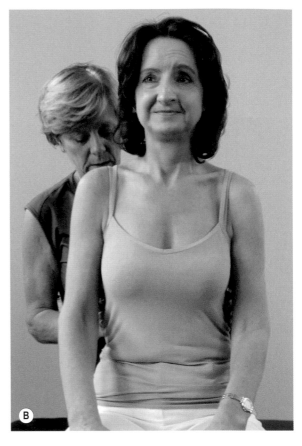

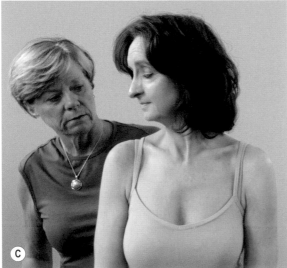

Figure 3.82

This woman has a structural scoliosis and reports that her ability to right rotate her head and neck has always been more limited than her ability to left rotate; however, after fracturing the left 5th metatarsal she has noticed that her ability to right rotate her head and neck is less and that the wrinkles on the left side of her forehead have increased. She has multiple translated and rotated thoracic rings that are consistent with her scoliosis: Her C7 is translated right and rotated left, her C2 is translated left and rotated right, and she has a congruent left ICT and left-rotated sphenoid. (A) Note the sickle shape of the left foot in sitting (elongation of the lateral side of the foot). (B) The persistent wrinkling of the left side of her forehead appears to be associated with overactivation of the frontalis muscle, which is innervated by the temporal branch of the facial nerve. (C) Note her ability to right rotate her head and neck without any corrections. No correction of her thorax, cervical or cranial regions improved her ability to right rotate her neck, although the activation of the frontalis muscle did subside somewhat with the correction of the cranium.

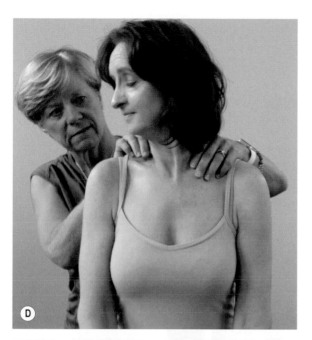

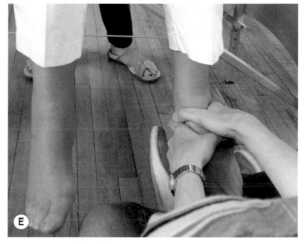

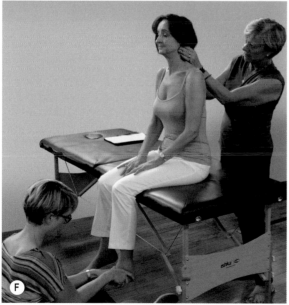

Figure 3.82 *continued*

(D) Note her improved right rotation, and the contribution of her upper thorax to this task, when her left foot was corrected. (E) The foot correction was simply to abduct the forefoot toward the hindfoot to reduce tension on the sural nerve. (F) A notable correction of the alignment of C2 (and C7) occurred when the foot was corrected. Further assessment of the right foot is required to address the subject's limited right rotation of the head and neck.

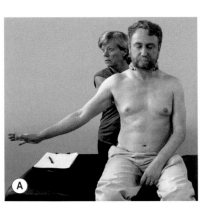
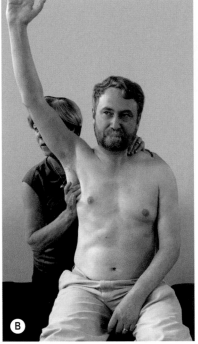
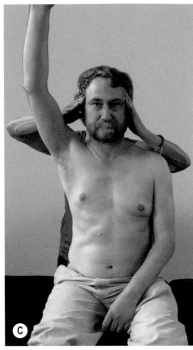

Figure 3.83

This man's meaningful complaint is neuralgia-type symptoms with elevation or abduction of the right arm, particularly movements that tense the right ulnar nerve. He presented with a left ICT and a congruently left rotated sphenoid, C7 translated right and rotated left, 2nd thoracic ring that alternated between left and right rotation and the 4th thoracic ring translated right and rotated left. (A) Since his symptoms appeared to involve the lower chord of the brachial plexus, C7 was palpated as he abducted his arm. At 45 degrees of abduction, the C7 translated further right and rotated further left. Individual corrections of each site of failed load transfer did not improve his ability to abduct the right arm. (B) The first correction to improve the range of motion was a co-correction of C7 and the 4th thoracic ring. However, this correction worsened the alignment of his cranium relative to his neck and did not change the ICT or the rotation of the sphenoid (note the left orbit is still deep). (C) The best correction which improved both his range of motion of arm elevation and the position of the 4th thoracic ring, C7 and the cranium was a correction of the cranium. This is an example of adverse neural tension being caused by suboptimal alignment of the skeletal system. Vector analysis of the cranium will determine the underlying system impairments and direct the treatment plan.

Clinical reasoning determines the relevance of each finding to the clinical picture, which subsequently directs management of the individual patient. While clinical reasoning can be taught through texts and online media, there will always be a need for hands-on practical courses; this is the art and skill of physiotherapy that is so difficult to measure with science.

This chapter has outlined the skills required to assess the thorax and its relationship to the whole body. Chapter 4 will outline the ISM principles for treatment, following which Chapter 5 will present several case reports that demonstrate this approach and its applicability to the biomechanically impaired thorax.

Introduction

After a comprehensive assessment, an individualized treatment plan follows certain principles that will be covered in this chapter. A variety of individual treatment plans for thoracic impairments will be highlighted in the case reports in Chapter 5. Specific treatment techniques and motor control and movement training for intrathoracic and interthoracic ring mobility and control will be described in Chapters 6 and 7.

The goal of treatment is to motivate a change in the patient's physical, cognitive and emotional behavior to improve the strategies they use for function and well-being. In a biopsychosocial, evidence-informed approach such as the Integrated Systems Model, this requires the identification of the primary barrier preventing change. What is stopping the patient from using strategies that are more functional and less painful? The barrier will determine whether the priority for initial treatment is:

- Education (hands-off); Explain Pain training (Moseley & Butler 2017) to align beliefs and language with knowledge and evidence; and motor learning and movement instruction; or

- Education (hands-on); Explain Pain training when necessary with manual therapy, release techniques, dry needling, and motor learning and movement instruction.

What is meant by 'Explain Pain training'? 'Explain Pain is not a singular and isolated therapy, but a range of conceptual change strategies based on current knowledge of the pain sciences' (Moseley & Butler 2017). There are many useful tools, graphics, models, nuggets, and suggestions in Moseley and Butler's book *Explain Pain Supercharged* to help clinicians educate and motivate patients to change behavior (both physical and cognitive). They suggest that: 'Combining two effective treatments should be useful as long as both subscribe to the biopsychosocial model ...' There are no formal studies that have

investigated the effectiveness of combining Explain Pain education and the Integrated Systems Model; I can only tell you that hundreds of trained physiotherapists in both methods combine them successfully in their practice. There are no recipes in either approach and they appear to integrate well.

While treatment for systemic inflammation and nutrition advice are not within the scope of physiotherapy practice, it is important to recognize the impact certain neurotoxins have on general health and healing. High blood glucose levels (sugar), alcohol, aspartame, gluten, and dairy are known to be inflammatory for some patients and those with chronic multiregional pain syndromes can potentially feel, and perform, better when these potential irritants are eliminated from their diet and their gut health has been addressed.

The Integrated Systems Model approach to treatment contains two components (Fig. 4.1):

- **Release** (reconceptualize) the barriers (cognitive, emotional, sensorial [physical]) that are creating suboptimal strategies for function, in conjunction with

- **Teach** optimal strategies for function that relate to the patient's goals and meaningful tasks.

Release – cognitive and emotional barriers

Cognitive barriers are addressed through education and, if possible, by providing a different experience in the body that potentially negates, or at least begins to challenge, cognitive beliefs. Education programs for changing persistent pain beliefs and catastrophizing language such as *Explain Pain* (Butler & Moseley 2003), *The Explain Pain Handbook: Protectometer* (Moseley & Butler 2015), and books that highlight the known potential of the brain to change such as *The Brain that Changes Itself* (Doidge 2007) and *Mindsight* (Siegel 2010) help patients understand the current theories and science of persistent pain and bioplasticity

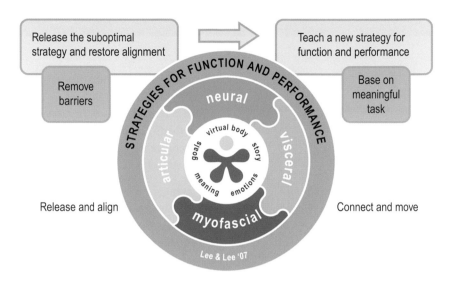

Figure 4.1

Principles of treatment of the Integrated Systems Model. Every ISM treatment session contains two components. The first component includes techniques and training to release the barriers that are creating suboptimal strategies for function and the second component includes motor control and movement training aimed to develop optimal strategies for function.

and the ability of the entire body to change over time, both of which play a key role in treatment. Providing a logical explanation for the pain experience, and how the various impairments (including thoughts and beliefs) may possibly be inputs to the cortical body matrix that result in undesirable outputs, can dampen the intensity of an individual's pain experience. Creating a biologically plausible, cohesive story of the overall experience helps to integrate the amygdala (emotional memories of an experience) and the hippocampus (autobiographical detail of that experience) and reduce threat (Siegel 2010). Pain that is better understood and explained is often less intense and less concerning than pain which is associated with fear or threat (Moseley & Butler 2017). The book *Explain Pain Supercharged* (Moseley & Butler 2017) presents an in-depth approach for the reconceptualization of beliefs around pain. It is not the intention of this text to do anything other than recommend that all clinicians who treat individuals in pain be familiar with their theories, evidence, concepts, and resources (www.noigroup.com).

Creating safe environments to explore cognitive barriers that have, in the past, resulted in kinesiophobia is critical for the patient whose beliefs and fears are impacting their recovery. A significant part of treating a complex patient is to restore hope and have a treatment plan that resonates and seems reasonable. This is a starting point for facilitating change (Bialosky et al. 2010). A primary goal of treatment is to 'illuminate a path to change' and to empower the patient to take control of that path and be responsible for their health. For the patient with central sensitization (sensitized cortical neurotags according to Moseley & Butler 2017), tools and techniques that help to reduce threat (activity of the sympathetic nervous system) and promote safety (activate the parasympathetic nervous system) are indicated. These can include various forms of meditation, mindfulness, yoga nidra, breathing (Nadi Shodhan or Anuloma Viloma pranayama), acupuncture, and education to reconceptualize their understanding of pain. These are helpful tools for empowering patients to take control and change the inputs to their cortical body matrix and thus the outputs.

Release – physical barriers

Physical barriers that perpetuate suboptimal strategies for function can be addressed with a wide variety of release techniques and motor control and movement training. Techniques that release specific system impairments help to change primary nociceptive input to the cortical body matrix from these sources. Treatment is directed initially to the primary system impairment noted on vector analysis of the driver.

The articular system includes the bones, joints, ligaments, and capsules. Release techniques for this system include vector-specific mobilization techniques and distraction manipulation techniques. These techniques are indicated when:

- Alignment and biomechanics of a specific body region cannot be manually or verbally corrected;

- Vector analysis reveals very short, firm vectors restricting joint mobility; and

- An underlying joint restriction is confirmed with specific arthrokinematic assessment techniques (see Chapter 3).

The myofascial system includes muscles and their tendinous, fascial and aponeurotic connections, as well as regular dense and loose connective tissue. Release techniques for this system include vector-specific elongation (stretching) techniques and intermuscular sliding techniques. These techniques are indicated when:

- Alignment and biomechanics of a specific body region are very difficult to manually correct;

- Vector analysis reveals long, resistant vectors restricting joint mobility; and

- Tight myofascial structures (resisting elongation or intermuscular sliding) are confirmed on palpation.

The neural system includes all components of the central and peripheral nervous systems, including the connective tissue and vascular components of these systems (dura and perineurium). Release techniques for this system include dry needling, release with awareness (Lee D 2001, Lee D & Lee L-J 2011a), neuromuscular recoil, muscle energy, or hold-relax, techniques and sustained vector-specific sustained holding (for dural and perineural mobility impairments). These techniques are indicated when:

- Alignment and biomechanics of a specific body region can be corrected;

- Vector analysis reveals short or long elastic vectors restricting joint mobility; and

- Overactive muscles are confirmed on palpation.

Dural and perineural release techniques are indicated when:

- Alignment and biomechanics of a specific body region can be corrected; however, every correction attempted results in worsening of alignment, biomechanics or control somewhere else in the body;

- Neurodynamic mobility tests (i.e., slump, upper limb tension tests, straight-leg-raise test, prone knee bend test, etc.) worsen when the alignment of the skeleton is improved.

The visceral system includes all the viscera. Specific release techniques for this system are not covered in this text; the reader is referred to the Barral Institute for further courses. The visceral techniques for the thorax presented in this text are not tissue specific. In short, the alignment of the skeleton (thorax, cranium and neck, pelvis) is maintained and various forms of breathing used to mobilize the intrathoracic visceral vectors. This technique is indicated when:

- Alignment and biomechanics of a specific body region can be corrected,

- Vector analysis reveals short or long elastic vectors restricting joint mobility that arise from inside the thoracic, abdominal, or pelvic canisters or cranium.

The clinical application of some of these system techniques is integrated in the case reports in Chapter 5. How to perform the techniques is described in detail in Chapter 6.

Chapter 4

Teach – optimal strategies for function

Following release of the primary and secondary system vectors, motor control and movement training (Stages 1 to 3, Levels 1 to 3) follows (see Chapter 7). This instruction facilitates a change in the input to the cortical body matrix from multiple tissues (articular, fascial, neural, visceral) and aims to change the motor output and strategies for function. All drivers are addressed and released in conjunction with motor control and movement training and they should change both within, and between, treatment sessions unless a major myofascial or articular system impairment is present. In conjunction with education and release techniques to address cognitive, emotional, and physical barriers to recovery, the patient should be taught better ways to move or sustain a static posture (in standing or sitting) that distribute load more efficiently. The goal of this part of the treatment session is to create new neural networks (brain maps) using the principles of bioplasticity and neuroplasticity for more efficient strategies.

Neuroplasticity is the 'ability of the nervous system to respond to intrinsic and extrinsic stimuli by reorganizing its structure, function and connections' (Snodgrass et al. 2014). The nervous system is embodied (Siegel 2010) and is therefore influenced by our thoughts, feelings and actions. Change is constantly occurring throughout life.

'There is overwhelming evidence that the brain is continuously remodelled in response to new or novel experiences ... Therefore, an appreciation of the influence of the central nervous system on all forms of movement as well as pain should underpin all forms of rehabilitation.' (Kleim & Jones 2008)

The assessment will have determined if specific motor control training for individual muscles is required. A muscle cannot be trained, strengthened or conditioned if the brain is not using it. The brain and nervous system are trained prior to giving exercises for strength and conditioning. Who needs specific motor control training? If correcting the driver results in immediate restoration of a better neuromuscular recruitment strategy that improves alignment, biomechanics and control of all sites that failed to transfer, or share, load optimally during the meaningful task, then specific motor control training for a muscle

noted to be performing poorly without correction of the driver is *not* necessary. These individuals tend to do well in yoga and Pilates classes where the focus is on release, lengthen, and move. If correcting the driver does not restore better neuromuscular recruitment strategies and one or more body regions continues to fail to transfer, or share, load optimally, then specific motor control training for the inhibited or atrophied muscle or muscles is indicated. These individuals tend not to do well initially in yoga or Pilates since releasing their suboptimal strategies leaves them feeling less controlled and more vulnerable.

Chapter 7 will describe in detail how to provide specific motor control training for both intrathoracic and interthoracic ring control as well as inter-regional mobility and control between the thorax, lumbopelvis–hip, shoulder girdle, head and neck. Specific taping techniques to facilitate intrathoracic and interthoracic ring control will be described in Chapter 7.

The key factors required for facilitating neuroplastic change include:

- Focused attention;
- Training tasks that have meaning;
- Massed practice of high quality repetitions;
- Provide sensory input that is not threatening;
- Provide positive feedback.

Changing habitual postures and movements is not easy and requires focused attention, or awareness, without distractions that take attention away from the body's experience when training. Learning and change can occur when there is awareness, and facilitated when tasks are trained that have meaning. Massed practice of high quality strategies that normalize the input to the cortical body matrix will increase the speed of synaptic connectivity and thus the ease of use of the strategy. How much is enough? Tsao's research (Tsao & Hodges 2007, 2008; Tsao et al. 2010) suggests the following prescription for training new strategies: the goal is to achieve three sets of 10, 10-second holds of the optimal strategy with a two-minute rest in between sets, and to perform this training at least twice, preferably three to four times, per day. When compliant, the brain map will be consolidated and less conscious effort is required to perform the task in as little as two weeks. The patient needs to have the awareness to know when they are using an optimal strategy for every training task (home self-check) and to only perform high quality movement patterns. Attending to the effort it takes to perform the task will inform the patient when the strategy is optimal or not, in that good strategies feel good (effortless, light, less symptomatic, etc.). The patient's experience improves when they train strategies that are better for their musculoskeletal health. Imagery, or visualization, of what a good strategy 'looks like' can also help.

Reinforce, strengthen, and condition – better strategies for function

Once the body has better alignment, biomechanics and control for multiple meaningful tasks, strength and conditioning can follow. There are many ways to do this with, for example, yoga, Pilates, gym exercises, and home exercises. Initially, exercises are prescribed according to a few specific meaningful tasks and from there a wide variety of movements and tasks should be included in the program. How exercise or movement training programs can be progressed will be covered in Chapter 7. When designing movement training for restoring musculoskeletal health, consideration must be given to the entire body since everything is relational. At minimum, the following should be monitored and provided during training:

- Local control of:
  - four pelvic joints
  - two hip joints
  - 15 lumbar joints
  - 130 thoracic joints (10 complete thoracic rings)

- Inter-regional control between the:
  - thorax and lumbopelvis
  - thorax and shoulder girdle
  - thorax and head and neck
  - thorax and shoulder girdle and upper extremity
  - thorax, lumbopelvis-hip and lower extremity

- Postural and motion control between the body and the environment: Add a higher level of challenge according to the patient's goals.

Conclusion – getting to WOW!

It is important to remember that for most patients, recovery is not linear. The game 'Snakes and Ladders' is a helpful metaphor for patients to understand that on the road to recovery, they may hit a 'snake' and regress. This is common and not to be catastrophized. A ladder is shortly ahead. The better they understand how to 'read their body' during training, the fewer 'snakes' they will encounter. Butler and Moseley (2003) refer to this as 'pacing.' When efficiency of movement, and not pain, is used as a barometer during training, the movement training progression appears to be facilitated.

Changing the patient's experience of their body in tasks that have meaning for them often brings comments like 'WOW! What just happened?' This is the first step to creating new, more efficient ways for them to live, move, and simply be in their body. Dan Siegel calls this 'SNAG the brain,' this being his acronym for Stimulate Neuronal Activation and Growth. In the Integrated Systems Model this is called 'Getting to WOW.' Chapter 5 will highlight specific conditions and case reports pertaining to the impact thoracic dysfunction can have both locally and at a distance, which will clarify the relationship of the thorax to the whole body in musculoskeletal, respiratory, and urogynecological health.

Diane Lee, Calvin Wong, Tamarah Nerreter

The case reports in this chapter highlight the clinical application of the Integrated Systems Model and the relationship of impaired thoracic function to the whole body. Detailed descriptions of the release techniques and stages of motor learning and movement training are provided in Chapters 6 and 7. Most of the case reports are accompanied by QR codes that link to videos on the www.learnwithdianelee.com website. The video quality is not always the best but the content of each video helps to consolidate the ISM concepts in this text. Instructions on how to access these clinical videos are found at the front of this text.

Thorax-driven pelvic girdle and hip pain

Diane Lee

Jennifer's story

At the time of this assessment, Jennifer was a 42-year-old physical therapy assistant attending a two-day course on the Integrated Systems Model and offered her story for the education of those in class. She had previously sustained multiple traumatic injuries as a competitive gymnast and from three motor vehicle accidents. It was her cognitive belief that these traumatic events caused her persistent bilateral pelvic girdle and hip pain in the groin region.

The left groin pain began insidiously after a foot injury sustained landing a jump in gymnastics at the age of 16. Jennifer also reported injuring her right shoulder in gymnastics at the age of 22. In her midthirties she was involved in two rear-end motor vehicle collisions, the first as a passenger and the second as a driver, and reported that her bilateral pelvic girdle pain began after these two accidents. Seventeen months ago, she was rear-ended again and all her symptoms were exacerbated. She felt that she had not recovered from this accident.

Jennifer has three children. The delivery of her first child failed to progress and, after a forceps attempt also failed, her daughter was delivered by emergency cesarean section (C-section). She experienced some right sciatica after this delivery that has since resolved. She delivered her subsequent two children by planned C-section. She did not report any subsequent symptoms of urinary incontinence or any symptoms suggestive of loss of pelvic organ support.

Jennifer's current meaningful complaints

Of primary concern for Jennifer was the persistent, intermittent, bilateral pelvic girdle pain that was aggravated by two tasks:

- sustained standing (doing dishes, standing to have a conversation), and

- tasks which required hip flexion (cycling, forward bending, and sitting).

She also experienced left groin pain that was aggravated by a deep squat.

Irritability: 15 minutes of standing was required to bring on her pain whereas a deep squat would cause pain in the left groin immediately. Ten minutes of walking would relieve the pain after prolonged standing or squatting.

Jennifer's cognitive beliefs

Imaging studies of Jennifer's hips revealed bilateral pincer-type femoral acetabular impingement associated with a tear of the left acetabular labrum. At the time of the initial assessment, she was scheduled for surgical exploration and repair of the left labral tear in approximately six weeks. She believed that the structural deficit of the left hip was the primary reason for her left groin pain.

Jennifer's emotional status

As Jennifer was telling her story there were no outward signs of anxiety, depression or anger that could provide barriers to her recovery; however, she was avoiding certain activities due to fears of further injuring herself (fear–avoidance behavior).

Meaningful tasks and screening tasks chosen for strategy analysis

Jennifer's meaningful tasks were to be able to stand, cycle, sit, and squat deeply pain free. Two initial screening tasks were chosen for analysis of strategy – standing and a deep squat. An assessment of the left hip was also planned to determine the role of the labral tear in her clinical picture, and thus support or negate her cognitive beliefs.

The key findings from Jennifer's story are noted in the center of her Clinical Puzzle (Fig. 5.1) and include:

- Meaningful complaint: Bilateral pelvic girdle and left groin pain;

- Cognitive belief: A labral tear in the left hip was responsible for the persistent hip, groin, and pelvic girdle pain;

- Meaningful tasks: Stand, cycle, sit, deep squat.

Screening task analysis – the standing postural screen

Video 5.1 (free code)

Jennifer's standing posture screen

The key clinical findings in standing were (Video 5.1):

- Pelvis: Right transverse plane rotation (RTPR) associated with a right intrapelvic torsion (RIPT).

- Hips: Both femoral heads were anterior relative to the acetabulum; the left hip was more anterior than the right. This finding is congruent with a RTPR associated with a RIPT of the pelvis.

- Lower thorax: Left transverse plane rotation (LTPR) associated with a 7th thoracic ring translated right and rotated left (congruent with the vertebrochondral transverse plane rotation and incongruent with the pelvis TPR and intrapelvic torsion (IPT)).

- Middle and upper thorax: The 2nd thoracic ring translated left and rotated right, the 3rd thoracic ring translated right and rotated left, and the 4th thoracic ring translated left and rotated right.

- Clavicles: The right clavicle anteriorly rotated and the left clavicle posteriorly rotated (congruent with the 3rd thoracic ring rotation as well as the lower neck).

- Cervical segments: C7 and C6 translated right and rotated left (congruent with the 3rd thoracic ring and the clavicles) and C2 translated left and rotated right (incongruent to C6 and C7, congruent with the 2nd and 4th thoracic rings).

- Cranial region: Left intracranial torsion (LICT) (congruent with C6 and C7, the clavicles, and the 3rd thoracic ring). The video says right and should say left! Her sphenoid is rotated congruently to the left.

- Feet: The right foot was twisted and the left foot was flattened (congruent with the RTRP of the pelvis).

Impact of corrections on standing posture – finding the drivers

Video 5.2 (free code)

Finding the drivers for Jennifer's standing posture

Correcting the alignment of Jennifer's pelvis made the alignment of her hips, feet and thorax worse (Video 5.2). Correcting her left hip made the alignment of the pelvis better; however, this correction made the alignment of the thorax worse. Correcting the feet made the alignment of both hips and the 7th thoracic ring worse. Correcting the alignment of the 2nd, 3rd, and 4th thoracic rings partially corrected the alignment of the pelvis, the right hip and both feet. This correction fully corrected the alignment of C6, C7, and the cranium. The left hip was only partially corrected with the thorax correction. Adding a left hip correction to the thorax correction resulted in complete correction of the pelvis, both hips, feet, neck, and cranium.

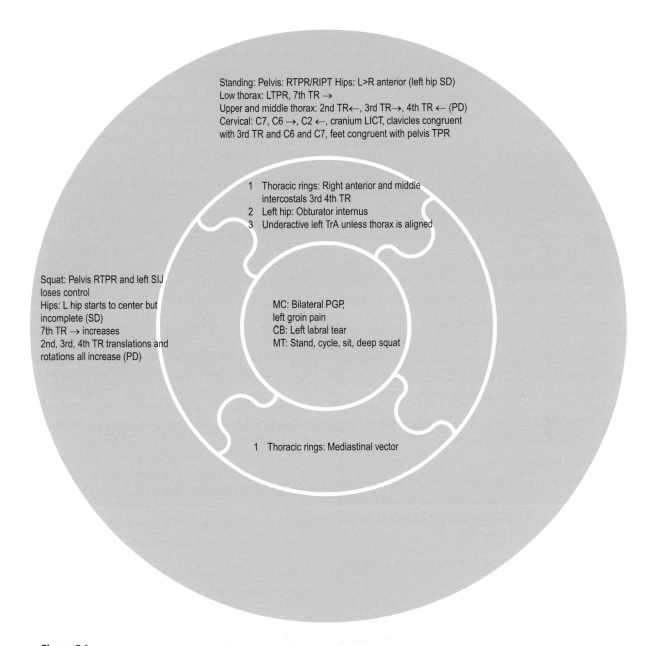

Standing: Pelvis: RTPR/RIPT Hips: L>R anterior (left hip SD)
Low thorax: LTPR, 7th TR →
Upper and middle thorax: 2nd TR←, 3rd TR→, 4th TR ← (PD)
Cervical: C7, C6 →, C2 ←, cranium LICT, clavicles congruent with 3rd TR and C6 and C7, feet congruent with pelvis TPR

1 Thoracic rings: Right anterior and middle intercostals 3rd 4th TR
2 Left hip: Obturator internus
3 Underactive left TrA unless thorax is aligned

Squat: Pelvis RTPR and left SIJ loses control
Hips: L hip starts to center but incomplete (SD)
7th TR → increases
2nd, 3rd, 4th TR translations and rotations all increase (PD)

MC: Bilateral PGP, left groin pain
CB: Left labral tear
MT: Stand, cycle, sit, deep squat

1 Thoracic rings: Mediastinal vector

Figure 5.1

Jennifer's completed Clinical Puzzle from the first assessment. CB = cognitive belief, LICT = left intracranial torsion, MC = meaningful complaint, MT = meaningful task, PD = primary driver, PGP = pelvic girdle pain, RTPR = right transverse plane rotation, RIPT = right intrapelvic torsion, SD = secondary driver, SIJ = sacroiliac joint, TR = thoracic ring, TrA = transversus abdominis, ← = left translation, → = right translation.

The primary driver for her standing posture was the thorax, specifically the alignment of the 2nd, 3rd, and 4th thoracic rings, and the secondary driver was her left hip.

Screening task analysis – the squat

Video 5.3 (free code)

Findings from Jennifer's squat task

The key clinical findings in Jennifer's squat task were (Video 5.3):

- Pelvis: The RTPR increased and the left sacroiliac joint (SIJ) lost control (the left innominate anteriorly rotated relative to the left side of the sacrum).

- Hips: The left hip centered slightly in the acetabulum but remained anterior to the right hip as the squat deepened. This finding is congruent with the increasing RTPR of the pelvis in the squat.

- Lower thorax: The 7th thoracic ring translated further right and rotated further left.

- Middle and upper thorax: The 2nd thoracic ring translated further left and rotated further right, the 3rd thoracic ring translated further right and rotated further left, the 4th thoracic ring translated further left and rotated further right.

Impact of corrections on the squat task – finding the drivers

The best correction for this task was also the 2nd, 3rd, and 4th thoracic rings combined with a verbal cue to correct the left hip. When the squat was performed with the thoracic rings in better alignment, the left SIJ remained controlled, the 7th thoracic ring alignment corrected and remained properly aligned during the squat, and Jennifer could go further into her squat before the left groin pain began. The left hip, however, still required additional correction and centering (via a verbal cue) for a full, deep, pain-free squat.

The primary driver for Jennifer's squat task was the thorax, specifically the alignment of the 2nd, 3rd, and 4th thoracic rings, and the secondary driver was her left hip.

Vector analysis of the drivers

Further assessment of the primary and secondary drivers (vector analysis) determines the underlying system impairments and the initial treatment plan.

Primary driver – the thorax (2nd, 3rd, and 4th thoracic rings)

Video 5.4 (free code)

Vector analysis of Jennifer's thorax

Both active and passive listening techniques were used to determine the underlying system impairments that were causing the suboptimal alignment and biomechanics of the 2nd, 3rd, and 4th thoracic rings in both standing and during a deep squat task (Video 5.4). A dominant vector was found in the anterior and middle intercostal muscles on the right between the 3rd and 4th ribs. Passive listening on release of the three-ring correction revealed that the right 3rd rib moved first into anterior rotation. The vector was in the midaxillary line, short, and between the 3rd and 4th ribs on the right (intercostals). Palpation of the right intercostals in the midaxillary line revealed marked tenderness. After anterior rotation occurred, the right 2nd, 3rd, and 4th ribs were pulled into the thorax by an intrathoracic visceral vector that appeared to impact all three thoracic rings simultaneously.

Secondary driver – the left hip

Video 5.5 (free code)

Vector analysis of Jennifer's left hip and its relationship to the thorax

In supine lying, the left femoral head remained centered up to 90 degrees of hip flexion. Beyond this point the femoral head translated anteriorly. At 90 degrees of hip flexion only 20 degrees of internal rotation was possible (Video 5.5). Passive listening on release of a femoral head correction at 90 degrees of flexion revealed an external rotation vector that was medial to the hip joint. The obturator internus was noted to be overactive and hypothesized to be responsible for displacing the femoral head anteriorly at 90 degrees of hip flexion and for limiting internal rotation. The anterior position of the left femoral head against the torn labrum could explain Jennifer's persistent groin pain, confirming part of her cognitive belief. The labrum and structures of the anterior left hip were a likely source of peripheral nociception in her clinical story; however, the hip was reacting, in part, to the suboptimal alignment and biomechanics of the upper and middle thorax since correcting the alignment of the 2nd, 3rd, and 4th thoracic rings allowed the left femoral head to partially center and restored a further 20 degrees of hip flexion and 25 degrees of internal rotation (a total of 45 degrees) in the supine position.

Impact of the thorax driver on abdominal wall recruitment strategy

Video 5.6 (free code)

Jennifer's abdominal wall assessment and its relationship to the thorax

In hook lying, increased resting activation of the right internal oblique was noted. When Jennifer contracted her levator ani, there was no response in the left transversus abdominis (TrA), and a slight contraction of the right TrA occurred (Video 5.6). When the alignment of the 2nd, 3rd, and 4th thoracic rings was corrected in this supine position, a symmetric, more robust recruitment response of the left and right TrA occurred. This suggests that when the alignment of the thorax is restored, Jennifer would be able to recruit her deep neuromuscular system for control of the pelvis with a better strategy. Following this, a release of the left obturator internus muscle (the dominant vector

found to be impairing the left hip) should correct the alignment and biomechanics of the left hip allowing her to achieve a deep squat without overloading the torn labrum.

ISM treatment for Jennifer's thorax-driven pelvis and hip

Release and align

Video 5.7 (free code)

Self-performed thoracic ring stack and breathe for releasing Jennifer's vectors

Thoracic ring stack and breathe (Lee L-J 2016) (see Chapter 6) is a general release and align technique that is not structure specific and can target multiple systems. This release technique was used to release and align the 2nd, 3rd, and 4th thoracic rings, and was followed by instruction on how to do this on her own at home to maintain the alignment (Video 5.7). The active bent leg raise was used as a home self-check for Jennifer to know when her thorax was aligned since her deep muscle system performed better when the upper and middle thorax were in alignment, and it was easier for her to lift her left leg. Note the range of left hip flexion Jennifer could achieve when she self-corrected her upper thorax in Video 5.7. The best breathing pattern for Jennifer to release the intercostals and the visceral mediastinal vector impacting alignment of her thorax was a lateral costal breath. This breathing pattern pulled the thorax out of alignment, therefore when the thoracic rings were prevented from translating and rotating as she breathed laterally, the vectors were lengthened. She was advised to repeat this breathing pattern with the thoracic rings corrected at least three to four times per day.

Connect, control, move

Specific motor control training for individual muscles of the thorax or abdominal wall was not required since correcting the alignment of the thoracic rings automatically restored a better recruitment strategy. The connect, control, move part of her treatment program started with

Stage 2 motor learning and movement training to build capacity for a better strategy (see Table 7.1).

After releasing the intercostals and the mediastinal visceral vector impacting the 2nd, 3rd, and 4th thoracic rings, the thoracic ring that failed to maintain optimal alignment during vertical loading was the 3rd thoracic ring. Static interthoracic ring control training was required for the 3rd thoracic ring (Stage 2 movement training) before movements of the thorax (Stage 3 movement training) could be introduced into her program. Initially, Jennifer was taught to manually correct the 3rd thoracic ring, then let the manual correction go and try to sustain the alignment of the 3rd thoracic ring as she breathed. This was progressed to finding a 'release and connect cue'; an image that would automatically correct the 3rd thoracic ring (see Chapter 7) without manual assistance. This is part of strategy capacity training – a key element of Stage 2 motor learning and movement training.

Video 5.8 (free code)

Stage 2 training for Jennifer's thorax in a squat task

With focused attention and some practice, Jennifer could progress to a more meaningful task, the deep squat (Video 5.8). Using both a manual and connect cue to correct the 3rd thoracic ring alignment, Jennifer then was instructed to squat only to the point where she began to feel the left hip impinge. At this point, she was advised to pause and think about letting her ischial tuberosities widen and the left hip soften. This is a release cue for the left hip and addressed the secondary driver for this task – the left hip. The thorax is not moving in this task, the pelvis is controlled, and the hips move. This is still Stage 2 motor learning and movement training for the thorax.

Video 5.9 (free code)

Taping Jennifer's vertebrosternal thoracic rings

To facilitate Jennifer's ability to maintain optimal alignment of the upper thoracic rings, the 3rd thoracic ring was taped (Video 5.9).

Conclusion

Jennifer had a primary thorax-driven hip and pelvic impairment with a secondary hip driver. After this initial session as a patient model during a conference, she was left with a Stage 2 motor learning home program aimed at restoring interthoracic ring control, pelvic control and hip alignment for standing, interthoracic ring control, pelvic control, and hip mobility for a deep squat.

Video 5.10 (free code)

Follow-up assessment and treatment for Jennifer

Jennifer was seen in my clinic for follow-up several months later and reported that she was pleased with her recovery (Video 5.10). She had proceeded with surgery to address the labral tear and pincer impingement of the left hip. While she felt her interthoracic ring alignment and control was better and that her overall range of left hip mobility had improved, she still noticed 'pinching' in the left groin with deep squat tasks. The 3rd thoracic ring alignment and control was much improved and her biomechanics for sagittal and transverse plane motions of the thorax (Stage 3 movement training) was optimal. Correcting the slight translation right and rotation left of the 3rd thoracic ring did not impact the alignment or the biomechanics of the left hip in the deep squat. A complete correction of the left hip was not possible for her squat task and suggested a postsurgical articular system impairment may exist.

The left hip was hypothesized to be the primary driver for the squat task and assessment of the left hip determined the underlying system impairment was articular. The dominant restrictive vector was localized to the anterior aspect of the hip capsule. Jennifer was taught how to use a strap to mobilize the anterior aspect of the capsule of the left hip and has continued to improve. She can participate in the active lifestyle she loves in addition to being able to stand, hike, cycle, sit, and squat deeply.

Pelvis-driven then thorax-driven recurrent hamstring injury

Diane Lee

Steve's story

At the time of his initial assessment, Steve was a 26-year-old premier league elite soccer player who two-and-a-half to three years ago had suffered an acute tear of the right proximal biceps femoris. His meaningful complaints were:

- a feeling of weakness in the right leg,

- feeling 'heavy on the field,' and

- reduced agility and speed since the hamstring injury.

He had received traditional soft tissue rehabilitation coupled with stretching and strengthening exercises for his right biceps femoris for six to eight weeks after the initial injury but still experienced frequent episodes of 'pulling pains' in his right upper thigh and lower buttock. He felt he could only exert himself to 80 per cent and that the upper hamstrings were always on the 'verge of grabbing.' Subsequent local treatment beyond the eight-week period had not restored his function, nor relieved his persistent symptoms.

Steve's current meaningful complaints

Of primary concern for Steve was his loss of performance on the soccer field (agility and speed) and the 'fear' that the hamstring would tear again if he 'goes as hard as he wants.'

Steve's cognitive beliefs

Steve believed that his right proximal hamstring was still weak and felt that more strengthening exercises were needed to help him reach his athletic goals. Although he had tried, he could not seem to improve the strength of his left leg. His exercises were not improving his speed and agility on the field.

Steve's emotional status

For Steve to maintain his position on both his team and in the league he felt his performance needed to improve substantially. This fear of losing 'his spot' on the team was creating some anxiety for him.

Meaningful tasks and screening tasks chosen for strategy analysis

Steve's meaningful tasks were to be able to run forward, backward, and sideways, manipulate the soccer ball with either foot, and do all this with speed and agility. Multiple screening tasks could be chosen for this sport, including:

- Double leg loading (squat);

- Weight shift to single leg standing, and stepping forward in a variety of directions;

- The same tasks with both congruent and incongruent rotation of the thorax and pelvis and the thorax and neck.

However, the first screening task chosen during the initial assessment was a prone hip extension task with resistance. This screening task was chosen to:

- Address Steve's cognitive belief that his right hamstring was weak;

- Provide information about his ability to control the pelvis during single leg extension; and

- Assess the impact that providing a controlled platform (i.e., the pelvis) could have on his hip extension strength.

The findings from this screening task alone were sufficient to begin to develop a treatment plan for Steve.

The key findings from Steve's story are noted in the center of his Clinical Puzzle (Fig. 5.2) and include:

- Meaningful complaint: Loss of speed and agility on the soccer field, feeling that the right upper hamstring is 'on the verge of grabbing.'

- Cognitive belief: The proximal upper right hamstring is still weak and will tear if he 'goes hard.'

- Meaningful tasks: Running and rotating in all directions, looking left and right, while manipulating a soccer ball with either foot.

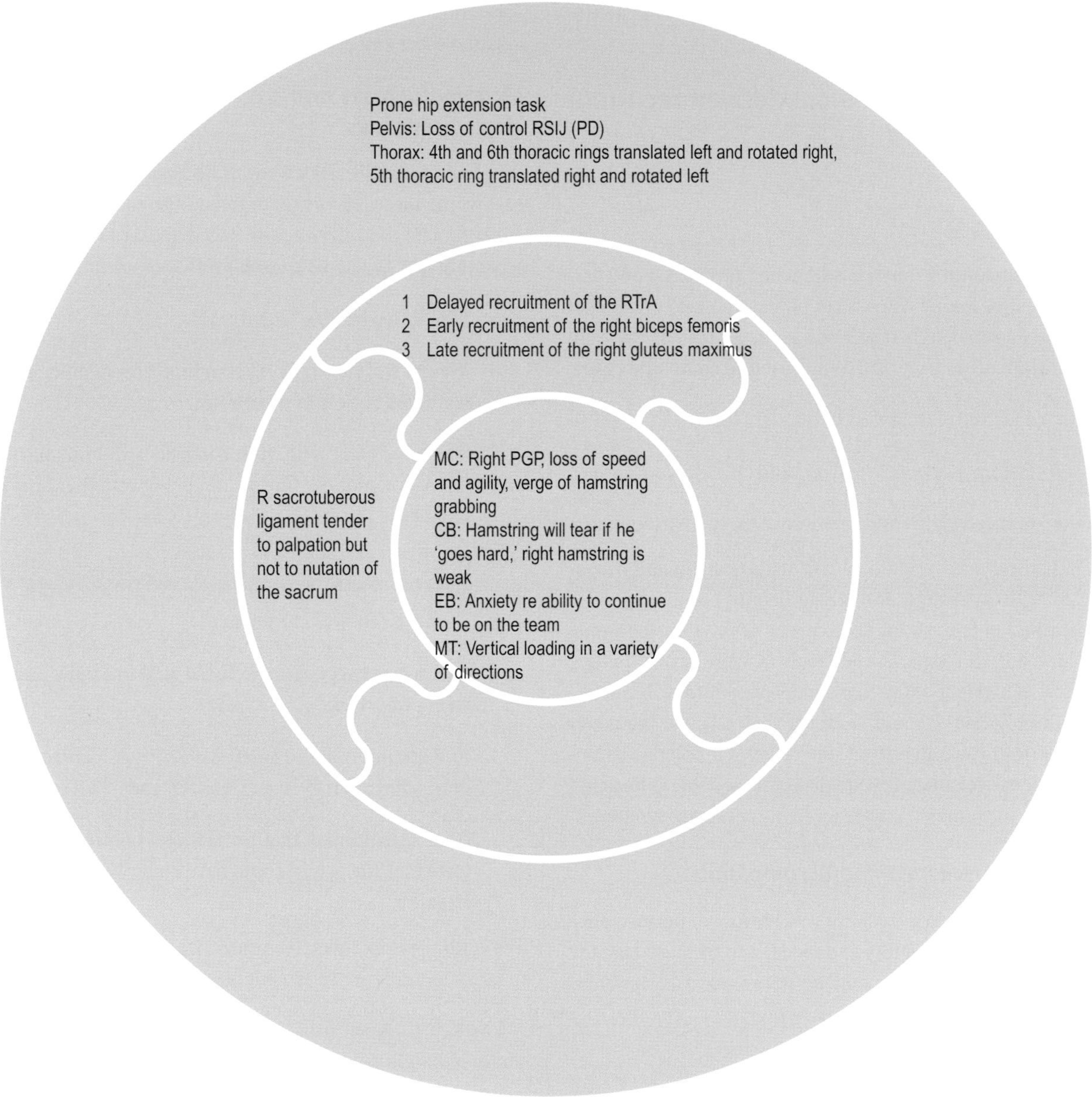

Prone hip extension task
Pelvis: Loss of control RSIJ (PD)
Thorax: 4th and 6th thoracic rings translated left and rotated right,
5th thoracic ring translated right and rotated left

1 Delayed recruitment of the RTrA
2 Early recruitment of the right biceps femoris
3 Late recruitment of the right gluteus maximus

R sacrotuberous
ligament tender
to palpation but
not to nutation of
the sacrum

MC: Right PGP, loss of speed
and agility, verge of hamstring
grabbing
CB: Hamstring will tear if he
'goes hard,' right hamstring is
weak
EB: Anxiety re ability to continue
to be on the team
MT: Vertical loading in a variety
of directions

Figure 5.2

Steve's completed Clinical Puzzle from the initial assessment. CB = cognitive belief, EB = emotional belief, MC = meaningful
complaint, MT = meaningful task, PD = primary driver, PGP = pelvic girdle pain, RTrA = right transversus abdominis,
RSIJ = right sacroiliac joint.

Screening task analysis – prone hip extension with resistance

During a single-leg-loading task in standing, Hungerford et al. (2003) reported that healthy subjects recruited the deep muscles responsible for control of the pelvis prior to the biceps femoris and the gluteus maximus (Fig. 5.3). Additionally, they noted that the healthy controls recruited the gluteus maximus prior to the biceps femoris in this task. In subjects with both pelvic girdle pain and an SIJ control impairment, a recruitment delay was noted in both the TrA and internal oblique and the multifidus. Additionally, a reversal of the timing of recruitment of the gluteus maximus and biceps femoris occurred (the biceps femoris contracted before the gluteus maximus).

Proximally, the biceps femoris attaches to the sacrotuberous ligament (Van Wingerden et al. 1993), which is a known contributor to the form closure mechanism of the SIJ (Vleeming et al. 1989a, 1989b). When the motor control strategy for control of the pelvis is suboptimal, it is common to find overactivation of the biceps femoris and delayed or absent activation of the gluteus maximus. If these findings were present, this could be a biologically plausible mechanism to explain Steve's sense of weak hamstrings.

Video 5.11 (free code)

Steve's prone hip extension task findings

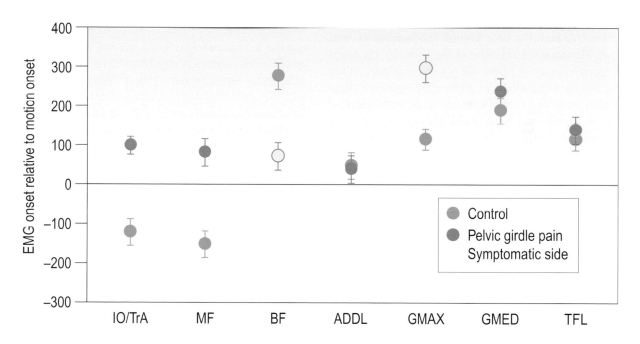

Figure 5.3

Mean EMG onset of IO and TrA (lowest fibers of internal oblique and transversus abdominis) for the supporting leg during single leg standing. Surface EMG was used in this study; therefore, recruitment of these muscles could not be differentiated. Healthy controls are shown in blue and subjects with pelvic girdle pain associated with ipsilateral SIJ control impairment are shown in orange. The subjects demonstrated delayed onset during a weight shift of IO and TrA and MF and a reversal of recruitment timing of BF and GMAX with BF being recruited earlier and GMAX later, shown in yellow. ADDL = adductor longus, BF = biceps femoris, GMAX = gluteus maximus, GMED = gluteus medius, IO = internal oblique, MF = multifidus, TFL = tensor fascia lata, TrA = transversus abdominis.

In prone, Steve could flex both the left and right knee independently without losing control of either his left or right SIJ (Video 5.11). However, he was unable to maintain control of his right SIJ when asked to extend his right hip with the knee straight (higher load task). His ability to generate force during single leg hip extension was much weaker on the right side. Without resistance, he noticed that the right leg was heavier to lift than the left. Was this weakness due to the prior right hamstring injury or due to his inability to control the right SIJ? When the right side of the sacrum was passively nutated, thereby increasing the form closure mechanism, which is a pelvic correction for this task, his ability to generate force during right single leg hip extension was much improved. This finding negates his cognitive belief that the hip extension weakness is due to a weak right hamstring.

In prone, the right TrA was not recruited when Steve contracted his pelvic floor. The left TrA response was normal. During active extension of the right hip, the biceps femoris contracted before the gluteus maximus. When he was cued specifically to activate the right TrA (Stage 1 intrapelvic ring control training), and then to maintain this recruitment as he extended his right leg, he could control the right SIJ and generate notably more right hip extension force. The recruitment sequencing of his biceps femoris and gluteus maximus reverted to a more optimal pattern (gluteus maximus before biceps femoris) when he contracted his deep system prior to extending his hip.

Steve's thorax was also noted to translate to the left when he extended his right hip (4th and 6th thoracic rings translated left and rotated right, 5th thoracic ring translated right and rotated left). Correcting and controlling his thorax prior to extending his right hip did not restore his right SIJ control, did not change the recruitment strategy of his abdominals or the timing of the biceps femoris and gluteus maximus, and did not improve his ability to generate more right hip extension force. The thorax was not the current driver for this task. Controlling the pelvis was the best correction for this task; therefore, the pelvis was considered the current primary driver and the best place to begin treatment. Further tests were required to determine specifically what would need to be treated or trained to restore pelvic control for right hip extension.

Steve believed that his pain was coming from the proximal insertion of his right hamstring. Palpation confirmed that the proximal hamstring was not tender to palpation; however, the right sacrotuberous ligament was, although nutation of the sacrum did not exacerbate his pain.

Vector analysis of the driver – the pelvis

There was no restriction of active or passive mobility of either the left or right SIJ; therefore, no vectors to release. This was a pelvic control impairment.

Hypothesis to explain Steve's pain and impairments

From this initial assessment, it was determined that the pelvis was Steve's primary driver for the screening task of prone hip extension. While his previous rehabilitation had likely addressed his initial acute right hamstring strain, a residual control impairment of his pelvis had remained, and may have preceded his injury. Without optimal strategies for pelvic control it is very difficult to generate force in either lower extremity and certainly difficult to perform with the speed and agility an elite athlete requires. Steve was attempting to gain control of his right SIJ by overusing the right biceps femoris to increase tension in the right sacrotuberous ligament to increase the form closure mechanism. The sacrotuberous ligament was possibly generating peripheral nociception and the overworked biceps femoris was likely creating the sensation that the 'hamstrings were on the verge of grabbing.'

Initial ISM treatment for Steve's pelvis-driven hamstring

Steve was prescribed Stage 1 motor control training for intrapelvic ring control specifically targeting the recruitment of the right TrA. The goal was to develop better neuromuscular recruitment strategies for load transfer through the pelvis. Stage 2 strategy capacity training for intrapelvic ring control (massed practice with focused attention on co-activation of the TrA, pelvic floor, and deep lumbosacral multifidus) with progressive leg loading (single bent leg lifts in supine, single leg extension in prone, circles both in supine and prone) and Stage 3, Level 1 motor control and movement training (small double leg squats with centered weight shifts) were prescribed over the next four weeks.

Follow-up – second session (one month later)

Steve was diligent with his home practice and felt some improvement in his hamstring strength but minimal change in his on-field speed or agility. The Stage 1, Stage 2, and Stage 3, Level 1 motor control training exercises prescribed are fundamental to intrapelvic ring control but are not whole-body tasks, nor were they specific to his sport. That is to come! The Clinical Puzzle in Figure 5.4 illustrates this follow-up session.

Screening task analysis – prone hip extension

Video 5.12 (free code)

Steve's squat and prone hip extension task findings one month later

Steve was now able to extend his right hip and maintain control of the right SIJ (Video 5.12, second half). The effort required to lift his right leg was now similar to the left. When the right SIJ was controlled with passive nutation of the sacrum, his ability to generate more force during right single leg hip extension was not different, which indicated that the pelvis was no longer the driver for this task. His 4th and 6th thoracic rings continued to translate further left and rotate right and the 5th thoracic ring (the primary ring of the three thoracic rings) translated further right and rotated further left during right hip extension. Correcting, and maintaining, the alignment of these three thoracic rings now markedly improved his right hip extension strength. For the prone hip extension task, the thorax was now the primary driver.

Screening task analysis – the squat task

Steve stood with a right transverse plane rotation (RTPR) of his pelvis associated with a right intrapelvic torsion (RIPT), and a left transverse plane rotation of his lower thorax (incongruent to his pelvis) (Video 5.12, first half). During a squat task the RTPR of his pelvis increased as did the right lateral translation and left rotation of the 5th thoracic ring. He could squat and maintain intrapelvic control, which indicated that the work he had done over the previous month was facilitating better function of his pelvis. The 4th and 6th thoracic rings translated left and rotated right (and approximated towards each other on the left) and the 5th thoracic ring translated further right and rotated further left during this squat task.

Correcting the pelvic alignment and biomechanics during the squat task made the alignment of the thorax worse and did not improve Steve's experience of strength or efficiency for the task. Correcting the alignment of the three thoracic rings (4th, 5th, and 6th) improved the alignment and biomechanics of the pelvis and while there was minimal change in his experience, it was noted to be easier to return to standing from the squat position. The thorax was now the primary driver for this task.

Screening task analysis – seated rotation of the thorax

Video 5.13 (free code)

Steve's seated trunk rotation findings

During seated rotation of the thorax, Steve noticed it was more difficult to rotate his thorax to the right and reported a 'pinching sensation' in his midthorax in the region of the 4th to 6th thoracic rings at the end of his available range (Video 5.13). Correcting the alignment and facilitating optimal biomechanics of the 4th to 6th thoracic rings improved the amplitude of right thoracic rotation and eliminated the pinching sensation in his midthorax.

Vector analysis of the driver – the thorax

Vector analysis of the 4th to 6th thoracic rings (passive listening on release of the correction) revealed the 5th thoracic ring to be the first to lose alignment. The first rib of the 5th thoracic ring to move was the left 5th rib, which posteriorly rotated. The entire 5th thoracic ring then translated right and rotated left followed by simultaneous left lateral translation and right rotation of the 4th and 6th thoracic rings. The vector was in the back, on the left and long. Palpation of the spinal extensors revealed overactivation

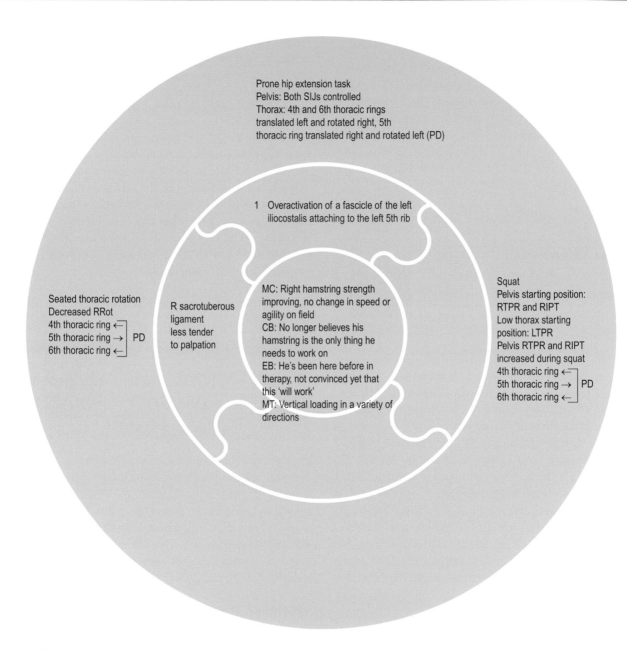

Figure 5.4

Steve's completed Clinical Puzzle from his second session. CB = cognitive belief, EB = emotional belief, MC = meaningful complaint, MT = meaningful task, PD = primary driver, RIPT = right intrapelvic torsion, RRot = right rotation, RTPR = right transverse plane rotation, SIJ = sacroiliac joint, ← = left translation, → = right translation.

of the right and left iliocostalis, the longissimus, and the segmental multifidus and rotatores.

ISM treatment – second session

The iliocostalis and longissimus were released using a muscle recoil technique (see Chapter 6) followed by segmental dry needling to T5–T6. Following this, the alignment and biomechanics of the 4th to 6th thoracic rings were improved and the effort to rotate the thorax to the right was less. Steve reported that the pinching sensation at the end of right rotation was gone. To maintain the alignment and the range of rotation gained from this release, thoracic ring stack, breathe and right rotate (Lee L-J 2016) (see Chapter 6) was given as home practice. Steve was to check his right thoracic rotation frequently during the day and to repeat this release exercise whenever he felt a reduction in his range, or a return of the pinching sensation (home self-check). In addition, he was advised to follow this with thoracic ring stack (manually first and then using imagery), connect (recruit the deep muscles responsible for lumbopelvic control with the cues taught in the first session, i.e., Stage 1 intrapelvic ring motor control training), and squat to begin to build a new 'brain map,' or motor control movement strategy for better alignment and biomechanics for his squat task. Combined, this movement practice is still Stage 2 motor control and movement training of two body regions. The thorax and pelvis are controlled in static alignment and the lower extremity moved (squat). Massed practice with focused attention was encouraged to facilitate the speed of synaptic connectivity and thus the ease of use of the strategy (principles of training using neuroplasticity).

Follow-up – third session (two weeks later)

Video 5.14 (free code)

Stage 3, Level 3 motor learning training for Steve

Once again, Steve was diligent with his home practice and this session could focus more on optimal strategies for the more complex movements required for his sport. On review of his current training regimen, it appeared that Steve had been taught to co-contract and brace his trunk while training (Video 5.14). While this strategy may be useful for aspects of some sports and tasks, it was not what he needed for speed or agility on the soccer field. He needed to be able to generate centered thoracopelvic rotation during single leg loading, which is a Stage 3, Level 3 task. He was encouraged to think about 'creating space between the middle thoracic rings' (release cue) and to initiate the rotation of his thorax from his chest and not his arms. The sensation or experience of performing this single leg thoracopelvic rotation task with different strategies and cues (bracing, floating, initiating the rotation using the thorax versus the arms, etc.) was repeated until Steve could determine which combination of movements and cues worked best for him to create fluid, easy movement. When he used his old strategy that limited his ability to rotate his thorax, the pinching sensation in the midthorax quickly returned and he also noticed more balance and control challenges (intermittent) when the task was performed with right single leg loading. The right biceps femoris would intermittently activate before the gluteus maximus on the times when he felt more control challenges in his pelvis. Steve was beginning to understand the role that his thorax was having on his pelvic control and persistent hamstring 'pulling.' The first step for motivating a change in behavior is to create awareness as to why behavior needs to change. Changing the experience of the body in a meaningful way is a powerful way to motivate behavioral change.

On-field visit (two weeks later)

Video 5.15 (free code)

Changing strategies in the context of sport for Steve

Chapter 5

I had the opportunity to watch and video Steve both during a field practice and in a game two weeks later (Videos 5.15, 5.16, 5.17). Immersed in the context of his sport, it was difficult for him to integrate the new strategies for thoracopelvic rotation and load transfer through his pelvis and right lower extremity and he tended to revert to a co-contraction bracing strategy for his trunk control. I shared the videos I had taken of his training and asked him how he felt during the practice. Here is his response.

'My hamstring and glut [sic] felt really good last night. I didn't notice any stiffness and it felt quite loose. I felt a few twinges very high up in the tendon just below the glut [sic] area a couple of times and I have some very minor soreness today. I can just tell I played last night but this is as good as I have felt after a session in a while. The last 20-30 minutes I really pushed as hard as I could so I am happy with how I feel today. My back was still a little stiff when I was doing the rotation exercises and I was trying to focus on keeping my upper body a little looser but it is still something I really need to be conscious of. Honestly, I don't realize how stiff my back is until I do the rotation exercises and I may need to spend a little more time loosening up my trunk before training.

'Thanks for the videos, it is awesome to have some visual footage to look at. Wow did I look rigid on Tuesday, even in the game footage there is a lot of room for improvement. I really took a lot of extra time loosening up my chest and back on Saturday so I think that helped a bit. I really appreciate all the work and effort you have put in so far. I can't tell you how many times I have gotten to where I was about 4 to 5 weeks ago and told different physiotherapists that it still doesn't feel right, only to have them tell me everything looks good, pelvis is way better and the strength in the hamstring is great, just keep stretching that hamstring every day. I really do feel like my chest/back is the final piece, the last week I have felt great and last night I felt the best I have felt physically in a game in a long, long time. I know I still have a lot of work to do going forward but I am feeling positive and hopeful that I will be able to stay healthy and continue to progress. I could feel the hamstring a bit last night but nothing like it has been over the last couple of years so that is progress and for once I am cautiously a little excited.'

Conclusion

Steve continued to work on his strategies for thoracopelvic rotation and load transfer through single leg loading to ensure that his right biceps femoris was not overworked and that loads were shared throughout his body. With focused attention, massed practice and training tasks that relate to meaningful goals, learning and change can occur. Over time, he learned to move better on the field and noticed his speed and agility returning. He also developed more confidence in his right hamstring and could 'go hard' at his sport. Stimulating neuronal activation and growth and then building up the speed of synaptic connectivity for ease and agility requires neuroplastic training. Steve's story is a good example of how poor strategies for pelvic control and thoracic biomechanics had created a persistent hamstring impairment.

Thorax-driven pelvic girdle pain and diastasis rectus abdominis

Diane Lee

The abdominal muscles receive motor innervation from the lower thorax and it has been clinically noted that translated and rotated lower thoracic rings can perturb the optimal sequencing of recruitment during a variety of tasks (Lee D 2016, Lee L-J 2016). This case report highlights the importance of assessing the alignment and biomechanics of the thorax for all individuals with abdominal muscle dyssynergies, regardless of the presence or absence of a diastasis rectus abdominis (DRA).

Amanda's story and current meaningful complaints

At the time of this initial assessment, Amanda was a 31-year-old Pilates instructor and mother of two children aged five years and five months. Her meaningful complaint was anterior pelvic girdle pain (pubic symphysis), which initially occurred during her first pregnancy, resolved between her two pregnancies and then recurred six to eight weeks after the delivery of her second child. Both deliveries were vaginal and no episiotomy was required. She reported no problems with her urinary continence, no pain with intercourse, and no issues with the function of her bowel. Her pubic symphysis pain was aggravated by tasks that involved jumping or rapidly shifting weight from one leg to the other in the coronal plane.

Amanda's cognitive beliefs and emotional status

Amanda believed that she needed to continue to strengthen her abdominal wall to support her pubic symphysis, was working with another Pilates instructor, who was also a physiotherapist, and was confident that she would achieve her goals. She presented as a patient model for a course I was teaching on the Integrated Systems Model and its application for rehabilitation of the abdominal wall in postpartum women.

Meaningful task and screening tasks chosen for strategy analysis

Amanda's meaningful task was to dance pain free; she identified her inability to rapidly shift weight in the coronal body plane as being her main barrier to this goal. The screening tasks chosen for this initial session were:

- Standing postural screen as a starting point for assessing change in alignment, biomechanics, and control for the next task;

- Standing weight shift in the coronal body plane.

If all findings were optimal for these two tasks, a lateral jump landing on one leg would be added.

The key findings from Amanda's story are noted in the center of her Clinical Puzzle (Fig. 5.5).

Screening task analysis – standing postural screen

Video 5.18 (free code)

Amanda's standing posture screen and single leg weight shift

The key clinical findings in standing were (Video 5.18):

- Pelvis and hips: Neutral in all planes.

- Thorax:

  ○ Lower thorax: Rotated to the right (RTPR) associated with an 8th thoracic ring translated left and rotated right;

  ○ Middle thorax: Rotated to the right (RTPR) and congruent and following the lower thorax with no notable individual thoracic ring translation and rotation;

  ○ Upper thorax: The 2nd thoracic ring translated right and rotated left, incongruent to the middle and lower thorax.

- Cervical: C7 translated left and rotated right; C2 translated right and rotated left.

Correction of the alignment of the 8th thoracic ring improved the alignment of all thoracic rings, C7, and C2. The 8th thoracic ring was the primary driver for standing.

Screening task analysis – standing weight shift

The key clinical findings in standing weight shift were:

- Pelvis: The right SIJ lost control (the right innominate anteriorly rotated relative to the right side of the sacrum) when Amanda shifted her weight to the right. The left SIJ retained control when she shifted her weight to the left leg.

- Lower thorax: During a weight shift to the right, the 8th thoracic ring translated further left and rotated

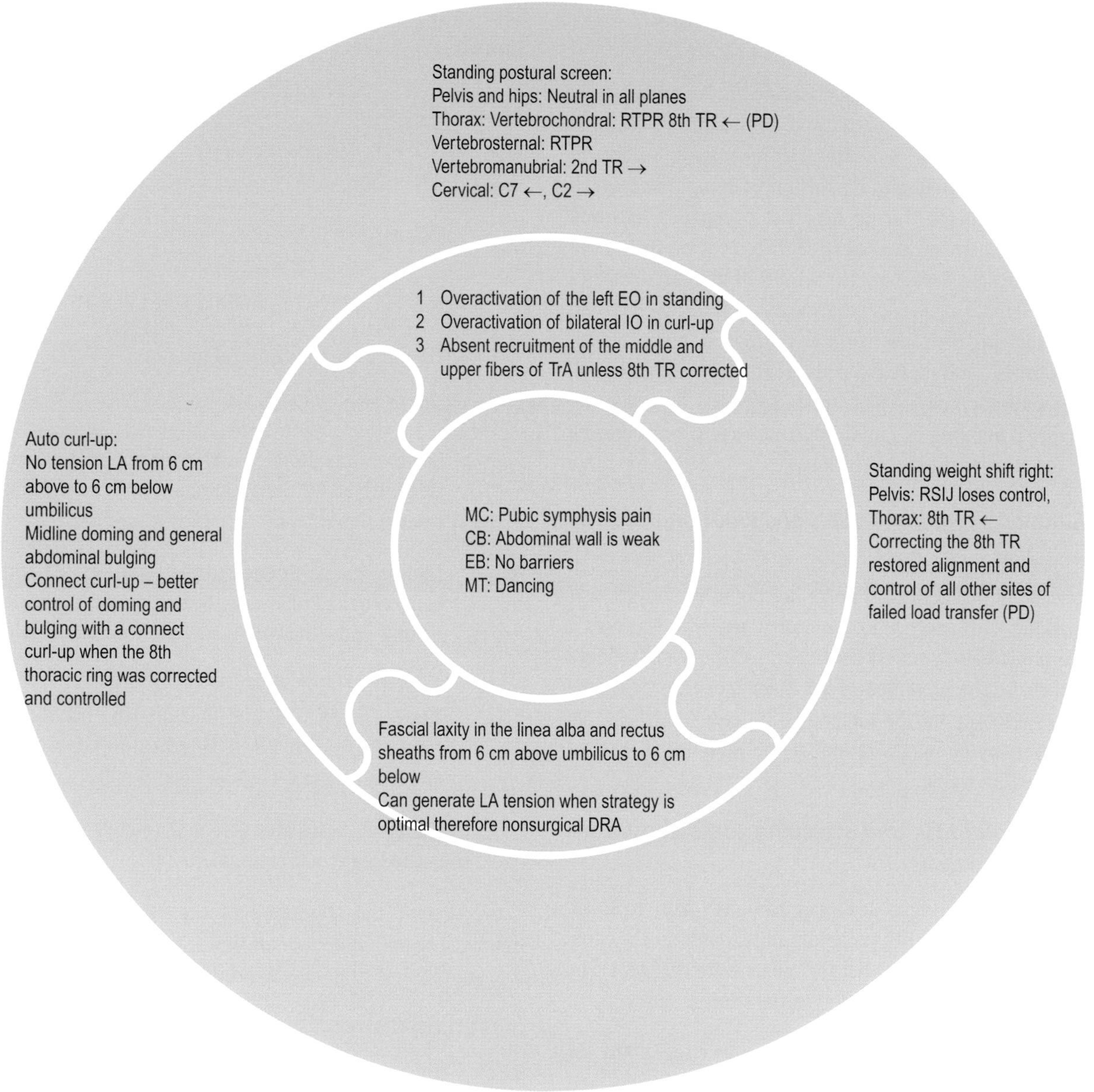

Standing postural screen:
Pelvis and hips: Neutral in all planes
Thorax: Vertebrochondral: RTPR 8th TR ← (PD)
Vertebrosternal: RTPR
Vertebromanubrial: 2nd TR →
Cervical: C7 ←, C2 →

1 Overactivation of the left EO in standing
2 Overactivation of bilateral IO in curl-up
3 Absent recruitment of the middle and
   upper fibers of TrA unless 8th TR corrected

Auto curl-up:
No tension LA from 6 cm
above to 6 cm below
umbilicus
Midline doming and general
abdominal bulging
Connect curl-up – better
control of doming and
bulging with a connect
curl-up when the 8th
thoracic ring was corrected
and controlled

MC: Pubic symphysis pain
CB: Abdominal wall is weak
EB: No barriers
MT: Dancing

Standing weight shift right:
Pelvis: RSIJ loses control,
Thorax: 8th TR ←
Correcting the 8th TR
restored alignment and
control of all other sites of
failed load transfer (PD)

Fascial laxity in the linea alba and rectus
sheaths from 6 cm above umbilicus to 6 cm
below
Can generate LA tension when strategy is
optimal therefore nonsurgical DRA

Figure 5.5

Amanda's completed Clinical Puzzle from the initial assessment. CB = cognitive belief, DRA = diastasis rectus abdominis,
EB = emotional belief, EO = external oblique, IO = internal oblique, LA = linea alba, MC = meaningful complaint, MT = meaningful
task, PD = primary driver, RTPR = right transverse plane rotation, RSIJ = right sacroiliac joint, TR = thoracic ring, TrA = transversus
abdominis, ← = left translation, → = right translation.

further right. When the alignment of the 8th thoracic ring was corrected and the biomechanics controlled during a weight shift to the right, the right SIJ was controlled and all other sites of failed load transfer noted in standing remained corrected. This suggests that the suboptimal alignment and biomechanics of the 8th thoracic ring was impacting the motor control strategy for intrapelvic ring control during right single leg loading. Amanda noted better balance and ease during the right weight shift with the 8th thoracic ring corrected.

The primary driver for a right weight shift task was also the 8th thoracic ring. Since the 8th thoracic ring can be corrected, the underlying system impairment was not articular but more likely neural or visceral.

Vector analysis of the driver – the thorax

The dominant vector creating the suboptimal alignment of the 8th thoracic ring during a right weight shift was apparent during passive listening on correction of the 8th thoracic ring, and on release of the correction. The vector was on the left, in the front, outside the thorax, and long. It was coming from overactivation of the left external oblique. Note that the external oblique crosses the pubic symphysis and excessive activation can create a 'shear stress' at this joint. As outlined in Chapter 1, the aponeurosis of the external oblique forms the inguinal ligament that runs from the anterior superior iliac spine of the ilium to the pubic symphysis, which it crosses to insert on the contralateral side (Stecco 2015).

Abdominal wall assessment

The following assessment was developed during the research study that investigated the behavior of the linea alba in healthy subjects and in those with DRA (Lee D & Hodges 2016). The text *Diastasis Rectus Abdominis: A Clinical Guide for Those who are Split Down the Middle* (Lee D 2017b) expands on this condition and the abdominal wall assessment, and provides extensive instruction for both release and training of the abdominal wall. Here is an abbreviated version of the assessment.

Abdominal profile and behavior in standing

Video 5.19 (free code)
Amanda's abdominal profile and behavior in standing

In standing, Amanda was asked to completely relax her abdominal and pelvic floor muscles (Video 5.19) and then to demonstrate what she had been practicing in Pilates to 'activate her deep system.' These words were familiar to her and I wanted to know what she thought was an optimal contraction of the deep muscles responsible for control of the lumbopelvis. The strategy she used produced a low belly lift; however, this lift was associated with a drawing in of the left lower rib cage (a sign of overflow into the left external oblique). This recruitment strategy did not control the right SIJ during a weight shift to the right and the 8th thoracic ring translated further left and rotated further right. Whatever she was recruiting with her 'connect strategy' was insufficient to provide control to her pelvic girdle and optimal alignment for her lower thorax.

The abdominal wall and thoracolumbar control

Amanda's automatic recruitment strategy was sufficient to control sagittal plane loading through her thorax and lumbar spine in the seated position but not a right rotation load through the vertebrochondral region. Her 'connect strategy' did not improve her ability to resist right rotation.

Supine single leg load – active bent leg raise test

Video 5.20 (free code)
Supine single leg load – Amanda's active bent leg raise test

Amanda found it harder to lift the left leg in hook lying and all three levels of her abdomen bulged, although the upper and middle abdomen appeared to bulge more than the lower abdomen (Video 5.20). When the 8th thoracic ring was corrected and controlled during the left leg lift task, there was a reduction in the effort required to perform the task and less bulging of the upper and middle abdomen was observed.

Behavior of the abdominal wall and linea alba in a curl-up task

Video 5.21 (free code)

Behavior of Amanda's abdominal wall and linea alba in a curl-up task

At rest, there was less tension in the linea alba from approximately 6 cm above the umbilicus to 6 cm below the umbilicus than above or below these points (Video 5.21). The rectus sheaths were more compliant in the transverse plane in the region where there was less tension in the linea alba.

When an automatic strategy was used to perform a short head and neck curl-up task, the following findings were noted:

- Dominance of the internal oblique over the external oblique. The lower rib cage widened during the curl-up. For this task, the internal oblique was dominating the previously found overactive left external oblique, which was noted to be dominant in a weight shift task.

- Doming of the linea alba occurred where less tension was noted at rest. The left and right rectus abdominis could be pulled apart in the curl-up position. This suggests that there was insufficient tension in the linea alba in this region of the abdominal wall. Ultrasound imaging confirmed increased distortion of the linea alba above and below the umbilicus and well up toward the xyphoid during the automatic curl-up (Fig. 5.6A&B). The middle and upper abdomen bulged during the automatic curl-up (Fig. 5.6C).

- There was no automatic recruitment response in the middle or upper fibers of the left or right TrA (Fig. 5.7A–D).

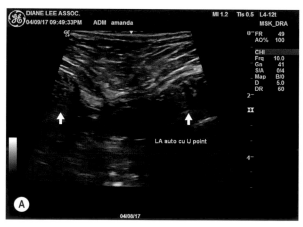
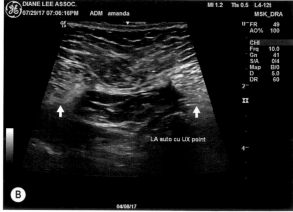

Figure 5.6

Behavior of the linea alba during an automatic curl-up task. (A) Just above the umbilicus (U point), the linea alba sagged as the left and right rectus abdominis approximated during the curl-up task when Amanda used an automatic strategy. Note the lack of echogenicity (tension) of the posterior rectus sheaths (arrows). This suggests that the transversus abdominis was not recruited in this strategy. (B) At 6 cm above the umbilicus (UX point), the behavior of the linea alba during the automatic curl-up was also suboptimal. No tension was apparent in either the posterior rectus sheaths (arrows) or the linea alba.

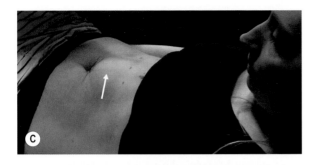

Figure 5.6 *continued*

(C) Note the doming of the midline abdomen just above the umbilicus when Amanda uses her automatic strategy for a curl-up task. LA = linea alba, auto = automatic, cu = curl-up.

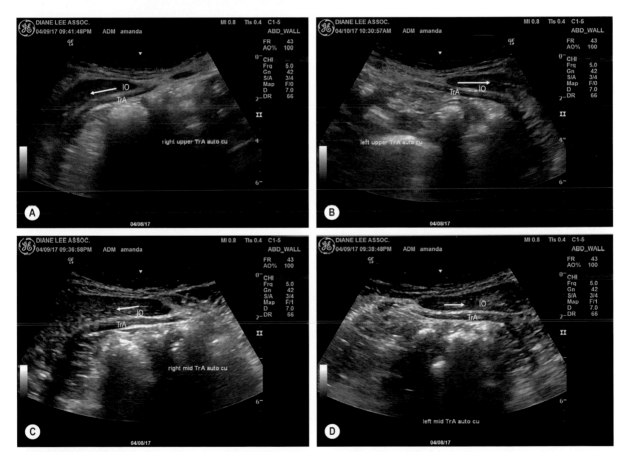

Figure 5.7

Behavior of the transversus abdominis during an automatic curl-up task. The upper fibers of the right (A) and left (B) transversus abdominis were not recruited in this strategy. Note how the internal oblique (IO) has slid laterally over the transversus abdominis (TrA) (arrows). The middle fibers of the right (C) and left (D) transversus abdominis were not recruited in this strategy. Note how the internal oblique has slid laterally over the transversus abdominis (arrows). This absence of recruitment explains the general bulging of the abdomen noted during Amanda's automatic curl-up and the increased distortion of the linea alba in this region. LA = linea alba, auto = automatic, cu = curl-up, IO = internal oblique, TrA = transversus abdominis.

- When the alignment of the 8th thoracic ring was manually corrected and controlled during the automatic curl-up task, the middle and upper fibers of the TrA were automatically recruited. This strategy eliminated both the doming of the linea alba and the bulging of the abdomen. Ultrasound imaging revealed less distortion of the linea alba; however, the inter-recti distance was greater with this strategy than the automatic strategy.

When Amanda was given a cue to contract her pelvic floor, an immediate recruitment of the lower fibers of the left and right TrA and the middle fibers of the right TrA could be felt. There was no response from the middle fibers of the left TrA or the left or right upper fibers. When the alignment of the 8th thoracic ring was manually corrected, there was an immediate improvement in the recruitment response of the middle fibers of the left TrA and both the left and right upper fibers of the TrA. Correcting the alignment of the 8th thoracic ring appeared to change the motor control strategy of the abdominal wall during this task as well as during the automatic curl-up. When the 8th thoracic ring was aligned, and controlled, Amanda could recruit all three levels of her TrA, maintain the contraction, and perform a short head and neck curl-up. This co-contraction strategy with improved 8th thoracic ring alignment produced the greatest tension in the linea alba

(Fig. 5.8A&B), eliminated the midline doming and general abdominal bulging (Fig. 5.8C).

For the short head and neck curl-up task, the 8th thoracic ring was the primary driver and was impacting the recruitment strategy of her abdominal wall, which in turn was impairing Amanda's ability to:

- generate force for rotation of her thorax, and

- control her pelvis during vertical loading tasks on the right leg.

ISM treatment for Amanda's thorax-driven abdominal wall and intrapelvic ring control

Release and align

Video 5.22 (free code)

ISM treatment for Amanda's thorax-driven abdominal wall and intrapelvic ring control

Release technique: 8th thoracic ring manual correction followed by left rotation of the thorax combined with a hold–relax technique to eccentrically lengthen the left external

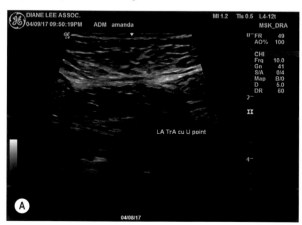

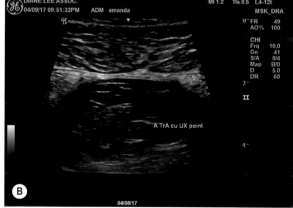

Figure 5.8

Behavior of the linea alba during a connect curl-up task (precontraction of the TrA) preceded by a manual correction of the 8th thoracic ring. Just above the umbilicus (U point) (A) and at the UX point (B) the linea alba was straight (with no distortion), although the inter-recti distance was greater when Amanda recruited the transversus abdominis bilaterally before initiating the curl-up task. cu = curl-up, LA = linea alba, TrA = transversus abdominis.

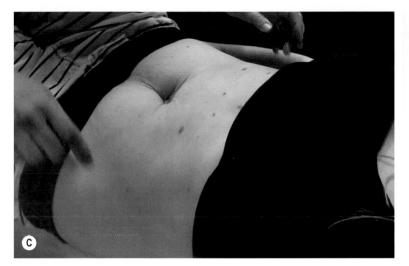

Figure 5.8 *continued*

(C) When the alignment of the 8th thoracic ring was corrected prior to her curl-up task, Amanda could recruit all her abdominals during the curl-up task and this strategy eliminated the general abdominal bulging as well as the midline distortion of the linea alba. Midline tension in the linea alba was palpable and notably different between the two strategies.

oblique (Video 5.22). A lateral costal breath was added to encourage further release the left external oblique. The phase of respiration was co-ordinated with the biomechanics of left rotation by rotating left on the inhale, holding on the exhale, and repeating three to four times. This movement practice for release of the left external oblique was given as a home exercise in addition to supine wipers with knees to the right, and a manual correction of the 8th thoracic ring.

Connect and control

After two to three repetitions of supine wipers for release of the left external oblique, a co-ordinated recruitment of the sides and layers of the abdominal muscles was added (Stages 1 to Stage 3, Level 1 motor learning). Amanda was instructed to connect to all three levels of the TrA (upper, middle and lower fibers) on the exhale breath, hold the contraction on the inhale, and on the next exhale breath take the knees to the right. The focus of this practice was to repattern the synchronization of recruitment of the entire abdominal wall. To return to neutral, she was instructed to initiate the derotation using her pelvis and not her knees. This exercise requires both eccentric and concentric recruitment of the left and right external and internal obliques in addition to a tonic, yet changing, activation of the left and right, upper, middle and lower fibers of the TrA. The active bent leg raise test was used as a home self-check for Amanda to determine if she was using an optimal strategy to connect. No abdominal bulging or midline doming should occur and her left leg lift should feel easy. Stage 1

to Stage 3, Level 1 motor learning training was advised for the next eight to 10 days until she had consolidated the new neural pathway for this task.

Conclusion

Follow-up with Amanda was via email correspondence only. This single session had broadened her awareness of what was impeding the postpartum recovery of her abdominal wall function, appearance, and strength. She was now aware of the relationship between her 8th thoracic ring alignment, her anterior pelvic girdle pain (pubic symphysis), and her inability to feel confident in her lateral jumps. Together with her physiotherapist and her Pilates program she is continuing to improve functionally with strategies that support both her thoracic alignment and biomechanics, and her intrapelvic ring control.

Thorax-driven persistent diastasis rectus abdominis and poor lumbosacral control

Diane Lee

Christine's story and current meaningful complaints

At the time of this initial assessment, Christine was a 41-year-old mother of five who had experienced urinary frequency and pelvic floor pain since her second pregnancy 12 years ago. All her babies were delivered vaginally and all deliveries required an episiotomy. In addition to urinary frequency and pelvic floor pain, she was getting up after

15 minutes of lying down for the night for a four-second void. She had been taught to 'boss her bladder' and could control the urgency during the day. In addition to her pelvic complaints, she experienced frequent low back pain episodes, which she described as her 'back going out.' She reported that she felt vulnerable and fragile when doing tasks that involved lifting and twisting and her back pain often came on insidiously over the subsequent 24 hours such that she was unable to move. She has had three such episodes each year of the last three years.

Christine was a model for a course I was teaching on the abdominal wall and the purpose of this assessment was to determine the role her abdominal wall and DRA had in her persistent pelvic floor and back pain. Her physical therapist Kathe Wallace (www.kathewallace.com) would be providing Christine's care with the recommended treatment based on this assessment.

Christine's meaningful complaints were persistent pelvic floor and back pain and a fragile, vulnerable feeling about the function of her back. Her meaningful tasks were lifting and twisting. The screening tasks chosen for analysis were:

- Standing postural screen;

- Standing weight shift progressing to single leg standing and then forward bending if the pelvis was controlled;

- Lumbar segmental control under load (seated loading through the upper extremities and supine loading through the lower extremities);

- Short head and neck curl-up task for assessment of the abdominal wall.

Screening task analysis – standing postural screen

Video 5.23 (free code)

Christine's standing postural screen, weight shift, and segmental lumbar loading tasks

The key findings from the standing postural screen included (Video 5.23):

- Pelvis: Left transverse plane rotation associated with a left intrapelvic torsion (LTPR and LIPT);

- Lower thorax: Right transverse plane rotation associated with an 8th thoracic ring translated left and rotated right;

- Middle thorax: Left transverse plane rotation associated with a 4th thoracic ring translated right and rotated left;

- Upper thorax: The 2nd thoracic ring translated left and rotated right.

Correcting the alignment of the 8th thoracic ring improved the alignment of the pelvis; however, the rotation of the upper thorax worsened. Correcting the alignment of the 4th thoracic ring improved the alignment of the lower thorax, pelvis, and upper thorax. The 4th thoracic ring was considered the primary driver for this task.

Screening task analysis – standing weight shift

The key findings from the standing weight shift included:

- Pelvis: Immediate loss of control of the right SIJ when shifting weight to the right leg;

- Thorax: No change in alignment of any of the thoracic rings.

No change in pelvic control was noted with correcting any site of failed load transfer including the 4th thoracic ring. Controlling the pelvis during the weight shift did not improve the alignment of the 8th, 4th or 2nd thoracic rings. As noted in standing, correcting the 4th thoracic ring improved the alignment of the 8th and 2nd thoracic rings. However, correcting the 4th thoracic ring did not restore control of the right SIJ during the right weight shift.

For the right weight shift task, the pelvis required passive control in addition to the 4th thoracic ring correction for improvement in both the experience and performance of the task; therefore, the pelvis and thorax were co-drivers.

Screening task analysis – lumbar segmental control under load

Video 5.24 (free code)

Assessment of Christine's deep lumbar multifidus

The key findings from the lumbar segmental control under load test were:

- Ability to control all lumbar segments during sagittal plane loading through the upper extremities;

- Inability to control the lower lumbar segments during resisted left rotation;

- Inability to control the lower thoracic rings during resisted right rotation;

- Inability to control the low lumbar segments (L5 and L4) during a right active bent leg lift (Video 5.24).

There was notable atrophy and fatty infiltration of the left sacral and lower lumbar multifidus with no automatic recruitment palpable when Christine lifted her right leg. Further investigation of the left deep multifidus and its ability to co-activate with the pelvic floor revealed no recruitment with Christine's attempt to contract her pelvic floor. The cue she used was to squeeze the muscles around the urethra and lift. When this cue was modified to involve the levator ani (i.e., gently contract the anal sphincter and then draw the anus to the back of the pubic bone), a co-activation response of the left deep multifidus occurred. The effort required to lift the right leg was reduced with this co-activation strategy of the pelvic floor and the deep multifidus. She was also able to control the low lumbar segments during this task with this strategy. The 4th thoracic ring did not require correction for this optimal change in the recruitment strategy of multifidus.

Christine was unable to control her pelvis, lumbar spine, and her lower thorax during a variety of tasks. Therefore, a complete examination of all three levels of her abdominal wall (upper, middle, and lower) would be required.

Screening task analysis – short head and neck curl-up

Video 5.25 (free code)

Assessment of Christine's abdominal wall: Fascial compliance and response to a verbal cue to contract the pelvic floor muscles

The key findings from the short head and neck curl-up task were:

- At rest, the linea alba could be easily distorted along its entire length (Video 5.25).

- During the automatic curl-up strategy, widening of the infrasternal angle occurred secondary to:

  ○ insufficient activation of the upper fibers of the TrA, and

  ○ overactivation of the internal obliques.

Video 5.26 (free code)

Assessment of Christine's abdominal wall: Behavior of the lateral abdominal muscles during a curl-up task

- During the automatic curl-up strategy, increased distortion (sagging) of the linea alba occurred (Fig. 5.9A&B) (Videos 5.26, 5.27). Sagging, or invagination, of the linea alba occurs when the strategy used for the curl-up task reduces the intra-abdominal pressure. This is often seen in individuals with DRA when there is dominance of the internal obliques along with the central tendon of the diaphragm remaining high on inspiration during the curl-up.

Video 5.27 (free code)

Assessment of Christine's abdominal wall: Behavior of the linea alba during a curl-up task

- During the connect (TrA) curl-up strategy initially no difference was noticed in the behavior of the linea alba when Christine was given a cue to connect to her deep system (TrA, pelvic floor, and multifidus) and then perform the head and neck curl-up. Further investigation revealed that

although she could recruit the middle and upper fibers of the TrA with cuing, she was not able to sustain this contraction during the curl-up task. When the alignment of the 4th thoracic ring was manually corrected, Christine could recruit and sustain the contraction of all three levels of her TrA and co-activate these muscles with her pelvic floor and deep multifidus. The distortion of the linea alba was reduced (Fig. 5.10) indicating that Christine should be able to regain a functional abdominal wall without a surgical repair of her DRA.

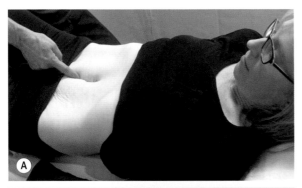

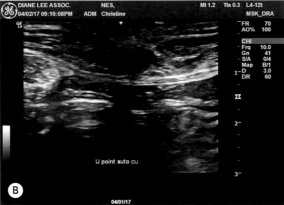

Figure 5.9

Behavior of the linea alba during a short head and neck curl-up task (the automatic curl-up strategy). (A) Note the invagination of the distorted linea alba and the widening of the infrasternal angle. These findings suggest insufficient recruitment of the upper fibers of the transversus abdominis and overactivation of the internal oblique (confirmed via ultrasound imaging), as well as insufficient activation of the middle fibers of the transversus abdominis (no tension of the linea alba). (B) Part of the right rectus abdominis and none of the left can be seen in this ultrasound image of the midline abdomen taken just above the umbilicus in the curl-up position. Note the sagging (distortion) of the linea alba. auto = automatic, cu = curl-up.

Video 5.28 (free code)

Testing the impact of changing the alignment of Christine's thorax and adding a connect cue for the deep muscles (transversus abdominis and multifidus) on her lumbar segmental and SIJ control

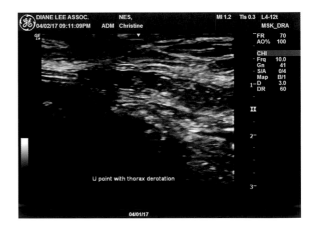

Figure 5.10

Behavior of the linea alba during a short head and neck curl-up task (the connect curl-up strategy). Neither the left or right rectus abdominis can be seen in this image since the contraction of the left and right transversus abdominis has reduced the distortion of the linea alba (reduced the sagging) and the inter-recti distance is wider than the ultrasound probe. The linea alba is much straighter in this image than in Figure 5.9B.

The 4th thoracic ring was determined to be the primary driver for the short head and neck curl-up task and the alignment of this thoracic ring was critical for recruitment of the middle and upper fibers of the TrA. See Video 5.28 to see the impact that correcting the alignment of the 4th thoracic ring and cuing a different recruitment strategy for her deep neuromuscular system had on her ability to control the right SIJ during a right weight shift task.

Vector analysis of the driver and relationship of the driver to motor control strategies – the thorax

Active and passive listening applied to the 4th thoracic ring upon correction and release of the alignment revealed a vector from a fascicle of the right external oblique and serratus anterior, which were collectively holding the 4th thoracic ring translated right and rotated left. The 8th thoracic ring and pelvis were compensating for this primary impairment. These twists were also having an impact on Christine's ability to recruit the upper and middle fibers of the TrA, which could be one mechanism for the loss of lower thoracic and lumbar segmental control during trunk rotation and lower extremity loading tasks. The 4th thoracic ring alignment did not seem to be contributing to the recruitment strategy of the deep multifidus since correction of the 4th thoracic ring was not required to activate the muscle. The deep fibers of the left multifidus were recruited with a cue to contract the levator ani (the 4th thoracic ring was still in suboptimal alignment). The combination of insufficient activation and capacity of the left deep lumbosacral multifidus, combined with insufficient activation and capacity of the upper and middle fibers of the TrA could explain Christine's multiple acute low back pain episodes and feeling of vulnerability when loading her low back.

ISM treatment for Christine's thorax-driven DRA and poor lumbosacral control

Treatment suggestions included:

- Release and align: Releasing the right serratus anterior and external oblique, specifically the fascicles pertaining to the 4th thoracic ring. It is interesting to note that the vector felt specific to the external oblique, yet most anatomy texts suggest that the external oblique does not attach to the 4th rib. Not everything found clinically can be easily explained!

- Connect and control training: Providing Stage 1 motor control training to activate and Stage 2 strategy training to build capacity in the:

  ○ left lumbosacral multifidus and

  ○ upper and middle fibers of the left and right TrA.

- Movement practice: Once Christine could automatically recruit her deep system with more reliability and control, exercises to further challenge and strengthen the capacity of the strategy (Stage 2 motor learning) were recommended, followed by exercises aimed at training movement control of the low thoracic rings, low back and pelvis (Stage 3 movement training).

Follow-up (four months later)

Video 5.29 (free code)

Follow-up of Christine four months later

Four months later, Christine was re-evaluated during another course. Her physical therapist, Kathe Wallace, informed the class that she had followed the treatment protocols suggested and that the first two to three sessions focused on releasing the vectors impacting the alignment and biomechanics of the 4th thoracic ring (right serratus anterior and the external oblique). Subsequently, Christine worked on the exercises and movement practice to build capacity in her left deep multifidus and middle and upper abdominal wall. She was feeling stronger and more confident in her ability to move and load her low back. She had regained both control and capacity of her left deep lumbosacral multifidus and thus could load her pelvis and low back much more. She could now automatically recruit all levels of her TrA in balance with her internal and external obliques. The invagination of the linea alba during her head and neck curl-up task was gone (Fig. 5.11; compare to Fig. 5.9A) and she was better able to generate tension in

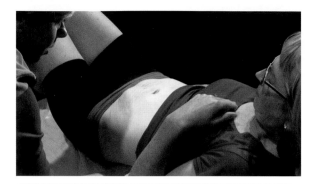

Figure 5.11

No invagination of the linea alba during the curl-up task suggests there is greater tension with this new strategy.

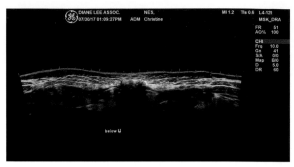

Figure 5.12

This is a panoramic view of Christine's abdominal wall at rest just above the umbilicus (U). Both the rectus sheaths and linea alba are still distorted at rest.

the linea alba even though the linea alba was still easily distorted and domed at rest (Fig. 5.12) (Video 5.29).

Thorax and cranial driven pelvis in a patient with stress urinary incontinence

Calvin Wong

Brad's story

At the time of the initial assessment, Brad was a 48-year-old truck driver and construction worker who had undergone radical prostatectomy for prostate cancer 10 months earlier. He reported experiencing symptoms of stress urinary incontinence throughout the day that caused him to use adult pads for absorption, but denied any symptoms of fecal incontinence. Brad experienced the most urinary leakage when lifting or bending to lift and rising from sitting and putting on his socks (lifting one leg). He reported that his urologist had counseled him on reducing the intake of potential bladder irritants that could exacerbate his urinary symptoms (caffeine and alcohol). Initially, Brad followed his urologist's instructions and began drinking less water, but found that he would still leak small amounts of urine despite his modified fluid intake. He realized that there was an underlying issue that he needed to address. Brad eventually began reintroducing small amounts of coffee and alcohol despite the urinary leakage that would result, and he began using absorbent pads again to cope. Currently, Brad reported that he usually had two cups of coffee per day and avoided water intake while at work. He

noted that he would normally use two to three absorbent pads through the day depending on his activity. He had returned to working out at the gym and reported noticing increased leakage from the workouts. Although months had gone by, and Brad was coping with his symptoms using pads and reducing his fluid intake, he was aware that he needed to take steps to address the underlying cause of his stress urinary incontinence.

Brad's meaningful complaints

Brad's primary concerns were centered around the movements that caused urinary leakage. It has been noted that individuals who experience stress incontinence are often affected by movements that increase intra-abdominal pressure (Stafford et al. 2015, Dorey 2006). Brad's symptoms were exacerbated by those movements thought to increase intra-abdominal pressure, primarily:

- rising from sitting,
- single leg standing (flexion of the contralateral hip), and
- squatting.

Brad's cognitive beliefs and emotional status

Brad was told by his attending physician that he likely had pelvic floor dysfunction that was causing his stress incontinence symptoms due to the length of time that had elapsed without resolution of his symptoms. This was his current cognitive belief. During the initial session, the effect of intra-abdominal pressure was explained and the potential inter-regional influence of the thorax on the function of the pelvic floor seemed a reasonable possible contributor to his current condition.

Over the 10 months of recovery from his prostatectomy, Brad had taken his own steps toward restoring normalcy to his life. This likely served to mitigate any outward signs of stress, anxiety or depression in his general demeanor. He was doing his best to cope despite knowing that he needed help to discover the reason for his persistent symptoms.

Screening task analysis

To address Brad's concerns, it was important to assess the meaningful tasks that he noted in his story that were related to the likely mechanism producing his stress incontinence – increased intra-abdominal pressure. Screening tasks were chosen to assess suboptimal movement strategies present during the performance of his chosen meaningful tasks.

Brad's meaningful tasks included:

- rising from sitting,
- single leg standing (putting on his socks), and
- squatting and lifting.

The screening tasks chosen for strategy analysis were standing postural screen, squat, and one leg standing (OLS).

Screening task analysis – standing postural screen

The key findings in standing were:

- Cranial region: Left intracranial torsion (ICT); the left temporal bone was posteriorly rotated, the right temporal bone was anteriorly rotated, and the occiput was rotated to the left. The sphenoid rotation was congruent with the ICT in that it was also rotated to the left.

- Cervical segments: C4 was translated right and side-bent and rotated left.

- Shoulder girdles: The right clavicle was anteriorly rotated and the left clavicle was posteriorly rotated.

- Upper thorax: The 2nd thoracic ring was translated left and rotated right. The manubrium was rotated to the left. The position of the manubrium was incongruent with the clavicles and the left and right 2nd ribs. A 'buckle' was evident at the right costochondral joint of the 2nd rib.

- Lower thorax: The 7th thoracic ring was translated left and rotated right, congruent with the 2nd thoracic ring.

- Pelvis: The pelvis was rotated to the left in the transverse plane (TPR) and this was associated with a congruent left IPT.

- Hips: The right femoral head was anterior to the left and congruent with the left TPR of the pelvis.

The right hip, pelvis, clavicles, C4 and cranial positional findings are congruent. The 2nd and 7th thoracic ring positions in standing posture are incongruent with all others.

Impact of corrections on standing posture – finding the drivers

Correction of the right hip did not improve the pelvis, thorax, C4 or cranium. Correction of the pelvis improved the hip, but not the thorax, C4 or cranium. Correction of the 7th thoracic ring improved the pelvis and hip but not the upper thorax, C4 or cranium. Correction of the 2nd thoracic ring improved the clavicles and manubrium but not the cranium, 7th thoracic ring, pelvis or hip. Correction of the 7th and 2nd thoracic rings improved C4, the clavicles, manubrium, pelvis and hip but not the cranium. Correction of the cranium improved the clavicles, manubrium and pelvis but not the 2nd ring, 7th ring or hip. Correcting the cranium with alignment cues for the 2nd and 7th thoracic rings produced the best overall standing alignment.

This is a cranial and thorax (2nd and 7th thoracic rings) co-driver for standing posture since no single regional correction totally improved the alignment of all other sites of suboptimal alignment.

Screening task analysis – the squat

The key findings in the squat were:

- Cranial region: The cranium remained in a left intracranial torsion (ICT), with a congruently rotated sphenoid.

- Cervical segments: C4 remained translated right and side-bent and rotated left.

- Shoulder girdle: The right clavicle remained anteriorly rotated and the left clavicle remained posteriorly rotated.

- Upper thorax: The 2nd thoracic ring translated further left and rotated further right. The manubrium remained incongruently rotated to the left. This is an intrathoracic ring positional finding.

- Lower thorax: The 7th thoracic ring translated further left and rotated further right, congruent with the 2nd thoracic ring.

- Pelvis: The pelvis rotated further to the left and the left SIJ unlocked (lost control) midway through the task.

- Hips: The right femoral head remained anterior to the left.

Impact of corrections on the squat task – finding the drivers

Similar to the standing task, correcting the 2nd and 7th thoracic rings improved the majority of areas of failed load transfer in the squat. However, the left SIJ still lost control (unlocked) midway through the squat and the cranium remained in a left ICT. Correcting the cranium improved the clavicles, manubrium, and the pelvis but not the 2nd thoracic ring, 7th thoracic ring, or hip, and the left SIJ still unlocked in the task.

Correction of the thorax (2nd and 7th thoracic rings) and cranium was tested next. Verbal alignment cues were used for correction of the cranium and the 2nd thoracic ring allowing manual correction of the 7th thoracic ring as well as monitoring of SIJ control during the squat. Brad was cued to 'create space in his upper chest between his rib cage and collarbones while finding the feeling of length from the back of his skull.' This imagery allowed Brad to stack and align his upper thorax and cranium. The 7th thoracic ring was then manually corrected while monitoring both the right and then the left SIJ for unlocking in the task. With the cranium, 2nd and 7th thoracic rings corrected, both SIJs remained controlled in the squat task.

This is a cranial and thorax (2nd and 7th thoracic rings) co-driver for the squat task since no single regional correction completely restored the alignment and control of all other sites of suboptimal performance.

Screening task analysis – right and left one leg standing

The key findings in the right and left OLS were:

- Cranial region: The cranium remained in a left ICT, with a left rotated sphenoid in both OLS tasks.

- Cervical segments: C4 remained translated right and side-bent and rotated right in both OLS tasks.

- Shoulder girdle: The right clavicle remained anteriorly rotated on the right and posteriorly rotated on the left in both OLS tasks.

- Upper thorax: The 2nd thoracic ring translated further left and rotated further right and the manubrium remained incongruently rotated to the left in both OLS tasks.

- Lower thorax: The 7th thoracic ring translated further left and rotated further right in both OLS tasks, congruent with the 2nd thoracic ring.

- Pelvis: The pelvis remained in a left TPR and the left SIJ unlocked in both OLS tasks. During left hip flexion and single leg loading on the right, the left innominate anteriorly rotated relative to the left side of the sacrum. During left single leg loading, the left SIJ lost control.

- Hips: The right femoral head remained forward compared to the left in both the standing and lifted leg (in both LOLS and ROLS).

Impact of corrections on the OLS tasks – finding the drivers

Again, correcting the 2nd and 7th thoracic rings corrected C4 and the right hip in both the right and left OLS task. This correction did not restore complete control to the left SIJ during the LOLS task, nor did it restore the biomechanics of the left SIJ during the ROLS task.

Correcting the cranium improved the clavicles and the manubrium but did not restore control of the left SIJ. Correcting the 2nd and 7th thoracic rings and the cranium produced the best overall alignment, biomechanics, and control in the ROLS task.

For both the left and right OLS task, the pelvis is an additional driver. Drivers for this task include the cranium, thorax, and pelvis.

Vector analysis of the drivers

Driver – the thorax (2nd and 7th thoracic rings)

Vector analysis was performed to determine the underlying system impairment for the drivers using a passive listening technique where the thoracic rings were corrected and released and the dominant vectors noted (see Chapter 3). The dominant vectors affecting the 7th thoracic ring were the left internal oblique and the left anterior diaphragm. The left anterior intercostals were the dominant vector for the 2nd thoracic ring producing a short pull on the left 2nd rib into anterior rotation.

Driver – the cranial region

Passive listening during correction and release of the cranium revealed a long right-sided dural vector that extended to the sacrum and coccyx.

Driver – the pelvis

Vector analysis of the pelvis (left and right SIJ) revealed no restrictive vectors within the pelvic girdle itself. The neutral zone motion of the left SIJ (passive arthrokinematic mobility testing) revealed greater motion at the middle part of the joint when compared to the right side. A connect cue aimed at increasing the recruitment of the pelvic floor muscles reduced the neutral zone motion at the left SIJ and restored control of the left and right SIJ during the OLS tasks when combined with a cranium and thorax driver correction.

Impact of drivers on pelvic floor recruitment strategies, strength, and endurance

When Brad first attended for care, he had been practicing pelvic floor contractions as instructed by his urologist months before. He did not remember the specific instructions his urologist had given him, but could recall that he was supposed to 'squeeze his Kegels.' On examination of this recruitment strategy, there was observable co-contraction of many superficial muscles including the oblique abdominals, glutes, and adductors. In the supine position, using real-time ultrasound to observe muscle activity, there was significant recruitment of the left and right internal oblique when Brad was asked to 'squeeze his Kegels.' This co-activation produced notable *descent* of the bladder, observed via transabdominal ultrasound imaging. While supine, using a cue to keep the abdomen relaxed and then gently and slowly think about 'shortening the penis,' a cue shown to recruit the pelvic floor muscles, (Stafford et al. 2015), Brad could produce a *lift* of the pelvic floor muscles and hold the contraction for more than 10 seconds. However, in standing, when the bladder and pelvic floor were observed via ultrasound, it was found that there was a lift of the pelvic floor but no significant ability to hold this lift (Fig. 5.13A&B).

Brad's experience of urinary leakage was his primary measure of improvement for his meaningful tasks. Thus, it was important to explore the effect of correcting the cranium and thorax on his pelvic floor function in these tasks. Correcting the 2nd and 7th thoracic rings and cranium improved his ability to sustain the recruitment of his pelvic floor although there was still an endurance deficit. This is consistent with the finding that when loads increased significantly (i.e., OLS tasks), Brad was unable to retain control of his left and right SIJ unless the thorax and cranium were corrected *and a connect cue for his pelvic floor muscles added* (three drivers for this task). There was also an improvement in co-ordination of his TrA and IO when the cranial and thorax drivers were corrected. This was observed using real-time ultrasound.

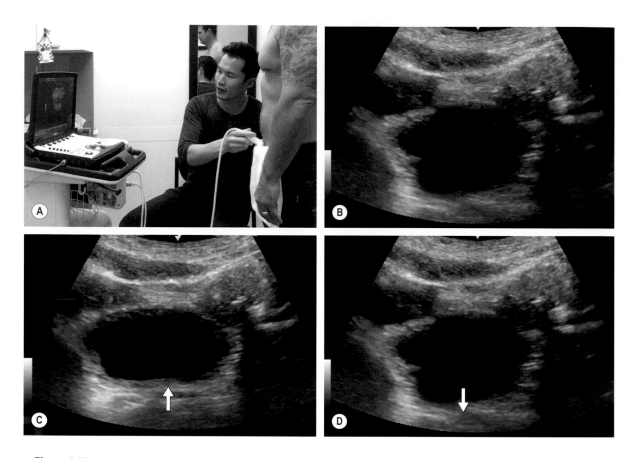

Figure 5.13

(A) Transabdominal imaging of the bladder and pelvic floor using ultrasound in standing during a pelvic floor contraction without any correction of the cranium or thorax. (B) Transabdominal ultrasound image of the bladder in standing prior to any instruction to contract the pelvic floor. Note the profile of the bladder and shape of its base. (C) Profile of the bladder during a pelvic floor contraction in standing. Note the lift of the base of the bladder (arrow). (D) Although Brad tried to keep his pelvic floor engaged, without correcting the alignment of his cranium and thorax, he was unable to sustain the contraction. Note the change in profile of the bladder and descent of the base, which occurred when the pelvic floor contraction reduced (arrow).

When all three drivers were corrected (cranial and thoracic alignment, pelvic control), Brad could squat further and lift his contralateral leg more easily and higher in the OLS tasks before he lost the ability to hold his pelvic floor muscles engaged. This is a Stage 2 training deficit (see Chapter 7) where the capacity (strength and endurance) of the pelvic floor muscles was the limiting factor to maintaining continence and control in higher loads of his meaningful tasks.

Figure 5.14 illustrates Brad's complete Clinical Puzzle for reflection of his findings.

A biologically plausible mechanism for thoracic and cranial contributions to incontinence

There are several biologically plausible mechanisms that may explain the impact of cranial and thoracic impairments on pelvic floor function and urinary continence.

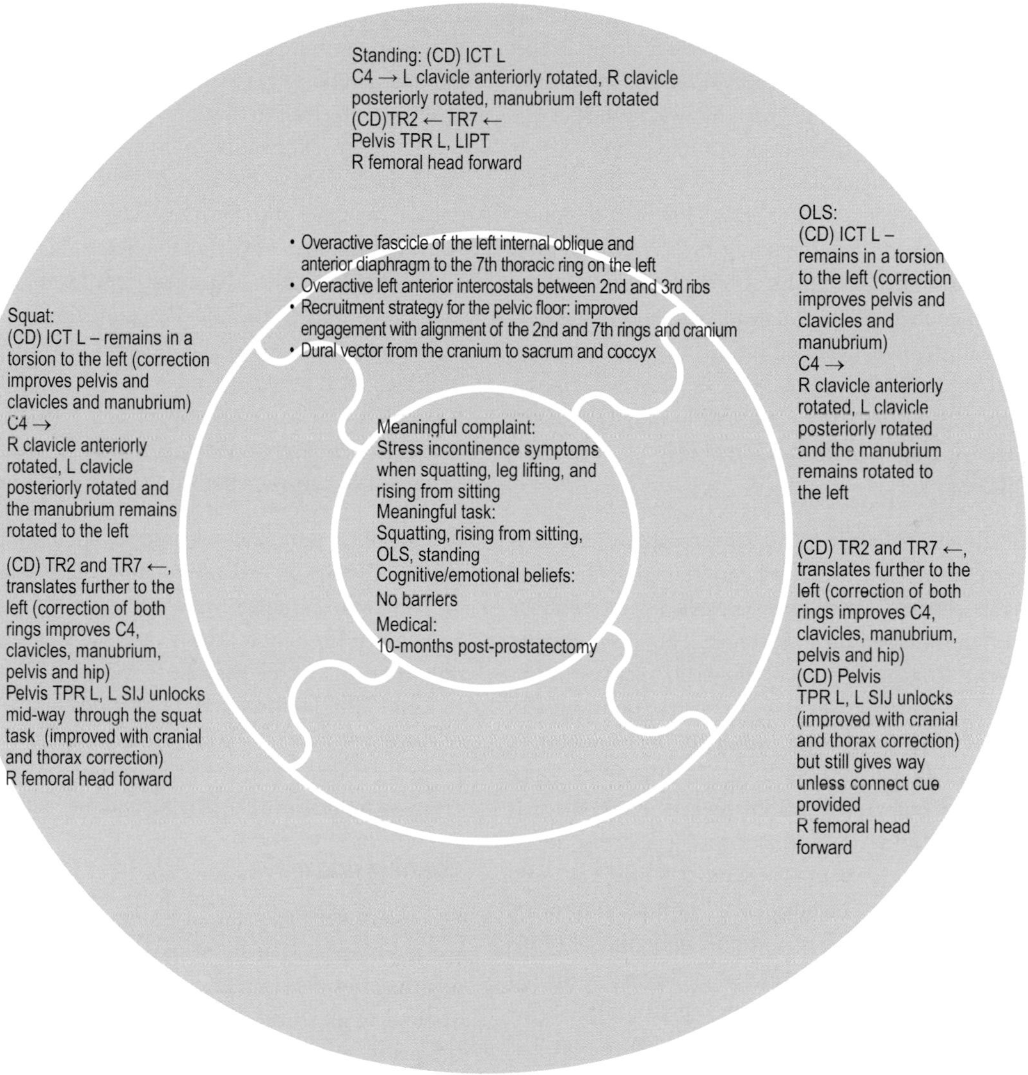

Standing: (CD) ICT L
C4 → L clavicle anteriorly rotated, R clavicle posteriorly rotated, manubrium left rotated
(CD)TR2 ← TR7 ←
Pelvis TPR L, LIPT
R femoral head forward

OLS:
(CD) ICT L – remains in a torsion to the left (correction improves pelvis and clavicles and manubrium)
C4 →
R clavicle anteriorly rotated, L clavicle posteriorly rotated and the manubrium remains rotated to the left

(CD) TR2 and TR7 ←, translates further to the left (correction of both rings improves C4, clavicles, manubrium, pelvis and hip)
(CD) Pelvis TPR L, L SIJ unlocks (improved with cranial and thorax correction) but still gives way unless connect cue provided
R femoral head forward

• Overactive fascicle of the left internal oblique and anterior diaphragm to the 7th thoracic ring on the left
• Overactive left anterior intercostals between 2nd and 3rd ribs
• Recruitment strategy for the pelvic floor: improved engagement with alignment of the 2nd and 7th rings and cranium
• Dural vector from the cranium to sacrum and coccyx

Squat:
(CD) ICT L – remains in a torsion to the left (correction improves pelvis and clavicles and manubrium)
C4 →
R clavicle anteriorly rotated, L clavicle posteriorly rotated and the manubrium remains rotated to the left

(CD) TR2 and TR7 ←, translates further to the left (correction of both rings improves C4, clavicles, manubrium, pelvis and hip)
Pelvis TPR L, L SIJ unlocks mid-way through the squat task (improved with cranial and thorax correction)
R femoral head forward

Meaningful complaint:
Stress incontinence symptoms when squatting, leg lifting, and rising from sitting
Meaningful task:
Squatting, rising from sitting, OLS, standing
Cognitive/emotional beliefs:
No barriers
Medical:
10-months post-prostatectomy

• Release: Unwind cranial ICT in crook-lying with wipers to lengthen the dural vector between the cranium and sacrum, RWA for the left IO and anterior diaphragm
• Stack and breathe for the 2nd ring to release intercostal vectors
• Align: Cued space behind the skull and elongation between the cranium and pelvis. Also alignment cues to breathe space laterally into the low ribs and upper chest with focus on breathing into the intercostal spaces around the 7th and 2nd rings
• Connect/control: Connect cues to 'shorten the penis' to engage pelvic floor in addition to alignment cues above to improve pelvic floor activation
• Move: Using the align and connect cues in the MTs - standing, squatting and OLS

Figure 5.14

Brad's completed Clinical Puzzle. CD = codriver, ICT = intracranial torsion, IO = internal oblique, LIPT = left intrapelvic torsion, MTs = meaningful tasks, OLS = one leg standing, RWA = release with awareness, SIJ = sacroiliac joint, TPR = transverse plane rotation, TR = thoracic ring, ← = left translation, → = right translation.

In Brad's case, it was hypothesized that the cranial correction reduced tension in the dura mater along the spinal canal to its distal end at the coccyx. Tension in the dura mater may extend through the perineurium to the peripheral nerves. As such, dural tension can impact pelvic floor function via its influence on the S2–S5 sacral nerve roots and the pudendal nerve. These structures provide innervation to the pelvic floor including the striated urethral sphincter and bulbospongiosus. Altered function of these muscles can contribute to urinary incontinence, especially in tasks that produce increased intra-abdominal pressure. Increased intra-abdominal pressure is known to impact the ability of the pelvic floor muscles to maintain continence against bladder neck descent (Delancey & Ashton-Miller 2004).

Clinically, it is observed that after prostatectomy men often have suboptimal recruitment strategies for pelvic control. Specifically, overactivation of the internal oblique (IO) is often observed on ultrasound. This IO-dominant recruitment strategy has been shown to increase intra-abdominal pressure greater than the pelvic floor muscles can support, resulting in a net descent of the bladder neck (Junginger et al. 2010). This highlights the importance of optimizing load transfer from regions above the pelvis while performing tasks that typically increase intra-abdominal pressure, such as squats, leg lifts and even standing, for men with incontinence. For Brad, improving alignment of his cranium and thorax and control of his pelvis improved the recruitment and endurance (capacity) of his pelvic floor muscles in his meaningful tasks. However, postoperative weakness was still apparent and it is likely that Brad will need to train the strength and capacity of his pelvic floor muscles in addition to addressing the alignment of his cranium and thorax.

ISM treatment for Brad's thorax and cranial driven pelvis

Release and align

A release with awareness technique was used to release the anterior costal fibers of the left side of the diaphragm and the left internal oblique, both of which were impacting the alignment and biomechanics of the 7th thoracic ring.

Thoracic ring stack and breathe (Lee L-J 2016) was used to release the anterior intercostal vector related to the 2nd thoracic ring. Cues to breathe into the left upper chest were given to bias release to the upper anterior intercostals. Brad was taught a self-practice to do at home for the 2nd and 7th thoracic rings with cues to breathe into the upper chest to bias the upper anterior intercostals and cues to breathe wide into the sides of thorax to release the left diaphragm and internal oblique. Alignment cues for the thorax were given to improve 2nd and 7th thoracic ring alignment including breath work and imagery. Imagery included 'think about creating space between the ribs, let the ribs float apart' particularly between ribs 2 to 7 on the left. Breath work imagery was thought to be pertinent as Brad's dominant vectors were both associated with breathing.

The spinal dura was released in hook lying with the pelvis initially in neutral rotation. The longer neural vectors into the pelvis were addressed by subsequently adding pelvic rotation (slowly take the knees to one side) only until the vector was felt to create more intracranial torsion. This position was maintained until the vector released (see Chapter 6). Release and alignment cues were given for the cranium with the intention to elongate and create space between the occiput and the sacrum.

Connect and move

A connect cue was required to improve the endurance of the recruitment strategy of the pelvic floor muscles once alignment of the cranium and thorax had been achieved. Stafford et al. (2015) suggested that a cue for 'shortening the penis' results in the greatest engagement of the striated urethral sphincter and bulbospongiosus muscles. As such, Brad was instructed to imagine shortening his penis to recruit his pelvic floor and lift the urethra. Brad began Stage 2 capacity training for his pelvic floor in supine and side lying (see Chapter 7) and quickly progressed to training in standing. He could use his pelvic floor connect cue in addition to his alignment cues for his thorax and cranium to produce a more sustainable contraction of his pelvic floor muscles without excessively increasing his intra-abdominal pressure. The result was improved range of movement in his meaningful tasks (squat and OLS) without significant bladder descent, urinary leakage or loss of SIJ control.

Conclusion

Brad was diligent with his home practice and applied the focused attention and massed practice required to change his posture, alignment, and motor control strategies. He has been able to improve his urinary incontinence symptoms in all his meaningful tasks. His use of absorption pads is reduced and they are regularly less saturated. He is continuing to work on improving his alignment and movement strategies into deeper ranges of his squat and continues to receive support with augmented training in clinic using real-time ultrasound as biofeedback. This helps to improve and refine his ability to align and control his thorax and cranium while engaging his pelvic floor. He is currently working on Stage 2 training of his meaningful tasks (see Chapter 7) to improve his inter-regional mobility and control of the thorax and cranium with limb loading. His program will progress into Stage 3 integrated whole body tasks with focus on multiple planes of movement in congruent and incongruent patterns.

Thorax and cranial driven pelvic floor in a patient with stress urinary incontinence

Tamarah Nerreter

Lisa's story and current meaningful complaint

At the time of this initial assessment, Lisa was a 40-year-old nulliparous, child development consultant who was referred by a gynecologist for ongoing stress urinary incontinence related to laughing and coughing. The gynecologist prescribed 'Kegels' and medication for treatment; however, this did not improve her condition.

Lisa's history of multiple minor motor vehicle accidents resulting in whiplash-associated disorder (ongoing neck pain) and headaches and other accidents (a fall onto her tailbone and an ankle sprain) could individually or collectively contribute to this pelvic floor dysfunction. That Lisa is also a cancer survivor is worthy of note. She was diagnosed with breast cancer in October 2009, treated with chemotherapy and, ultimately, a right mastectomy with a full breast reconstruction. She has been working with a naturopathic doctor to re-establish her precancer hormone function. Lisa is an avid dragon boat racer since being diagnosed with cancer and races with a group of women who are all survivors. She is not sexually active and requested that an internal pelvic floor examination not be carried out.

Lisa's meaningful complaint was persistent urinary incontinence, which was aggravated by two tasks: Laughing and coughing.

Urinary leakage would occur with laughing or coughing in both the standing and seated positions.

Lisa did not experience pain; however, she did report ongoing tension and tightness throughout her upper back and neck both during her meaningful tasks (laughing and coughing) and in daily life.

Lisa's cognitive beliefs

Lisa believed that her bladder was the main problem and that her pelvic floor was not strong enough. She did occasionally experience stress urinary incontinence as a child and adolescent; however, the episodes were less frequent than the past few years. When medication did not yield any results, and the 'Kegels' prescribed by the gynecologist did not seem to strengthen the pelvic floor, she thought her condition might somehow be related to her breast cancer experience.

Lisa's emotional status

Lisa did not show any signs of distress, anxiety, depression or anger regarding her meaningful complaint. We spoke about her breast cancer experience, and she did disclose that the experience was 'beyond words.' With the help of her naturopathic doctor and counseling provided by the BC Cancer Agency, she felt she had confidently dealt with the emotional side of the experience.

Meaningful task and screening tasks chosen for strategy analysis

Lisa's meaningful task was to be able to laugh or cough in any social setting without leaking urine. The screening tasks chosen for the analysis of strategy were standing and squat to sit.

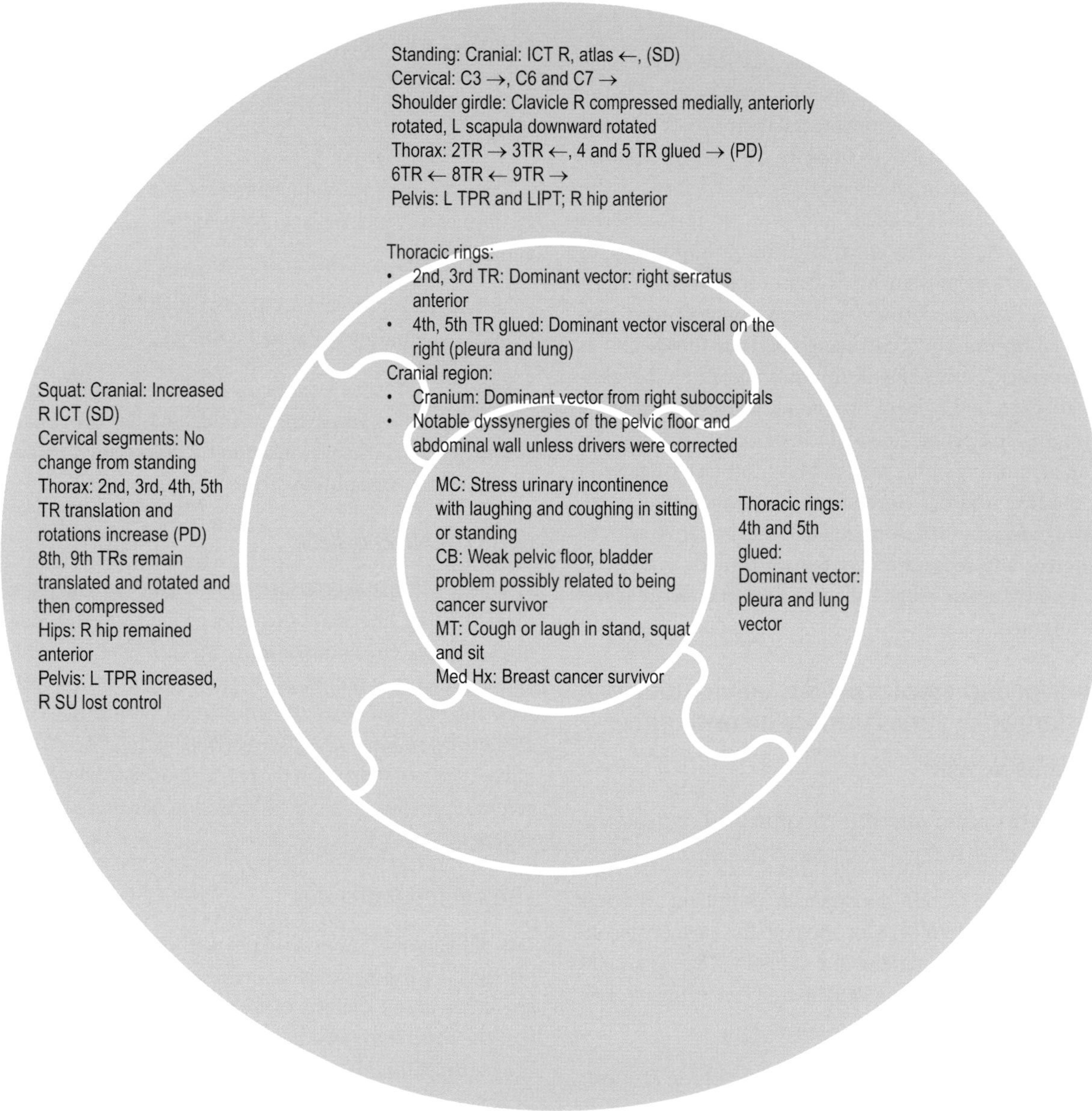

Standing: Cranial: ICT R, atlas ←, (SD)
Cervical: C3 →, C6 and C7 →
Shoulder girdle: Clavicle R compressed medially, anteriorly rotated, L scapula downward rotated
Thorax: 2TR → 3TR ←, 4 and 5 TR glued → (PD)
6TR ← 8TR ← 9TR →
Pelvis: L TPR and LIPT; R hip anterior

Thoracic rings:
- 2nd, 3rd TR: Dominant vector: right serratus anterior
- 4th, 5th TR glued: Dominant vector visceral on the right (pleura and lung)

Cranial region:
- Cranium: Dominant vector from right suboccipitals
- Notable dyssynergies of the pelvic floor and abdominal wall unless drivers were corrected

MC: Stress urinary incontinence with laughing and coughing in sitting or standing
CB: Weak pelvic floor, bladder problem possibly related to being cancer survivor
MT: Cough or laugh in stand, squat and sit
Med Hx: Breast cancer survivor

Thoracic rings:
4th and 5th glued:
Dominant vector: pleura and lung vector

Squat: Cranial: Increased R ICT (SD)
Cervical segments: No change from standing
Thorax: 2nd, 3rd, 4th, 5th TR translation and rotations increase (PD)
8th, 9th TRs remain translated and rotated and then compressed
Hips: R hip remained anterior
Pelvis: L TPR increased, R SU lost control

Figure 5.15

Lisa's completed Clinical Puzzle. CB = cognitive belief, ICT R = intracranial torsion right, LIPT = left intrapelvic torsion, LTPR = left transverse plane rotation, MC = meaningful complaint, Med Hx = medical history, MT = meaningful task, PD = primary driver, SD = secondary driver, SIJ = sacroiliac joint, TR = thoracic ring, ← = left translation, → = right translation.

The key findings from Lisa's story are noted in the center of her Clinical Puzzle (Fig. 5.15) and included:

- Meaningful complaint: Stress urinary incontinence with laughing and coughing in sitting or standing.

- Cognitive belief: Weak pelvic floor or possible contributing effects from the mastectomy and chemotherapy.

- Meaningful tasks: To be able to laugh or cough without urinary leakage in any social situation.

Screening task analysis – standing

The key clinical findings were:

- Cranial region: Right intracranial torsion (ICT); atlas translated left and rotated right (congruent with the 3rd thoracic ring and the 6th and 8th thoracic rings).

- Cervical segments: C3 translated right and rotated left (congruent with 2nd thoracic ring, 4th, 5th, and 9th thoracic rings); C6 and C7 translated right and rotated left (congruent with 2nd thoracic ring and 4th, 5th, and 9th thoracic rings).

- Shoulder girdle: Left scapula downward rotated, right clavicle compressed medially and anteriorly rotated.

- Thorax – upper and middle regions: 2nd thoracic ring translated right and rotated left; 3rd thoracic ring translated left and rotated right; glued 4th and 5th thoracic rings translated right and rotated left; 6th thoracic ring translated left and rotated right.

- Thorax – lower region: 8th thoracic ring translated left and rotated right; 9th thoracic ring translated right and rotated left.

- Pelvis: Left transverse plane rotation associated with a congruent left intrapelvic torsion (LTPR and LIPT).

- Hips: The right femoral head was anterior relative to the acetabulum, which is congruent with the LTPR of the pelvis.

Impact of corrections on standing posture – finding the drivers

Correcting the alignment of Lisa's pelvis improved the alignment of her right hip; however, it made the alignment of her thorax, neck, and cranial region worse. Correcting the alignment of the right hip improved her pelvis; however, this correction did not change or improve her thorax, neck or cranial region. Correcting the alignment of the 8th and 9th thoracic rings improved the alignment of her pelvis, hip, and neck, worsened the alignment of her upper thorax, and did not change the cranial region. Correcting the alignment of the 2nd, 3rd, 4th, and 5th thoracic rings collectively resulted in complete correction of alignment of the cervical segments, pelvis and hip, and a partial correction of the cranial region. A correction of the right ICT (cranium) and cranium over the atlas facilitated further correction of the 2nd to 5th thoracic rings.

In addition to improved alignment, Lisa reported feeling lighter, and she could take a bigger breath when her thorax and cranial regions were corrected (her experience improved). These findings suggest that Lisa's primary driver in standing was the thorax with a secondary cranial region driver.

Screening task analysis – squat to sit

The key clinical findings in the squat-to-sit task were:

- Cranial region: The right ICT noted in standing increased during the squat task.

- Cervical segments: C3 remained translated right and rotated left; C6 and C7 remained translated right and rotated left.

- Thorax – upper and middle regions: The 2nd to 6th thoracic ring translations and rotations all increased.

- Thorax – lower region: The alignment of the 8th and 9th thoracic rings did not change; however, increased internal oblique activation and upper abdominal bracing added more compression of both thoracic rings medially.

- Hips: The right hip remained slightly anterior as the squat deepened (failed to center).

- Pelvis: LTPR increased and the right sacroiliac joint (SIJ) lost control (the right innominate was noted to anteriorly rotate relative to the right side of the sacrum) and this occurred late in the task.

Impact of corrections on the squat task – finding the drivers

The best correction for this task was correcting the alignment of the 2nd to 5th thoracic rings, which in turn corrected the alignment and control of the cervical segments, pelvis, and right hip. An additional verbal cue to facilitate correction of the cranial region improved the ability to completely restore the alignment of the thoracic rings. This combined cranial region and thorax correction resulted in a better strategy for control of the right SIJ, which remained controlled throughout the squat. Less abdominal bracing was noted, and reported, during the squat.

The primary driver for this task is the thorax and the secondary driver is the cranial region.

Vector analysis of the drivers

Vector analysis, or assessment of active and passive mobility and active and passive control, determines the underlying system impairments and is done only at the regions of the driver or drivers.

Primary driver – the thorax (2nd, 3rd, 4th, and 5th thoracic rings)

Passive listening during correction and release was used to determine the underlying system impairments causing the suboptimal alignment and biomechanics of the 2nd, 3rd, 4th, and 5th thoracic rings in both the standing and squat-to-sit task. This test revealed a dominant vector of pull from the right serratus anterior (the vector was short and lateral) to both the right 2nd and 3rd ribs. Another (later) vector of pull was felt from the right posterior scalene, which attaches to C5, C6, C7, and the anterior aspect of the 2nd rib. Given the position of the right 2nd rib (anteriorly rotated), this later vector is likely a reactor to the dominant vector arising from a fascicle of the right serratus anterior.

Passive listening of the glued 4th and 5th thoracic rings during both correction and release revealed a dominant vector of pull that went inside the thorax to the pleura and lung (a visceral vector).

Secondary driver – the cranial region

Passive listening during release of the right ICT revealed a dominant vector of pull on the right, which was posterior and deep. This vector was extracranial (outside the cranium) between the cranium and upper neck arising from the deep suboccipital muscles.

Impact of the thorax driver on the abdominal wall and pelvic floor recruitment strategy

Using real-time ultrasound, a transabdominal view of the bladder and pelvic floor revealed asymmetric overactivity of the pelvic floor muscles; the right side was greater than the left (Fig. 5.16). Minimal elevation of the bladder base occurred with a cue aimed to recruit the pelvic floor muscles. Furthermore, there was minimal response of the lower or middle fibers of the transversus abdominis to this cue. The internal oblique, however, responded to the pelvic floor cue with increased activation on both the right and left, with greater activation on the right than on the left. When the alignment of the thorax (2nd to 5th thoracic rings) and cranial region was corrected, an immediate improvement in the resting tone of the pelvic floor occurred (Fig. 5.17A). A notable increase in the bladder base lift (produced by contraction of the levator ani) occurred when Lisa was then given the same verbal cue to contract her pelvic floor (Fig. 5.17B). The lower and middle fibers of the transversus abdominis responded appropriately to this cue and the response of the internal oblique was diminished. This improved response of the deep muscles is likely why her SIJ control was restored in the squat task when the cranial and thorax regions were corrected.

Lisa reported that the combined correction of her thorax and cranial regions allowed her to breathe more easily, and she felt this allowed her to relax her superficial abdominal muscles and pelvic floor. She reported improvement in the sensation of her pelvic floor recruitment and that it did not feel 'as labored.'

ISM treatment for Lisa's thorax and cranial driven pelvic floor

Release and align

Release with awareness was used to reduce the overactivation of the right serratus anterior, specifically the fascicles

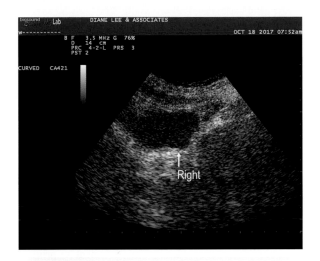

Figure 5.16

Before treatment: Transabdominal view of the bladder and pelvic floor using real-time ultrasound imaging. Note. This image does not follow the usual convention in ultrasound in that the right side of the image is the right side of the patient's body. Optimally, the base of the bladder should be a convex shape toward the *bottom* of the image. Note how the bottom of the bladder is concave, lifted more on the right than the left (arrow). This suggests overactivation of the pelvic floor muscles, more so on the right than on the left.

pertaining to the right 2nd and 3rd ribs. (see Chapter 6). Subsequently, thoracic ring stack and breathe (a general, multiple system release technique [Lee L-J 2016]) was used to release the visceral vectors 'gluing' the 4th and 5th thoracic rings. Self-release techniques were taught for home practice: Thoracic ring stack and breathe with a focus on the 4th and 5th thoracic rings and a ball release home practice in side lying for the right serratus anterior fascicles to the 2nd and 3rd ribs. The right suboccipital muscles were released using release with awareness.

Concurrently, a home practice aimed at improving cranial and thoracic alignment in conjunction with relaxation and recruitment of the pelvic floor and transversus abdominis was given. Lisa was instructed to sit on a soft ball (placed at the perineum, between the ischial tuberosities), to align her thorax (2nd to 5th thoracic rings) and cranial region with both manual and imagery cues, and then to practice both relaxing and contracting her pelvic floor and transversus abdominis. This is a Stage 1 motor learning practice.

Once Lisa could master this home practice, she was instructed to maintain her cranial and thoracic alignment and then anteriorly and posteriorly tilt her pelvis. This is a progression to Stage 2 strategy capacity training for static

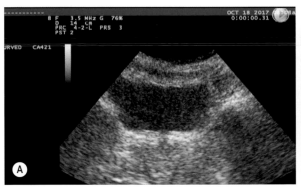

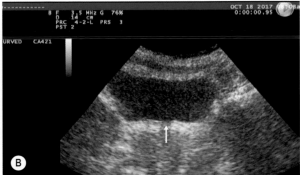

Figure 5.17

After treatment: Transabdominal view of the bladder and pelvic floor using real-time ultrasound imaging. (A) At rest. Compare the shape of the bladder base at rest to Figure 5.16. Note how the shape is less concave, flatter and more symmetrical between sides. (B) When Lisa was given a cue to contract and then relax all three layers of her pelvic floor muscles, a midline lift of the bladder base (arrow), followed by relaxation, was seen. This is a better recruitment and relaxation strategy of the pelvic floor muscles and could only be produced when the alignment of her cranial and thorax regions was corrected.

alignment since neither the thorax nor cranial regions are moving.

Connect and control

Once Lisa could maintain alignment of the cranial region and thorax, diaphragmatic breathing, co-ordinated with pelvic floor descent on the inhale, was encouraged to restore synergy between the respiratory and pelvic diaphragms (Stage 2 strategy capacity training). Both release and connect cues were incorporated into this practice. Release cues aimed at facilitating further release of the pelvic floor included: Imagine your sitting bones widening, your tailbone growing long, and space between the front, back and sides of your pelvis.

Once Lisa began to feel a sensation of lightness through her thorax, abdomen, pelvis, and hips, she was taught to correctly activate (connect to) all three muscular layers of the pelvic floor. The connect cues included:

- Bring the clitoris to the anus (layer 1 – superficial urogenital diaphragm);

- Compress the urethra by 'holding the pee' (layer 2 – deep urogenital diaphragm);

- 'Close your curtains' meaning bring the labia together (layers 1 and 2 including superficial and deep transverse perineal muscles); and

- 'Lift the elevator' meaning bring the anus to the pubic bone (layer 3 – levator ani).

Lisa was instructed to hold this co-contraction for three breaths and then relax for three breaths. This was progressed to holding the pelvic floor contraction for five to eight breath cycles and then relaxing for two to three breath cycles. Co-activation of the transversus abdominis was encouraged. This motor learning practice was initially done in supine and then progressed to more vertically loaded positions, such as sitting, standing, and squat (Lisa's meaningful task positions).

Move

Lisa's initial movement practice was to integrate her release, align and connect cues while standing. Once this was mastered, she practiced maintaining optimal alignment of her thorax and cranial regions and a gentle recruitment of the deep system (pelvic floor and transversus abdominis) without breath holding as she moved from standing through a squat to sit (Stage 2 movement training).

In sitting, Lisa was instructed to practice her release, align, and connect cues and then cough and giggle. To associate this new strategy for alignment and control to a variety of social contexts, Lisa was advised to add watching funny shows (in private) while training. This is meaningful task training and meets the requirements of both cognitive and associative motor learning (see Chapter 7). Over time, and with practice, the strategy should become automatic.

Conclusion

Lisa's story is not uncommon when assessment for primarily pelvic floor complaints includes the whole body and person using the Integrated Systems Model. Her primary impairment is a thorax-driven pelvic floor impairment, with a secondary cranial region driver. She continues to intermittently attend for treatment, especially through the dragon boating season, which is highly compressive on the thorax and can result in loss of alignment, which then leads to increased frequency of urinary leakage. Leakage can also occur when she has a significant chest cold associated with strong coughing. Overall, Lisa reports that her episodes of urinary incontinence continue to decrease as her whole-body alignment and strategies for managing increased abdominal canister pressure improve.

Short case reports

What follows are not complete case reports but rather clinical examples that highlight key elements of assessment not covered in the case reports above.

Thorax-driven head and neck in a patient with restricted left rotation

Diane Lee

Video 5.30 (free code)

Miyuki: A thorax-driven head and neck in restricted left rotation

Miyuki's story and current meaningful complaint and task (Video 5.30)

Miyuki had restricted left rotation of her head and neck.

Meaningful task analysis – left head and neck rotation in sitting

Sites of suboptimal alignment, biomechanics or control for left rotation of the head and neck:

- Clavicles: Loss of anterior rotation in the right clavicle and posterior rotation in the left clavicle.

- Left scapula: Was protracted and anteriorly tilted.

- Upper and middle thorax: The 2nd, 3rd and 4th thoracic rings were all translated left and rotated right in sitting and remained translated left and rotated right during left rotation of the head and neck.

- Cervical segments: C7 and C2 were both translated left and rotated right in sitting; however, both C2 and C7 could translate right and rotate left during left rotation of the head and neck (suboptimal position in sitting but optimal biomechanics for the left head and neck rotation task).

The corrections carried out during the meaningful task of left head and neck rotation had the following results:

- Correction of the 3rd thoracic ring corrected the alignment of the 2nd and 4th thoracic rings and C7 in sitting. This correction restored the biomechanics of both the left and right clavicles and improved the amplitude and Miyuki's experience of left head and neck rotation.

- Correction of the left scapula corrected the alignment of the 2nd, 3rd, and 4th thoracic rings but did not have the same impact on the amplitude of left head and neck rotation, nor did it improve the experience of this task as much as correcting the 3rd thoracic ring.

The primary driver for Miyuki's left head and neck rotation task was the thorax, specifically the 3rd thoracic ring.

Vector analysis of the driver – the thorax (3rd thoracic ring)

Passive listening during correction of the 3rd thoracic ring

When correcting the 3rd thoracic ring, there was a sensation that the vector impeding the correction was coming from beneath the scapula. A metaphor for this sensation is that it feels like you are 'stuffing your foot into a shoe with a sock in the toe.' This is often a vector from a specific fascicle of serratus anterior.

Passive listening on release of the correction of the 3rd thoracic ring

When the 3rd thoracic ring correction was released, both the left 3rd rib and the scapula moved simultaneously; the left 3rd rib into anterior rotation and the scapula into protraction. This suggests that the left serratus anterior may be overactive and palpation of the fascicle overlying the body of the left 3rd rib confirmed this hypothesis.

ISM treatment

Release with awareness for the specific fascicle of the left serratus anterior related to the left 3rd rib (see Chapter 6) followed by a specific myofascial stretch of the interface between the serratus anterior and the subscapularis. Reassessment of left head and neck rotation revealed improved amplitude of motion and a reduction in the sense of restriction for Miyuki. More myofascial mobilization of the interface between the left subscapularis and serratus anterior would be needed for complete restoration of function.

Thorax-driven thorax in restricted rotation of the thorax – articular system impairment

Diane Lee

Video 5.31 (free code)

Ayami: Articular system impairment of the costotransverse joint impacting rotation of the thorax

Ayami's story and current meaningful complaint and task (Video 5.31)

Ayami continued to present with restricted right rotation of the thorax with no improvement in the performance or experience of this task after multiple neural system releases were carried out during a four-day course on the thorax in Japan.

Meaningful task analysis – right rotation of the thorax in sitting

The following were sites of suboptimal alignment, biomechanics or control for right rotation of the thorax:

- The 3rd thoracic ring remained translated right and rotated left;

- The alignment of the 3rd thoracic ring in neutral sitting could not be corrected and the correction was met with an immediate hard resistance indicative of an articular system impairment.

The hypothesis was that there was a stiff joint within the 3rd thoracic ring that was impacting right rotation and left translation. Further analysis of the articular system specific to the 3rd thoracic ring was required to confirm or negate this hypothesis.

Vector analysis of the driver – the thorax (3rd thoracic ring)

- Active osteokinematic mobility: The 3rd thoracic ring was unable to rotate actively or passively to the right.

- Passive arthrokinematic mobility:

  ○ Inferior glide of the right 3rd costotransverse joint: Restricted;

  ○ Superior glide of the left 3rd costotransverse joint: Mobile;

  ○ Inferior glide of the right zygapophyseal joint T2–T3: Mobile;

  ○ Superior glide of the left zygapophyseal joint T2–T3: Mobile.

ISM treatment

A vector-specific inferior glide mobilization technique (see Chapter 6) was applied to the right costotransverse joint (sustained hold until the vector released). An immediate improvement in the amplitude of right thoracic rotation occurred as well as an improvement in Ayami's experience of the task. The biomechanics of the 3rd thoracic ring were now congruent with the thoracic ring above and below and the 3rd thoracic ring was now aligned with those above and below in sitting.

Articular system impairments prevent correction of alignment of a thoracic ring and do not respond to general or specific neural system release techniques.

Pelvis-driven thorax in a patient experiencing pain in sitting

Diane Lee

Video 5.32 (free code)

Leah: Pelvis-driven thorax in pain in sitting

Leah's story and current meaningful complaint and task (Video 5.32)

Meaningful complaint: Burning in the midthorax, and pain which radiated up the right side of her neck within minutes of sitting on a portable treatment table. Leah noted that using her arms did not change her experience during sitting. The symptoms appeared regardless of what she did with her arms, head or neck. She also experienced the same symptoms when she squatted to sit on a chair; however, for the 'portable treatment table sitting task' a squat is not a useful screening task.

Meaningful task analysis – sitting using a weight-bearing-arm strategy

Leah used her arms to 'vault' into sitting on the portable treatment table during class. During this meaningful task, she lost control of her right SIJ and her pelvis ended up in a left transverse plane rotation with the right SIJ unlocked. There was notable overactivation of the right longissimus and when the specific fascicle was traced superiorly, the tendon inserted into the right transverse process of T6. This was consistent with the location of her midthoracic burning symptoms. This strategy could be an attempt to nutate her sacrum and thus provide more force closure to her pelvis.

Correction of the 7th thoracic ring reduced the activation of the right longissimus; however, correction of this thoracic ring did not provide control to the right SIJ when she repeated her meaningful task. A squat task for sitting in a chair without weight bearing through her arms was also tested. Her right SIJ lost control early in the squat and she sat in a chair with the same postural pattern and the same overactivation of the right longissimus. Correction of the 7th thoracic ring did not result in a controlled pelvis during her squat task to sit in a chair. Providing compression to her pelvis to control the right SIJ as she 'vaulted' onto the table, and as she squatted to sit in a chair, corrected both the pelvis and the alignment of the 7th thoracic ring in sitting and resulted in reduced activation of the right longissimus. Leah was then able to sit for longer without midthoracic burning or radiation of symptoms into her neck. The pelvis is the driver for both tasks and loss of control and the resultant suboptimal neuromuscular strategy for sitting was the likely cause of her midthoracic and neck pain.

Vector analysis of her pelvis (active and passive mobility, active and passive control) would be required to determine the underlying system impairment perturbing control of her right SIJ when she sat.

Thorax-driven loss of cervical control for left arm elevation

Diane Lee

Video 5.33 (free code)

Elayne: Thorax-driven loss of cervical control for left arm elevation

Elayne's story and current meaningful complaint and task (Video 5.33)

Meaningful complaint and task: Difficulty with elevation of the left arm; it feels weak.

Meaningful task analysis – left arm elevation

The following were sites of suboptimal alignment, biomechanics or control for elevation of the left arm:

- The 5th thoracic ring started translated left and rotated right, the 4th thoracic ring started translated right and rotated left and the position of both thoracic rings did not change when Elayne elevated her left arm to 90 degrees.

- C7 started translated left and rotated right and did not change with left arm elevation.

With added load the results were as follows:

- When resistance was added to this task (increased load) the 4th thoracic ring translated further right and rotated further left, the 5th thoracic ring translated further left and rotated to the right, and C7 translated further left and rotated further right.

The impact of corrections was as follows:

- Correction of the 4th and 5th thoracic rings resulted in an automatic correction in the alignment of C7.

- Correction of the 4th and 5th thoracic rings resulted in reduced effort to lift her left arm and C7 remained controlled when load was added to her arm

- Correcting the alignment of C7 did not improve the alignment of the 4th and 5th thoracic rings, nor did it improve the performance of the arm elevation task.

Hypothesis

The suboptimal alignment and control of the 4th and 5th thoracic rings were perturbing the alignment and control of C7. Collectively, poor alignment and control of all three segments was impairing Elayne's ability to lift her left arm effortlessly. Vector analysis (active and passive mobility and control) of the 4th and 5th thoracic rings was required to determine the underlying system impairment and direct the treatment plan.

Summary

Individual case reports, while not ranked as high level evidence, contribute significantly to our body of knowledge. As mentioned in Chapter 3, current evidence and clinical experience (Garner 2016, Hodges 2015, Hodges et al. 2013, Jones & Rivett 2004, Kent & Hartvigsen 2015, Moseley & Butler 2017, O'Sullivan et al. 2015, Sahrmann & van Dillen 2015) support an individual, clinically reasoned, biopsychosocial approach for complex patients. This chapter has provided several case reports for complex and less complex cases to illustrate how the Integrated Systems Model helps to structure individualized care, and the role the thorax plays across multiple musculoskeletal conditions.

Release techniques for system impairments

Note to reader: It is not the intention of this chapter to describe every release technique possible for all system impairments. An overview of an integrated approach to release techniques, some of which are specific and others more general, are described in this chapter. The focus is on articular and neural system restrictive impairments, recognizing that the myofascial and visceral systems are also important. This author's strengths are in the articular and neural systems and she prefers to refer readers to alternate resources for structure-specific myofascial and visceral releases.

Introduction

The Integrated Systems Model (ISM) helps the clinician to organize all the information from the assessment to develop prescriptive, individual treatment programs. The ISM acronym for treatment is RACM: Release, Align, Connect and Control, Move. ISM treatment is initially directed toward the driver or drivers and each session contains components of techniques, exercises, and education to *release* and *align* the driver (region of the body that when corrected has the biggest impact on the function of other regions). Following release, reassessment of the screening task determines whether motor control training – *connect and control* – for specific muscles pertaining to the driver (primary or secondary) is necessary. The final and critical part of each session is training to *move*. The aim is to build new 'brain maps' and movement strategies that transfer load, and control excessive cranial, thoracic, abdominal or pelvic pressure in a way that sustains tissue structure, blood flow and drainage, function, and overall health. This chapter describes specific techniques for releasing barriers to change.

Release and align

Treatment begins by addressing the variety of barriers (cognitive, emotional, sensorial and physical) that are contributing to the suboptimal strategies for the meaningful task and goals. Motor control and strategies for movement are influenced by multiple mechanisms and the goal of assessment is to determine the primary barrier to change. Cognitive, emotional, and physical barriers are considered relevant in biopsychosocial approaches such as ISM; however, gut health is not regularly addressed as part of physiotherapy practice. However, ingesting potential neurotoxins such as excessive gluten, dairy, alcohol, sugar, hydrogenated oils, and aspartame can impact inflammation and pain as well as the ease with which new motor pathways are developed. Gut health, and its role in inflammatory and chronic pain states, is sometimes the primary barrier to restoring overall movement health. If this is not a 'tool in your toolbox,' find someone in your community who is able to educate your patients on the role of nutrition (acidic versus alkaline diets, elimination diets, hydration, etc.) in musculoskeletal health.

Cognitive barriers

Cognitive barriers (thoughts and beliefs) are addressed with education through conversations, videos, books, websites or referral to other professionals (counselors, psychologists, etc.). A powerful way to change thoughts and beliefs is to offer a logical hypothesis derived from the assessment that explains the pain experience, and the problem, in understandable and nonthreatening language. This can help to reduce anxiety and threat, restore self-confidence and hope for the future by giving back control. Always avoid catastrophizing language, and if you verbalize your findings during an ISM assessment be sure to put them in context ensuring that the patient leaves with a positive understanding of their problem and the plan for change. Make sure you have agreement on what will be used to monitor change (function versus pain), in other words, agreement on what they will reflect on (the meaningful complaint) before the next session to answer the question 'how are you?'

Emotional barriers

Emotional barriers (fear, anger, threat, sadness, depression) can be addressed by changing the body's reaction to thoughts or social contexts. Techniques to dampen the sympathetic nervous system (SNS) and augment the parasympathetic nervous system (PNS) are helpful for those whose SNS has been 'hijacked' and is in a high state of threat. Many treatment techniques can help, including:

- craniosacral therapy

- acupuncture

- salt float tanks

- meditation

- conscious breathing or relaxing pranayama (controlled breath practices)

- counseling.

The technique chosen depends on the skill set of the practitioner, the referral network, and the effect of the technique or practice on the patient. For all techniques and practices, creating a safe environment to practice is critical for success.

Sensorial and physical barriers

Sensorial and physical barriers are those created by the various system impairments underlying the suboptimal alignment, biomechanics and control of the driver, determined through vector analysis. Once the driver for the meaningful task is determined, further assessment, including active and passive mobility tests (including vector analysis) and active and passive control tests of the driver or drivers differentiates the order and system for release. After each release technique, the screening task is repeated to assess the impact of the intervention. Commonly, four to six vectors are present; however, only two to three are dominant and the others are reactive. Passive listening during correction and release of the driver identifies the specific system and structure within that system, which then determines the relevant release technique. The screening task that is related to the meaningful task is repeated after complete release of the driver to determine if control of the driver is required, or if motor control has been automatically restored after release. If the alignment, biomechanics, and control of the driver are now optimal, no specific motor control training is required and the movement training practice can

focus on maintaining the alignment and biomechanics of the driver in task-specific movements (see Stage 2 and 3 training in Chapter 7). If after release, or after a few repetitions of the screening task, suboptimal alignment, biomechanics or control of one or more drivers persist, and passive listening does not reveal any limiting vectors impacting the driver, then the underlying impairment is one of motor control, strength and endurance. Specific motor control training (Stage 1 motor learning), followed by Stage 2 strategy capacity training and then Stage 3, Levels 1 to 3 movement training of more complex tasks that require mobility and control of multiple body regions are then required (see Chapter 7). Expect the drivers to change both during a treatment session and between sessions, especially if the system impairment is neural or visceral. The neural and visceral release techniques effect a change quickly, whereas articular and myofascial system impairments (structural changes in anatomy) sometimes, but not always, require more time and intervention for change. The order of techniques and systems in this chapter is random; vector analysis determines the system of priority for intervention.

Articular system impairments

A restrictive articular system impairment prevents complete correction of the driver (see Ayami's story in Chapter 5). Restricted joint motion can result from articular pathology secondary to habitual postures, degeneration, trauma or an autoimmune disorder (e.g., rheumatoid arthritis, psoriatic arthritis, diffuse interstitial skeletal hyperostosis, ankylosing spondylitis, etc.). The common result is fibrosis with dehydration of the connective tissue components of the articular capsule. Joints that are fused by osteophytosis cannot be mobilized, whereas the fibrosed or dehydrated joints can, and require vector-specific mobilization. Neural system impairments will affect the arthrokinematic mobility of the joints if the starting position of the joint is not considered when interpreting the mobility findings. The key difference between joints that are restricted by articular versus neural system impairments is that the articular system impairment prevents manual correction of the alignment and biomechanics for the task. Neural system impairments can be corrected. Myofascial system impairments can also restrict the correction; however, the vectors produced by myofascial system impairments have a different quality and end feel. Other than surgical scarring of the intercostals, myofascial vectors are longer and softer than articular vectors, which are short and firm. Visceral vectors create pulls to the inside of the thorax, abdomen, pelvis, or cranium on release of the correction.

Loss of anatomical integrity of articular structures secondary to joint degeneration or trauma can cause excessive joint mobility and a control impairment. Intrathoracic ring control training is indicated for this condition (see intrathoracic ring motor control training, Stage 1 in Chapter 7). If the motor control strategy cannot produce enough force closure to control unwanted motion of the joint, then prolotherapy is indicated.

Thoracic zygapophyseal joints

If fibrosis or dehydration has impaired mobility of the left and right zygapophyseal joints of a thoracic ring equally, the alignment of the thoracic ring may be optimal in standing or sitting and the limitation of motion only apparent during sagittal, coronal or transverse plane movements.

An individual with a unilaterally fibrosed or dehydrated zygapophyseal joint presents often with:

- A persistent translated and rotated thoracic ring that cannot initially be brought into neutral with a manual correction.

- Restricted active and passive unilateral osteokinematic and arthrokinematic mobility:

  ○ a restricted superior glide limits flexion and contralateral rotation and side bending of the thoracic ring (Fig. 6.1A–G);

  ○ a restricted inferior glide limits extension and ipsilateral rotation and side bending of the thoracic ring (Fig. 6.2A-F).

- Short and firm vectors on vector analysis.

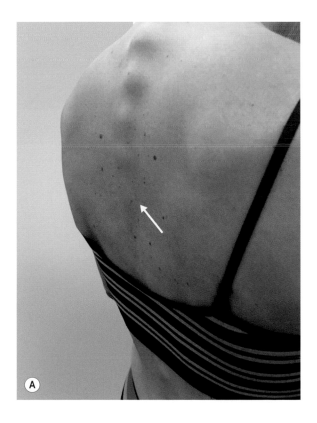

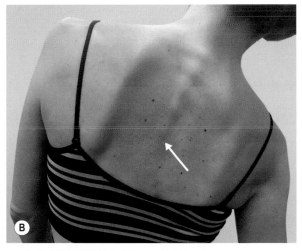

Figure 6.1

(A) This woman presented with an inability to flex her midthoracic spine below the 4th thoracic ring (arrow). (B) Note the segmental kink in the midthoracic region during right side bending (arrow) and also in right rotation (arrow) (C, overleaf). *Continued*

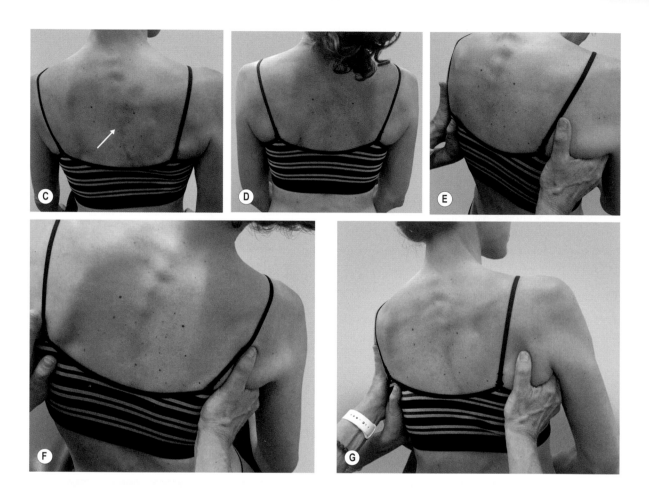

Figure 6.1 *continued*

(D) The patient could extend the midthoracic region although the persistent right 5th thoracic ring shift noted in sitting did not change when she extended. (E) Her 5th thoracic ring was translated right and rotated left and could not be manually corrected. An attempt to correct the alignment and biomechanics of the 5th thoracic ring was met with hard firm articular vectors and the correction did not improve her ability to flex, right side-flex (F) or right rotate (G). Arthrokinematic analysis of the spinal joints at T4–T5 revealed a restriction of superior glide of the left zygapophyseal joint.

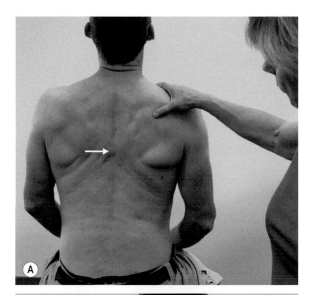

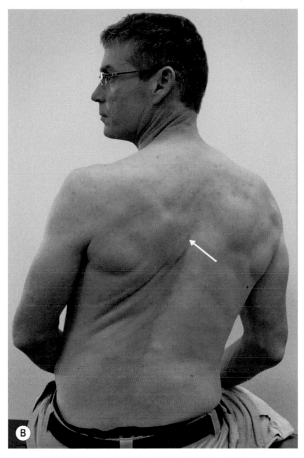

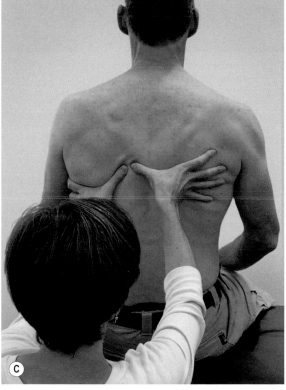

Figure 6.2

(A) This man presented with an articular system impairment of the 8th thoracic ring that impaired his ability to extend his thorax (arrow). The 8th thoracic ring was translated left and rotated right. (B) Left rotation of the thorax produced a segmental kink at T7–T8 (arrow). (C) Active physiological mobility testing during inhalation revealed a limitation of the anterolateroinferior glide at the left 8th costotransverse joint. The left rib was anteriorly rotated and could not posteriorly rotate. *Continued*

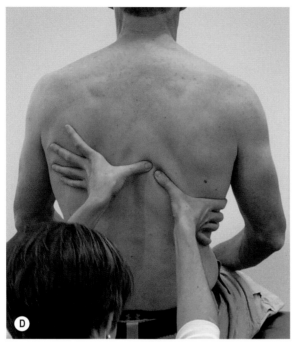

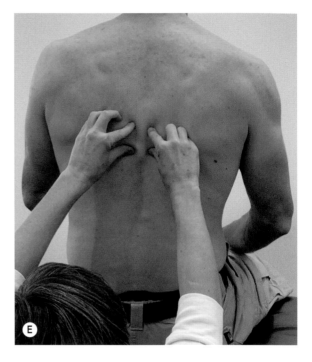

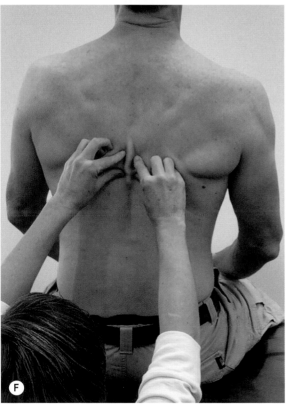

Figure 6.2 *continued*

(D) Active physiological mobility testing during exhalation revealed ample mobility of the posteromediosuperior glide at the right 8th costotransverse joint. The right rib was posteriorly rotated and could anteriorly rotate. (E) T7–T8 was right side-bent and right rotated. (F) Extension revealed a limitation of an inferior glide of the left zygapophyseal joint at T7–T8.

The two passive arthrokinematic glides that confirmed that this is an articular system restriction were: an inferior glide of the left zygapophyseal joint T7–T8 and an anterolateroinferior glide of the left 8th costotransverse joint. Both joints were restricted. Specific vector mobilization restored both the alignment and mobility of the 8th thoracic ring.

Vertebromanubrial region

Bilateral restriction of flexion and bilateral superior glide (e.g., T1–T2)

This technique addresses a bilateral restriction of flexion, and superior glide, of the zygapophyseal joints at T1–T2. The patient is supine, and the therapist is seated at the patient's head. With the lateral aspect of the metacarpophalangeal (MCP) joint of the index finger, fix the spinous process of T2 (Fig. 6.3A). With the opposite hand, support the head and neck down to T1 (Fig. 6.3B). Localize the flexion barrier by flexing the neck and T1–T2 until the articular vector is felt. Fix T2 and apply a bilateral superior glide to T1 that is vector specific. Feel for the 'line' of greatest resistance and hold until the vector releases.

A general regional technique can be done with the patient sitting or standing with both hands behind the neck, fingers interlaced and thumbs or fingers placed in the interspinous space between T1–T2. The therapist stands behind the patient. Wind both arms beneath the patient's axillae and through the triangular space created by the flexed elbows. Interlace your fingers and place them over the patient's hands or wrists (Fig. 6.4). Localize the technique to T1–T2. Apply a sustained, vector-specific, longitudinal traction force with the arms and hands and give the vector sufficient time to release.

To maintain the mobility gained, the patient is instructed to perform the following exercise. With the fingers interlaced behind the neck and the index fingers in the interspinous space at T1–T2, have the patient flex the head and neck. The fingers may assist the motion by applying a superior glide to the inferior aspect of the spinous process of T1. The amplitude of the exercise should be in the pain-free range and should not aggravate any symptoms.

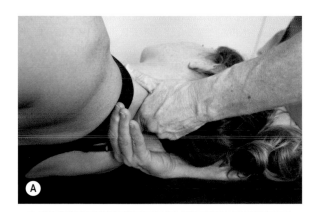

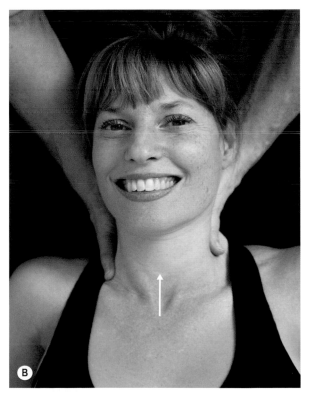

Figure 6.3

This is a vector-specific mobilization technique to restore bilateral superior glide of the zygapophyseal joints and flexion at T1–T2 in supine. (A) The right hand is stabilizing T2. (B) The left hand localizes the technique to T1–T2 by flexing the neck to this segment and then applies longitudinal distraction.

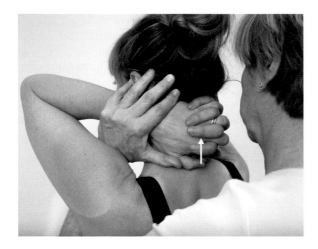

Figure 6.4

General regional distraction to restore bilateral superior glide of the zygapophyseal joints and flexion at T1–T2.

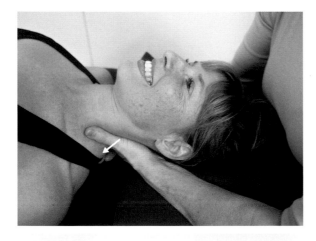

Figure 6.5

This is a vector-specific mobilization technique to restore bilateral inferior glide of the zygapophyseal joints and extension at T1–T2 in supine. The right hand is stabilizing T2. The left hand localizes the technique to T1–T2 by extending the neck to this segment and then applies a dorsal inferior glide bilaterally with the left hand (arrow).

Bilateral restriction of extension and bilateral inferior glide (e.g., T1–T2)

This technique addresses a bilateral restriction of extension, and inferior glide, of the zygapophyseal joints at T1–T2. The patient is supine, and the therapist stands at the patient's head. With the lateral aspect of the metacarpophalangeal (MCP) joint of the index finger, fix the spinous process of T2 (Fig. 6.3A). With the opposite hand, support the head and neck down to T1–T2. Localize the extension barrier by allowing T1 to glide dorsally (toward the table) followed by segmental extension of T1–T2 to the barrier (Fig. 6.5). Try to be vector specific with both the dorsal glide and extension and sustain the hold until release is achieved.

Maintaining the mobility gained usually requires postural instruction that corrects the alignment of both the shoulder girdles and the upper thoracic rings as opposed to an exercise that merely moves T1–T2 into extension. Useful images and cues include those that encourage:

- decompression of the sternoclavicular joints (broadening along the line of the clavicles),

- alignment of the scapulae followed by

- creation of space between the upper thoracic rings as the manubrium is lifted and the cervical spine gently glides dorsally such that the upper thoracic segments extend.

Unilateral restriction of flexion and unilateral superior glide (e.g., right T1–T2)

This technique addresses a unilateral restriction of flexion, and superior glide, of the right zygapophyseal joint at T1–T2. The patient is supine, and the therapist stands at the patient's head. With the lateral aspect of the left index finger, palpate the left transverse process of T2. Wrap the tip of this index finger around the spinous process of T2. With the other hand, support the head and neck with the right thumb over the anterior aspect of the transverse process of T1 and the index finger of this hand over the lamina of T1. Fix T2 with the left hand and localize the unilateral flexion barrier of the right T1–T2 zygapophyseal joint

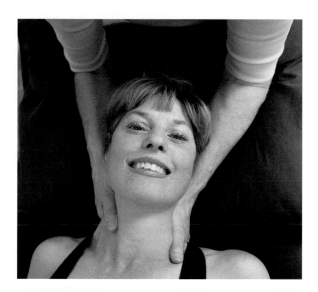

Figure 6.6

This is a vector-specific mobilization technique to restore unilateral flexion (superior glide) of the right zygapophyseal joint at C7–T1.

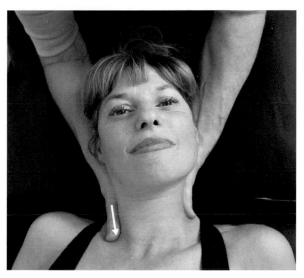

Figure 6.7

This is a vector-specific mobilization technique to restore unilateral extension (inferior glide) of the right zygapophyseal joint at T1–T2.

with segmental left side bending, left rotation, and superior glide using the right hand. Vector specificity is critical for effective release. Sustain the hold until the vectors release. Figure 6.6 illustrates the same technique applied to C7–T1.

Maintain the mobility gained with the following home exercise. Instruct the patient to palpate the right transverse process and lamina of T1 with the index and middle fingers of the left hand. As they turn their head to the left, unilateral flexion, or superior glide, of the right T1–T2 zygapophyseal joint is facilitated by pulling T1 superiorly and to the left.

Unilateral restriction of extension and unilateral inferior glide (e.g., right T1–T2)

This technique addresses a unilateral restriction of extension, and inferior glide, of the right zygapophyseal joint at T1–T2. The patient is lying supine, the therapist stands at the patient's head. With the lateral aspect of the right index finger, palpate the right transverse process of T1. With the other hand, support the head and neck.

Localize the unilateral extension barrier of the right zygapophyseal joint at T1–T2 with segmental right side bending and inferior glide using the right hand (Fig. 6.7). Vector specificity is critical for effective release. Sustain the hold until the vectors release.

Maintain the mobility gained by instructing the patient to elevate the right arm above 90 degrees and simultaneously right rotate the head and neck. Both tasks require unilateral extension of the right zygapophyseal joint at T1–T2.

Vertebrosternal and vertebrochondral regions

Bilateral restriction of flexion – supine roll-down technique

This technique addresses a segmental bilateral restriction of flexion, and superior glide, of the zygapophyseal joints in the vertebrosternal and vertebrochondral regions. The patient is right side lying with their head supported on a pillow and arms crossed such that the bottom arm grasps the scapular

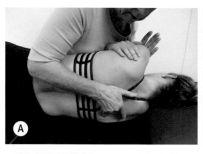
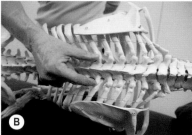
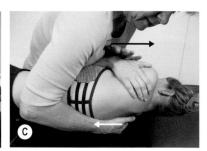

Figure 6.8

This is a vector-specific mobilization technique to restore bilateral flexion (superior glide) of the zygapophyseal joints at any segment from T2–T3 to T9–T10. (A) The inferior vertebra of the segment to be mobilized is stabilized through the scaphoid and flexed PIP of the middle finger. (B) The index finger and thumb are landmarking the transverse processes on this image to be stabilized with the scaphoid and the middle finger of this hand. (C) The segment is localized by flexing the thorax to the segment of interest with the left arm and hand. The inferior vertebra is further stabilized by pulling the right arm and hand inferiorly (short arrow). The mobilization is achieved by shifting weight from the back to the front foot (long arrow) while maintaining the vector-specific localization.

region of the thorax. The therapist stands facing the patient. Extend the thumb and index finger of the right hand and palpate the left and right transverse processes of the inferior vertebra of the segment to be mobilized with the tubercle of the scaphoid and flexed proximal interphalangeal (PIP) joint of the middle finger ('pistol' grip) (Fig. 6.8A & B). The other hand and arm lie across the patient's bottom arm. Localize the segmental bilateral flexion barrier by flexing the thorax to the vector-specific barrier with the hand and arm on the patient's bottom arm. Maintain this localization and roll the patient toward supine only until contact is made between the table and the therapist's dorsal hand (Fig. 6.8C). Maintain the segmental flexion barrier, adduct the dorsal arm (i.e., prevent lateral translation) and fix the inferior vertebra by gently pulling the transverse processes inferiorly. Further bilateral flexion is achieved by shifting weight from the back leg and foot to the front leg and foot. The hand and arms localize the technique to the specific segment while the trunk and legs produce the mobilization force. The goal is to achieve vector specificity then sustain the hold until the vectors release.

Bilateral restriction of flexion – seated distraction technique

A general regional technique for a bilateral restriction of flexion, and superior glide, can be carried out with the patient sitting with the arms crossed to opposite shoulders.

The therapist stands behind the patient. Place a small towel against the spinous process of the inferior vertebra of the segment to be mobilized. Fix a towel against your sternum and wrap both arms around the patient's thorax and grasp the bottom elbow (Fig. 6.9). Some localization can be achieved by flexing the thorax until the segmental articular vector is felt. Apply a sustained, vector-specific, longitudinal traction force with your arms and hands, allowing gravity to facilitate the segmental distraction. Hold and wait for the vector to release.

For both techniques, the mobility gained can be maintained with the following home exercise. In sitting, have the patient bring their chin to the chest and then specifically articulate each thoracic segment into flexion with cues to soften the sternum and lengthen the spine into a C-curve.

Unilateral restriction of flexion – supine roll-down technique (e.g., left T5–T6)

This technique addresses a unilateral restriction of flexion, and superior glide, of the left zygapophyseal joint at T5–T6. The patient is right side lying with their head supported on a pillow and arms crossed such that the bottom arm grasps the scapular region of the thorax. The therapist stands facing the patient. Extend the thumb and index finger of

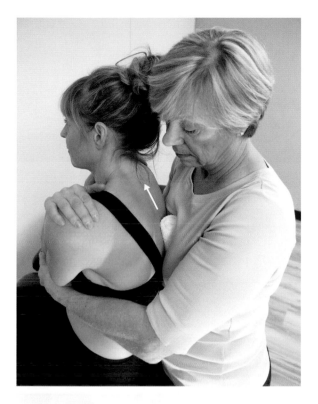

Figure 6.9

General regional distraction to restore bilateral superior glide of the zygapophyseal joints and flexion in the vertebrosternal and vertebrochondral region. The towel fixes the inferior vertebra of the targeted segment to be mobilized.

Further unilateral flexion is achieved by shifting weight from the back leg and foot to the front leg and foot. The hand and arms localize the technique to T5–T6 while the trunk and legs produce the mobilization force. The goal is to achieve vector specificity, find the vector of greatest resistance and sustain the hold until the vector releases.

Unilateral restriction of flexion – prone arthrokinematic technique (e.g., right T3–T4)

This technique also addresses a unilateral restriction of flexion, and superior glide, of the right zygapophyseal joint at T3–T4. The patient is prone with the head and neck in neutral rotation. The therapist stands at the patient's side. Palpate the inferior aspect of the left transverse process of T4 with one thumb. Palpate the inferior aspect of the right transverse process of T3 with the other thumb. Fix T4 with a gentle superior force and apply a superoanterior glide to T3 (Fig. 6.11A & B). Vary the direction of the glide to identify the specific direction that is limited (i.e., be vector direction specific – look for a string within a spring). Find the vector of greatest resistance and sustain the hold until the vector releases.

For both techniques, the mobility gained can be maintained with the following home exercise. In sitting, have the patient bring their chin to the chest and then specifically articulate each thoracic segment into flexion with cues to soften the sternum and lengthen the spine into a C-curve. Once the segment of interest is reached, side-bending to the opposite side will facilitate further unilateral flexion (superior glide) of the relevant joint.

Unilateral restriction of extension – supine roll-down technique (e.g., left T5–T6)

This technique addresses a unilateral restriction of extension, and inferior glide, of the left zygapophyseal joint at T5–T6. The patient is right side lying with their head supported on a pillow and arms crossed such that the bottom arm grasps the scapular region of the thorax. The therapist stands facing the patient. Extend the thumb and index finger of the right hand and palpate the left transverse processes of T6 with the tubercle of the scaphoid and the right transverse process of T5 with the flexed proximal interphalangeal (PIP) joint of the middle finger

the right hand and palpate the left transverse process of T6 with the tubercle of the scaphoid and the right transverse process of T5 with the flexed proximal interphalangeal (PIP) joint of the middle finger (Fig. 6.10A & B). Place the other hand and arm across the patient's bottom arm. Localize the unilateral flexion barrier by flexing then right side bending the thorax to the T5–T6 segment with the hand and arm on the patient's bottom arm. Maintain this localization and roll the patient toward supine only until contact is made between the table and the therapist's dorsal hand (Fig. 6.10C). Maintain the segmental unilateral flexion barrier, adduct the dorsal arm (i.e., prevent lateral translation) and fix the inferior vertebra by gently pulling the left transverse process of T6 inferiorly.

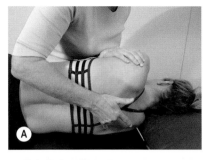
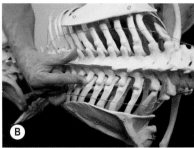
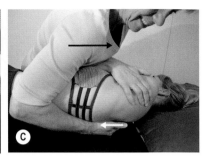

Figure 6.10

This is a vector-specific mobilization technique to restore unilateral flexion (superior glide) of the left zygapophyseal joint at T5–T6.
(A) Stabilize the right T5–T6 zygapophyseal joint by fixing the left transverse process of T6 and the right transverse process of T5.
(B) The index finger and thumb are landmarking the transverse processes on T5–T6 to be stabilized with the scaphoid and the middle finger of this hand. (C) The segment is localized by flexing and right side bending the thorax to the segment of interest with the left arm and hand. T6 is further stabilized by pulling the right arm and hand inferior (short arrow). The mobilization is achieved by shifting weight from the back to the front foot (long arrow) while maintaining the vector-specific localization.

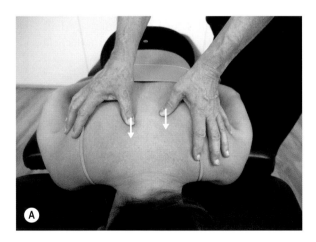
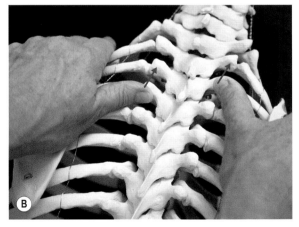

Figure 6.11 A & B

This is a vector-specific mobilization technique to restore the ability of the right inferior articular process of T3 to glide superiorly relative to the superior articular process of T4.

(Fig. 6.10B, 6.12A). Place the other hand and arm across the patient's bottom arm. Flex the thorax down to T4–T5 to localize the technique to T5–T6, and roll the patient toward supine only until contact is made between the table and the dorsal hand. Maintain this localization with your chest and move your left hand to the patient's left shoulder.

Laterally flex T5–T6 to the left (inferiorly glide the left zygapophyseal joint at T5–T6 to the barrier) with the left hand on the patient's left shoulder. Maintain the extension barrier at T5–T6, and fix the inferior vertebra by gently pushing the left transverse process of T6 superiorly. Further unilateral extension is achieved with both arms (Fig. 6.12B). The goal

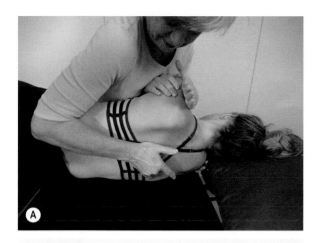

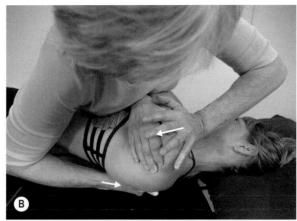

Figure 6.12

This is a vector-specific mobilization technique to restore unilateral extension (inferior glide) of the left zygapophyseal joint at T5–T6. (A) Stabilize the right T5–T6 zygapophyseal joint by fixing the left transverse process of T6 and the right transverse process of T5 (see also Fig. 6.10B). (B) After localization, the mobilization is achieved by stabilizing the left transverse process of T6 with a superior force (short arrow) and applying an inferoposterior force to the left zygapophyseal joint at T5–T6 through the patient's left shoulder using the left hand (long arrow).

is to achieve vector specificity, find the vector of greatest resistance, and sustain the hold until the vector releases.

Unilateral restriction of extension – prone arthrokinematic technique (e.g., right T6–T7)

This technique addresses a restriction of extension, and inferior glide, of the right zygapophyseal joint at T6–T7. The patient is prone with the head and neck in neutral. Palpate the inferior aspect of the right transverse process of T7 with one thumb. Palpate the superior aspect of the right transverse process of T6 with the other thumb. Fix T7 with a gentle superior force and apply an inferior glide to T6 (Fig. 6.13). Vary the direction of the glide to identify the specific direction that is limited (i.e., be vector direction specific – look for a string within a spring). Find the vector of greatest resistance and sustain the hold until the vector releases.

Mobility gained can be maintained with the following home exercise. In sitting, have the patient specifically articulate each thoracic segment into extension with cues to lift the sternum. Once the segment of interest is reached, side bending to the ipsilateral side will facilitate further unilateral extension (inferior glide) of the relevant joint.

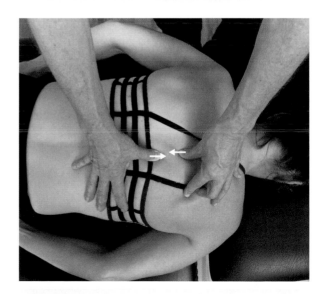

Figure 6.13

This is a vector-specific mobilization technique to restore the ability of the right inferior articular process of T6 to glide inferiorly relative to the superior articular process of T7.

Thoracic costotransverse joints

An individual with a unilaterally fibrosed or dehydrated costotransverse joint presents with:

- A persistent laterally translated and rotated thoracic ring that cannot initially be brought into neutral with a manual correction.

- Restricted active and passive unilateral osteokinematic and arthrokinematic mobility:

  ○ a restricted superior glide (VM and VS: superior glide and anterior roll, VC: posteromediosuperior glide) limits anterior rotation of the rib and therefore flexion and contralateral rotation of the thoracic ring and results in lateral translation and rotation of the entire thoracic ring on exhalation;

  ○ a restricted inferior glide (VM and VS: inferior glide and posterior roll, VC: anterolateroinferior glide) limits posterior rotation of the rib and therefore extension and ipsilateral rotation of the thoracic ring and results in lateral translation and rotation of the entire thoracic ring on inhalation (see Ayami's story in Chapter 5).

- Short and firm vectors on vector analysis.

Vertebromanubrial region

Unilateral restriction of anterior rotation (e.g., right 1st rib)

This technique addresses a unilateral restriction of anterior rotation, superior glide and anterior roll, of the right 1st costotransverse joint. The patient is supine with the head supported on a pillow. The therapist stands or sits at the patient's head. Palpate the superior aspect of the right transverse process of T1 with the right thumb (Fig. 6.14A). Palpate the inferior aspect of the right 1st rib with the index and middle fingers of the right hand (6.14B). Support the head and neck with the other hand. Localize the barrier by applying a posteroinferior glide to the transverse process of T1. This results in a relative superior glide and anterior roll (anterior rotation) of the 1st rib at the costotransverse joint. The middle and index fingers of the right hand fix the inferior aspect of the 1st rib. The

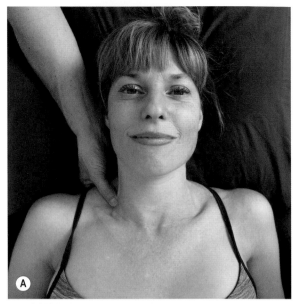

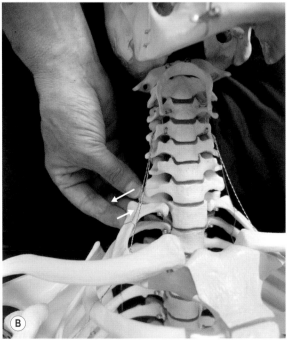

Figure 6.14

This is a vector-specific mobilization to restore the ability of the right 1st rib to glide superiorly relative to the transverse process of T1 and thus facilitate anterior rotation of the right 1st rib.

goal is to achieve vector specificity, find the vector of greatest resistance, and sustain the hold until the vector releases.

Unilateral restriction of posterior rotation (e.g., right 1st rib)

This technique addresses a unilateral restriction of posterior rotation, inferior glide and posterior roll, of the right 1st costotransverse joint. The patient is supine with the head supported on a pillow. The therapist stands or sits at the patient's head. Palpate the superior aspect of the right 1st rib with the lateral aspect of the MCP of the index finger of the right hand (Fig. 6.15A & B). Support the neck and upper thorax with the other hand. The segment is localized with side bending of C7, T1 and T2 to the right and rotation to the left. The articular vector barrier of the 1st costotransverse joint is localized and mobilized by applying an inferior glide and posterior roll to the tubercle of the rib. The goal is to achieve vector specificity, find the vector of greatest resistance and sustain the hold until the vector releases.

Vertebrosternal region

Unilateral restriction of anterior or posterior rotation – supine roll-down technique

This technique addresses a unilateral restriction of anterior or posterior rotation, superior glide and anterior roll or inferior glide and posterior roll, at the left 6th costotransverse joint. The patient is right side lying, the head supported on a pillow and the arms crossed such that the bottom arm grasps the scapular region of the thorax. The therapist stands facing the patient. Palpate the left 6th rib just lateral to the transverse process of T6 with the proximal phalanx of the right thumb (Fig. 6.16A & B). Place the other hand and arm across the patient's bottom arm. Localize the thoracic ring by flexing the thorax to T5–T6. Maintain this localization and roll the patient toward supine only until contact is made between the table and the therapist's dorsal hand. From this position, adduct the dorsal arm (i.e., prevent lateral translation) and rotate the thorax over the right thumb. This will

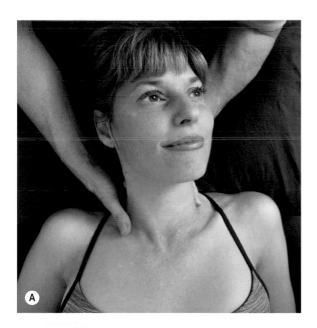

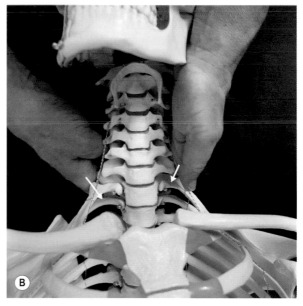

Figure 6.15

(A) This is a vector-specific mobilization to restore the ability of the right 1st rib to glide inferiorly and roll posteriorly relative to the transverse process of T1 and thus facilitate posterior rotation of the rib. (B) Points of hand contact.

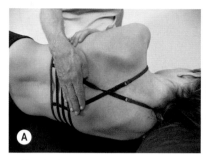
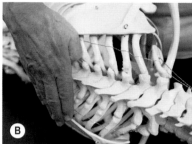
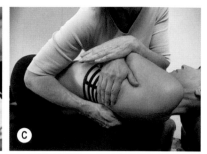

Figure 6.16

This is a vector-specific mobilization for the left 6th costotransverse joint. (A) The rib is stabilized with the proximal phalanx of the right hand with the PIP joint flexed. (B) Points of contact. (C) The vector is localized with side bending of the thorax after the patient is rolled to supine only until contact is made with the table with the dorsal hand. Right side bending produces a relative inferior glide and left side bending produces a superior glide at the costotransverse joint since the rib is fixed and the transverse process is moving.

result in distraction of the costotransverse joint. Find the specific articular barrier by adding slight left or right side bending of the thorax for superior glide and anterior roll or inferior glide and posterior roll of the rib respectively at the left 6th costotranverse joint (Fig. 6.16C). Find the vector of greatest resistance and sustain the hold until release occurs.

Unilateral restriction of anterior rotation – prone arthrokinematic technique (e.g., right 4th rib)

This technique addresses a unilateral restriction of anterior rotation, superior glide and anterior roll, of the right 4th rib at the costotransverse joint. The patient is prone with the head and neck in neutral. The therapist stands at the patient's side. Palpate the superior aspect of the transverse process of T4 with one thumb. Palpate the inferior aspect of the right 4th rib just lateral to the tubercle with the other thumb. Fix T4 with a gentle inferior force and glide the 4th rib superiorly allowing the conjunct anterior roll to occur (Fig. 6.17A & B). Vary the direction of the glide to identify the specific direction that is limited (i.e., be vector direction specific – look for the string within a spring). Find the vector of greatest resistance and sustain the hold until the vector releases.

Unilateral restriction of posterior rotation – prone arthrokinematic technique (e.g., right 4th rib)

This technique addresses a unilateral restriction of posterior rotation, inferior glide and posterior roll, of the right 4th rib at the costotransverse joint. The patient is prone with the head and neck in neutral. The therapist stands at the patient's side. With one thumb palpate the inferior aspect of the right transverse process of T4. Palpate the superior aspect of the right 4th rib just lateral to the tubercle with the other thumb. Fix T4 with a gentle superior force, and with the other thumb distract the costotransverse joint slightly and glide the 4th rib inferiorly allowing the conjunct posterior roll to occur (Fig. 6.18A & B). Vary the direction of the glide to identify the specific direction that is limited (i.e., be vector direction specific – look for a string within a spring). Find the vector of greatest resistance and sustain the hold until the vector releases.

Vertebrochondral region

Unilateral restriction of anterior rotation – prone arthrokinematic technique (e.g., right 9th rib)

This technique addresses a unilateral restriction of anterior rotation and posteromediosuperior glide of the right 9th rib at the costotransverse joint. The patient is

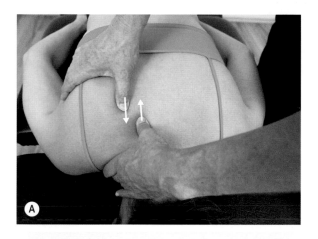

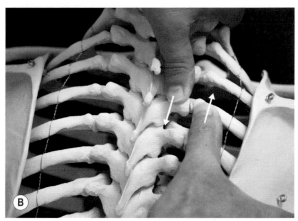

Figure 6.17 A & B

This is a vector-specific mobilization technique to restore the ability of the right 4th rib to glide superiorly relative to the transverse process of T4 at the costotransverse joint and thus facilitate anterior rotation of the right 4th rib.

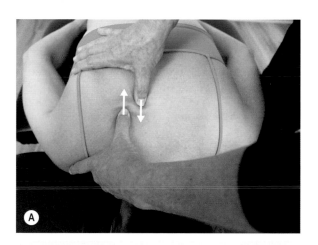

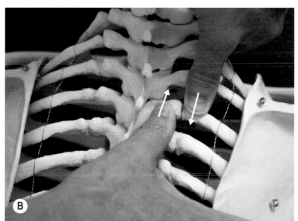

Figure 6.18 A & B

This is a vector-specific mobilization technique to restore the ability of the right 4th rib to glide inferiorly relative to the transverse process of T4 at the costotransverse joint and thus facilitate posterior rotation of the right 4th rib.

prone with the head and neck in neutral rotation. The therapist stands on the opposite side to be mobilized. With the left thumb palpate the right transverse process of T9. With the right hand, palpate the 9th rib with the thumb just lateral to the transverse process of T9 and the index or middle finger along the body of the 9th rib. Fix the transverse process by gently pushing

T9 anterolaterally and inferiorly and glide the 9th rib posteromedially and superiorly (Fig. 6.19A & B) at the costotransverse joint. Vary the direction of the glide to identify the specific direction that is limited (i.e., be vector direction specific – look for a string within a spring). Find the vector of greatest resistance and sustain the hold until the vector releases.

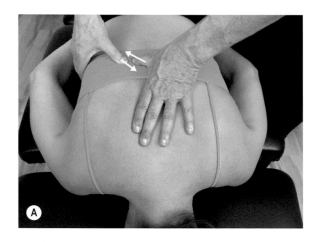

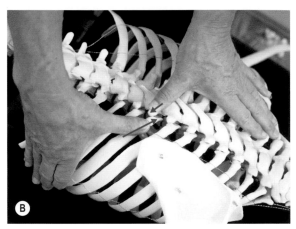

Figure 6.19 A & B

This is a vector-specific mobilization technique to restore the ability of the right 9th rib to glide posteromedially and superiorly relative to the transverse process of T9 at the costotransverse joint and thus facilitate anterior rotation of the right 9th rib.

Unilateral restriction of posterior rotation – prone arthrokinematic technique (e.g., right 9th rib)

This technique addresses a unilateral restriction of posterior rotation and anterolateroinferior glide of the right 9th rib at the costotransverse joint. The patient is prone with the head and neck in neutral rotation. The therapist stands on the opposite side to be mobilized. With the left thumb palpate the right transverse process of T9. With the right hand, palpate the 9th rib with the thumb just lateral to the transverse process of T9 and the index or middle finger along the body of the 9th rib. Fix T9 by applying a gentle posteromediosuperior force to the transverse process of T9 and glide the 9th rib anterolaterally and inferiorly (Fig. 6.20A & B). Vary the direction of the glide to identify the specific direction that is limited (i.e., be vector direction specific – look for a string within a spring). Find the vector of greatest resistance and sustain the hold until the vector releases.

Mobility of the costotransverse joints in all regions of the thorax can be maintained using targeted breathing practice combined with specific movements of the thorax:

- Inspiration combined with extension will facilitate posterior rotation of the ribs;

- Expiration combined with flexion will facilitate anterior rotation;

- Inspiration combined with right rotation will facilitate posterior rotation of the right ribs;

- Expiration combined with right rotation will facilitate anterior rotation of the left ribs.

Manual self-mobilization and movement integration can be combined with this home release practice (Fig. 6.21).

Vertebrosternal and vertebrochondral regions

Fixation of the left 5th costotransverse joint

Note to reader: High-velocity, low-amplitude thrust techniques require special hands-on, in-class, training. Do not attempt these techniques if you are not certified or trained to do so.

This technique addresses a fixation of the left 5th costotransverse joint. A fixated joint is one that is held compressed at the end of, or just beyond, the physiological motion barrier by overactivation of muscles. No arthrokinematic motion is possible when the joint is fixated.

To be clear, these joints are not 'out' or 'subluxed'; the protective response of the neuromuscular system is responsible for the lack of articular mobility. The passive joint restraints (capsule and ligaments) are often lengthened, or stretched, during the trauma that caused this

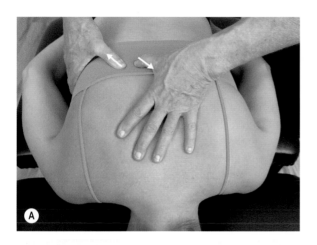
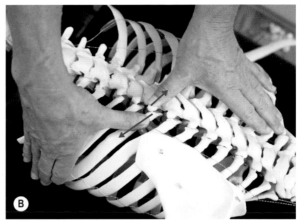

Figure 6.20 A & B

This is a vector-specific mobilization technique to restore the ability of the right 9th rib to glide anterolaterally and inferiorly relative to the transverse process of T9 at the costotransverse joint and thus facilitate posterior rotation of the right 9th rib.

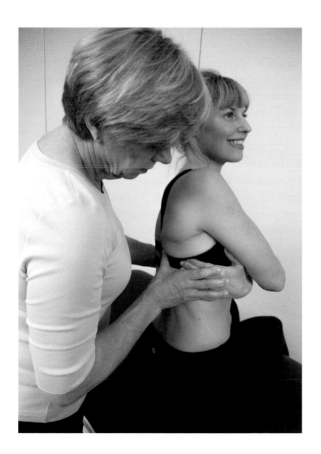

Figure 6.21

Home release practice to maintain mobility of the right 8th costotransverse joint and posterior rotation of the right 8th rib after manual mobilization. The patient is correcting, and monitoring, her 8th thoracic ring in the midaxillary line. She is then instructed to inhale and rotate to the right only as far as the right 8th rib can posteriorly rotate. When the rib has reached the limit of the available range of motion, the entire 8th thoracic ring will begin to translate right and rotate left. The patient is taught to not push past this point, but rather to maintain the correction (posterior rotation of the right 8th rib) and inhale directly into the region of the right 8th rib. This process can be repeated two to three times.

condition and therefore the two joint surfaces can move slightly beyond their physiological end range.

The patient is right side lying, the head supported on a pillow and the arms crossed such that the bottom arm grasps the scapular region of the thorax. The therapist stands facing the patient. Palpate the left 5th rib just lateral to the left transverse process of T5 with the proximal phalanx of the right thumb, flex the PIP. Place the other hand and arm across the patient's arms. Localize the 5th thoracic ring by flexing the thorax down to, but not including, this level. Maintain this localization and roll the patient toward supine only until contact is made between the table and the therapist's dorsal hand. From this position, adduct the dorsal arm (i.e., prevent lateral translation) and rotate the thorax slightly over the right thumb. This will result in slight distraction of the costotransverse joint. A very low-amplitude, high-velocity thrust applied through the thorax into left axial rotation will produce a cavitation of the joint and a neural response that results in a reduction

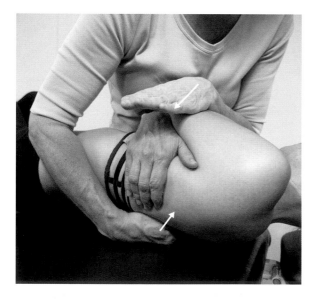

Figure 6.22

High-velocity, low-amplitude thrust technique to reduce a fixation of the costotransverse joint. The axial rotation force is delivered with the therapist's the left hand and arm while the right thumb stabilizes the rib.

of activation of the segmental muscles restricting all movement (Fig. 6.22). The arthrokinematic mobility of the joint should now be restored; however, the passive control test – anterior distraction costotransverse joint (intrathoracic ring) may be positive (see Chapter 3). Alternately, or in addition, active control of the costotransverse joint may not automatically return. If the biomechanics are still suboptimal for seated rotation of the thorax, it is prudent to tape the left 5th costotransverse joint for intrathoracic ring alignment and control (see Chapter 7) until motor control training can begin.

Thoracic ring lateral translation and rotation fixation

Note to reader: High-velocity, low-amplitude thrust techniques require special hands-on, in-class training. Do not attempt these techniques if you are not certified or trained to do so.

This fixation involves the entire thoracic ring, and was initially described in 1996 (Lee D G 1996). This articular system impairment occurs primarily in the vertebrosternal region and occasionally in the vertebrochondral region. It can occur when the thorax is forced into excessive rotation or when rotation of the thorax is forced against a fixed rib cage (seat belt injury). At the limit of right rotation, the superior vertebra has translated to the left relative to the inferior vertebra, the left rib has translated posterolaterally relative to the left transverse process of the inferior vertebra and the right rib has translated anteromedially relative to the inferior vertebra. Further right rotation results in a right lateral tilt of the superior vertebra. Fixation of the superior vertebra occurs when the left lateral translation exceeds the physiological motion barrier and the vertebra is unable to return to its neutral position due to a protective neuromuscular response.

Left lateral translation and rotation fixation (e.g., 6th thoracic ring)

The following findings are present when the 6th thoracic ring is fixated in left lateral translation and right rotation:

- Standing or sitting posture of the thorax: T5 is right rotated and side-bent relative to T6, the right 6th rib is anteromedial relative to the right transverse process of T6 and posteriorly rotated and the left 6th rib is posterolateral relative to the left transverse process of T6 and anteriorly rotated. The 6th thoracic ring is excessively translated left and rotated right.

- Active segmental mobility: All movements of the thorax produce a kink in the spinal curve at T5–T6; the most affected movement is left rotation.

- Passive segmental mobility: There is a complete block to both left and right lateral translation of the left and right 6th ribs and T5 relative to T6.

- Passive segmental control: It is not possible to test lateral translation control when the thoracic ring is fixated. After mobility is restored, the passive control tests reveal excessive left lateral translation of the left and right 6th ribs and T5 relative to T6 (form closure impairment) and active control tests reveal loss of segmental thoracic ring control when loaded (force closure impairment).

The following technique addresses a left lateral translation and right rotation fixation of the 6th thoracic ring. The patient is left side lying, the head supported on a pillow and the arms crossed such that the bottom arm grasps the scapular region of the thorax. The therapist stands facing the patient. With the proximal phalanx of the left thumb, palpate the right 7th rib posteriorly just lateral to the right transverse process of T7. T6 is controlled by compressing the right 7th rib toward the midline into the vertebral bodies of T7 and T6 (Fig. 6.23A). Care must be taken to avoid limiting the mobility of the 6th ribs, which must be free to glide relative to the transverse processes of T6. Place the other hand and arm across the patient's arm. Localize the 6th thoracic ring by flexing the thorax to this level. Maintain this localization and roll the patient toward supine only until contact is made between the table and the therapist's dorsal hand. From this position, T5 and the left and right 6th ribs are translated laterally to the right through the thorax to the motion barrier (Fig. 6.23B). Strong longitudinal traction is applied through the thorax by shifting weight from the therapist's back leg and foot to the front leg and foot. This traction is maintained and

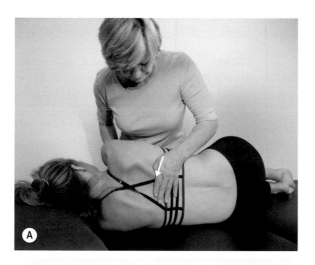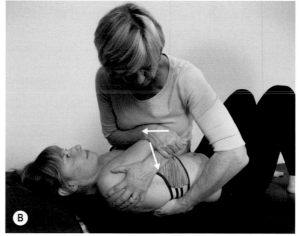

Figure 6.23

High-velocity, low-amplitude thrust technique to reduce a left lateral translation fixation of the 6th thoracic ring. (A) Medial compression of the right 7th rib into the vertebral bodies of T6 and T7 stabilizes T6. (B) The right lateral translation barrier for T6 and the left and right 6th ribs is localized first, followed by strong longitudinal traction. The direction of the high-velocity, low-amplitude thrust is right lateral translation while maintaining the strong distraction.

a high-velocity, low-amplitude thrust is applied to the 6th thoracic ring in a right lateral direction. The goal of the technique is to distract and laterally translate T5 and the left and right 6th ribs relative to T6.

The arthrokinematic mobility of the joint should now be restored; however, the passive control test (lateral translation of the intrathoracic ring) may be positive (see Chapter 3). Alternately, or in addition, active inter-thoracic ring control may not automatically return. If the biomechanics are still suboptimal for seated rotation of the thorax, it is prudent to tape the 6th thoracic ring for intrathoracic ring alignment and control (see Chapter 7) until motor control training can begin.

Neural system impairments

Unlike an articular system impairment, a restrictive neural system impairment does not prevent complete correction of the driver. This is a key differentiating feature between articular and neural system impairments. Overactivation of any muscle that attaches to any part of the thoracic ring secondary to increased neural drive can initiate a chain of events that without vector analysis is difficult to interpret. An overactive muscle can be tender to palpation yet may not require release if it is reacting to a vector of pull from an antagonistic muscle or another system vector. How does the Integrated Systems Model facilitate clinical reasoning to determine which tender, 'tight' muscles to release? Passive listening during both manual correction and release of the driver provides information relating to the vector, such as its:

- location (left or right, front or back, inside or outside the thorax, abdomen, pelvis or cranium),

- length (long or short), and

- quality (firm or soft).

For example, if a fascicle of the right external oblique (EO) attaching to the anterior aspect of the right 7th rib was the dominant vector causing the 7th thoracic ring to be translated right and rotated left with an associated overactive fascicle of the right iliocostalis to the posterior aspect of the right 7th rib, releasing the iliocostalis (the reactor)

would cause the thoracic ring to translate and rotate further (Fig. 6.24A). This mistake in clinical reasoning can be avoided by paying attention to the analysis of the vectors during correction and release of the 7th thoracic ring. In this scenario, passive listening during manual correction would reveal a vector of pull from the right and anterior aspect of the thorax (from the EO) and passive listening during release of this correction would confirm that the vector was coming from the right and anterior aspect of the thorax. The right rib would not be pulled into the thoracic or abdominal canisters (i.e., is not a visceral vector) and the length would be long and the quality relatively soft compared to a vector from an articular system impairment.

Alternately, understanding the biomechanics of the thoracic ring and how each muscle impacts its mobility can be used to determine the dominant (acting) and secondary (reacting) vectors. In the same scenario above, the right iliocostalis would posteriorly rotate the right rib if it was the dominant vector and therefore, the 7th thoracic ring would be translated left and rotated right (Fig. 6.24B). Clinically, it is prudent to use both clinical reasoning of the biomechanics and passive listening to interpret the findings from vector analysis and determine which vectors to release to achieve a neutral position of the thoracic ring (Fig. 6.24C).

Often multiple neural vectors are present and it is difficult to discern the dominant vector. In this case, the preferred release technique is a multisystem general technique that begins with thoracic ring stack and breathe (Lee L-J 2016), combined with hold–relax and possibly specific arthrokinematic articular mobilization. This technique addresses multiple vectors from all systems simultaneously and will be described under neural system impairments. It could equally be described in any of the other systems. The techniques described in the neural section of this chapter include:

- Release with awareness

- Dry needling

- Muscle recoil or muscle manipulation (Hartman 1996)

- Specific techniques for individual muscles

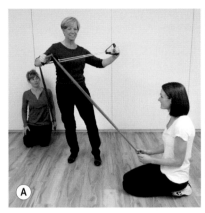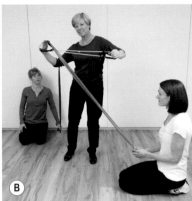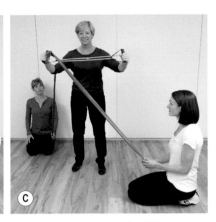

Figure 6.24

(A) When a fascicle of the right external oblique is the dominant vector perturbing the thoracic ring, the thoracic ring will be translated right and rotated left. The right iliocostalis often reacts to this vector of pull; however, releasing the iliocostalis would merely permit the external oblique to translate and rotate the thoracic ring further. (B) When a fascicle of the right iliocostalis is the dominant vector, the thoracic ring will translate left and rotate right. The right external oblique often reacts to this vector of pull. In this scenario releasing the right iliocostalis would result in less activation of both muscles and a neutral thoracic ring (C).

- General, non-structure-specific technique for multiple system impairments (thoracic ring stack and breathe (Lee L-J 2016).

- Dural and perineural system release techniques.

Principles of the release with awareness technique

This technique was first introduced in 2001 (Lee D 2001) to treat 'butt grippers,' i.e., individuals who habitually overactivate the ischiococcygeus as part of their strategy to control the pelvis. The concept was expanded, and several techniques published, for the fourth edition of *The Pelvic Girdle* (Lee D & Lee L-J 2011a). Release with awareness can be used on any muscle in the body that is overactive due to increased neural drive. There is often a latent trigger point in the relevant muscle that the patient may not be aware of until the muscle is palpated. The trigger point is monitored with one hand with just enough pressure to increase the patient's sensory awareness but not so much that it provokes pain. The joint, or the muscle itself, is moved to approximate the origin and the insertion of the muscle. This immediately reduces the afferent input to the

spinal cord from the primary annulospiral ending in the intrafusal muscle fiber by reducing tension on the muscle spindle (Fig. 6.25). Within 10 to 15 seconds a reduction in the activation of the muscle will be felt.

The second part of the technique (awareness) engages the patient in the release process. They are asked to bring their attention to any sensation in the muscle being palpated while being given verbal cues that facilitate relaxation or letting go. Provide cues that 'stop them from doing something' as opposed to 'doing something in addition to what they are already doing.' For example, to release the ischiococcygeus, give cues such as 'let my fingers sink into this muscle; let the sitting bones widen and your tailbone float' as opposed to 'pull the sitting bones apart.' The goal is to reduce activation; therefore, they must figure out how to stop doing something as opposed to adding on another layer of muscle activation that will further compress and restrict the joint. When the nervous system responds to the manual and verbal cues, encourage them with positive reinforcement that they are on the right path. They will often say 'but I didn't do anything' to which you can reply 'I don't want you to do something; I want you to stop

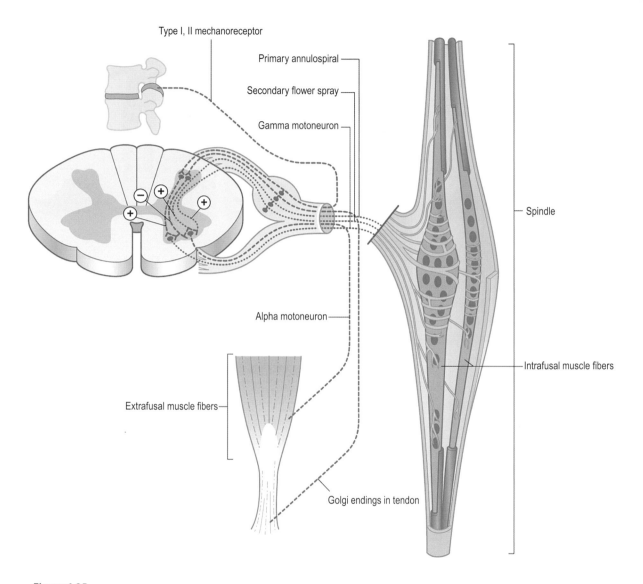

Type I, II mechanoreceptor

Primary annulospiral

Secondary flower spray

Gamma motoneuron

Spindle

Alpha motoneuron

Intrafusal muscle fibers

Extrafusal muscle fibers

Golgi endings in tendon

Figure 6.25

Activation of a muscle is influenced and controlled by many neural feedback loops involving the brain, spinal cord, and peripheral receptor systems. Changing the position of the joint and its associated muscles, tendons, and fascia can alter afferent input and thus efferent output to the related extrafusal muscle fiber. The result can be a decrease in activation of the targeted muscle at rest. This is called a positional release. Imagery and awareness can activate the higher centers that have a descending inhibitory influence on the efferent output to the extrafusal muscle fibers and can further reduce a muscle's activation.

Redrawn by Elsevier from an original artwork by Diane Lee (Lee D 2016). Reproduced with permission.

doing something.' Meanwhile, you continue to move the joint in various combinations of movements that facilitate further relaxation of the muscle until no further release is obtained. If you move the joint, or muscle, from this point in any direction, you often engage another barrier. The osteopathic physicians call this a 'still point.' After a short period of time an expansive release occurs, following which the muscle will relax further allowing more lengthening and greater range of joint motion.

The third part of the release with awareness technique addresses any myofascial restrictions within the perimysium, epimysium or endomysium of the muscle. The muscle (and the relevant joint) is taken into the newly gained range and stretched. Following this technique, the alignment, biomechanics and control of the driver are reassessed in the screening task that pertains to the meaningful task.

Principles of dry needling

Note to reader: Dry needling requires special hands-on, in-class, training. Do not attempt these techniques if you are not certified or trained to do so, or if dry needling is not within the scope of practice for your state or country.

Dry needling targets active trigger points in overactive muscles and is a useful tool when used in conjunction with other manual release techniques and followed with a home release practice. If a latent or active trigger point in a peripheral muscle is associated with over-activation of the relevant segmental paraspinal muscle, then both the peripheral muscle and the spinal segment are needled (Gunn 1996).

Principles of muscle recoil or muscle manipulation

This is a release technique which relies on the golgi tendon organ (GTO) in the muscle to facilitate relaxation of the extrafusal muscle fibers. The GTOs are inhibitory to these fibers and are activated when stretched quickly (Hartman 1996).

What follows are descriptions of specific release techniques for individual overactive muscles, which vector analysis has determined to be dominant. The order presented in this chapter is random; vector analysis determines the order of intervention.

Transversus thoracis

Excessive neural drive to the transversus thoracis (Fig. 1.23A & B) can impact the alignment and biomechanics of the 2nd to 6th thoracic rings collectively or individually. Passive listening during correction of the alignment of a thoracic ring reveals a vector of pull from the anterior thorax. Passive listening during release of the correction reveals a vector that is anterior, inside the thorax, not very deep and often oblique. The relevant rib of the thoracic ring is held in anterior rotation; therefore, the thoracic ring is translated to the same side as the overactive fascicle of the transversus thoracis. The following technique is an example of how to use release with awareness to reduce the activation of a fascicle of the transversus thoracis attaching to the right 3rd rib.

Release with awareness: The patient is left side lying with the right arm alongside the thorax. The therapist stands behind the patient. With one hand, palpate the 3rd rib in the right axilla or anterior thorax. With the other hand stabilize the xyphoid. Approximate the right 3rd rib toward the xyphoid and wait approximately 10 to 15 seconds (Fig. 6.26A). Cue the patient to imagine broadening, or expansion of the anterior chest and on the inhale breath, fix the xyphoid and take the right 3rd rib into posterior rotation, and right rotate the 3rd thoracic ring (myofascial release part of the release with awareness technique) (Fig. 6.26B). Repeat two to three times, then reassess the alignment, biomechanics and control of the 3rd thoracic ring during the relevant screening task.

The release can be maintained with the following home practice. Instruct the patient to self-correct the 3rd thoracic ring through the right rib (gently lift the anterior aspect of the rib and push it back toward the right axilla). Hold this correction with the right hand and teach them to palpate the xyphoid with the left hand (Fig. 6.26C). On the inhale breath, stabilize the xyphoid and facilitate posterior rotation of the right 3rd rib and right rotation of the 3rd thoracic ring (Fig. 6.26D). Repeat three to four times and retest the screening task. There should be a change in the experience of performing the task.

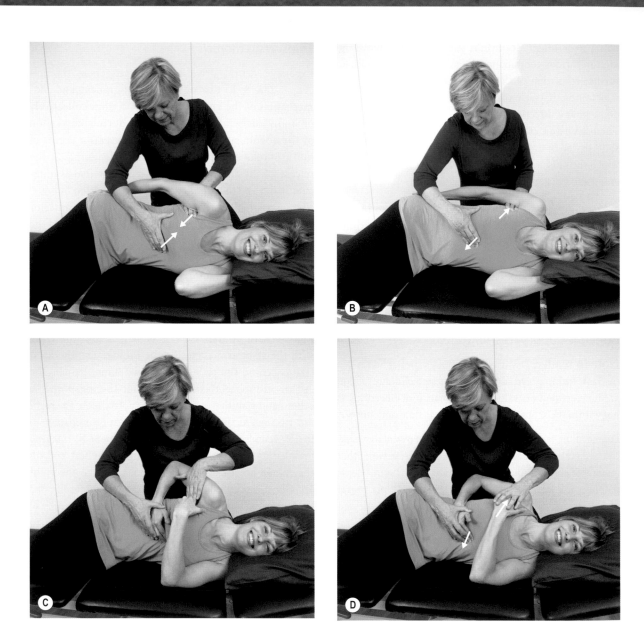

Figure 6.26

Release with awareness for a fascicle of transversus thoracis attaching to the right 3rd rib. (A) The right 3rd rib is approximated towards the xyphoid and held for 10 to 15 seconds. (B) After release of the neural component, a myofascial stretch follows by fixing the xyphoid and rotating the right 3rd thoracic ring to the right on the inhale breath. (C) Home practice: The patient is taught to self-correct the 3rd thoracic ring and stabilize the xyphoid. (D) On the inhale they are instructed to right rotate the 3rd thoracic ring while continuing to stabilize the xyphoid.

Diaphragm

Excessive neural drive to the diaphragm (Figs 1.23, 1.30, 1.31) may require that the cranium or cervical spine (or both) be treated prior to specifically releasing the diaphragm. If the vector of pull from the cranium or upper thorax is coming from the diaphragm, then a specific release technique for the diaphragm may help.

Release with awareness: The patient is sitting with their arms crossed to opposite shoulders. The therapist stands behind the patient. To release the left side of the diaphragm, place your right arm over the patient's right shoulder to palpate the left lower ribs. The left arm reaches the same area of the rib cage from the left side. The diaphragm flexes and ipsilaterally rotates the lower thorax; therefore, flex and left rotate the lower thorax to shorten the anterior costal fibers (Fig. 6.27A): Gently approximate ribs 7 to 10 toward the central tendon and wait. Cue the patient to imagine an expansive space between the lower ribs and to widen their lower rib cage on the exhale breath. As the rib cage

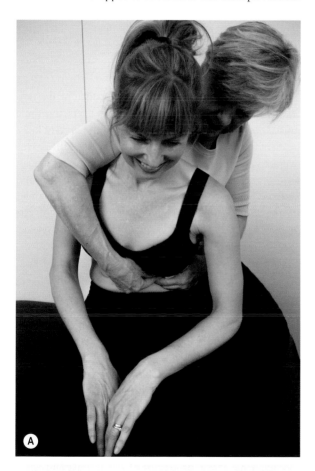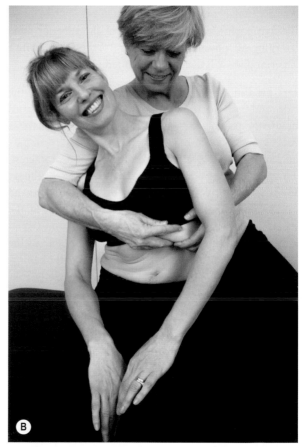

Figure 6.27

Release with awareness for the left anterior costal fibers of the diaphragm. (A) The fibers are initially shortened with flexion and left rotation of the lower thorax. Approximate the lower ribs toward the central tendon of the diaphragm. (B) The patient is cued to imagine their lower rib cage widening as they exhale (when the diaphragm relaxes). When the rib cage begins to expand, extend and right rotate the lower thorax.

starts to expand laterally, extend and right rotate the lower thorax (Fig. 6.27B). Repeat two to three times and repeat the screening task. If successful, there should be a change in the experience of performing the task.

Multifidus and rotatores

Unlike the low back and cervical regions, no studies have investigated the motor control adaptation response of the rotatores (Fig. 1.30) and multifidus (Fig. 1.33) to pain in the thoracic spine. Clinically, both muscles can present with overactivation or underactivation with or without atrophy. An overactive multifidus and rotatores will compress the zygapophyseal joint and prevent the superior glide (flexion). All movements of the thoracic ring that require a superior glide will therefore be limited.

Dry needling: The patient is prone with the arms by the sides and the head in neutral rotation. The therapist stands beside the patient. With one hand palpate the transverse process and part of the spinous process that is directly parallel to the transverse process at the segment of interest. This landmarking is critical when dry needling the thorax to avoid inadvertently needling the intercostal space and risking a pneumothorax. The needle is inserted in the space between the transverse and spinous process and aimed toward the lamina of the superior vertebra of the segment (Fig. 6.28). The depth of insertion is to the lamina.

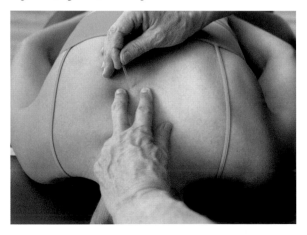

Figure 6.28

Dry needling of the thoracic multifidus and rotatores.

When there is overactivation of multifidus or rotatores (or both) either a muscle-grab or twitch response will occur before the bone is reached. When the muscle grabs the needle, leave the needle inserted until the grab response subsides. The grab response is still occurring if it is difficult to remove the needle. When it has subsided, the needle will be easy to remove. Following this release, reassess the alignment, biomechanics, and control of the thoracic ring during the relevant screening task. Interthoracic ring mobility and control achieved through sagittal plane movement training targeted to the restricted segment is given for a home exercise practice to maintain the release gained (see Stage 3, Levels 1 or 2 in Chapter 7).

Intercostals

The intercostals (Fig. 1.34A & B) are supplied by the ventral rami of the intercostal nerves. When overactive these muscles tend to 'glue' two thoracic rings and prevent independent movement between them (Lee L-J 2016). This overactivation can be reduced with many techniques; however, the preferred technique is thoracic ring stack and breathe (Lee L-J 2016), which will be described later under the heading: General, non-structure-specific technique for multiple system impairments. Following this release, reassess the alignment, biomechanics and control of the glued thoracic rings during the relevant screening task. Multidirectional range of motion exercises for the thorax (see Stage 3, Level 1 in Chapter 7) combined with breathwork (inhalation and exhalation) targeted to the restricted segment are given for a home exercise practice to maintain the release gained.

Serratus anterior

The serratus anterior (Fig. 1.35A & B) is commonly overactive and responsible for 'gluing' the scapula to the thorax (often to a specific thoracic ring) and for preventing independent movement between the scapula and the relevant thoracic ring. It is a protractor of the scapula and when the alignment of the thorax is easier to perturb than the scapula, the overactive fascicle posteriorly rotates the relevant rib. More often, the scapular alignment is easier to perturb such that when a fascicle of the serratus anterior is overactive, the scapula protracts and the rib anteriorly rotates. The thoracic ring, therefore, tends to be translated to the same side and rotated to the opposite side as the overactive fascicle of the serratus anterior. This neural system impairment often produces a co-driver between the thoracic ring and the shoulder girdle (scapula). Passive listening during correction of the relevant thoracic ring reveals a vector of pull from beneath the scapula. It feels like you are trying to 'stuff your foot into a shoe that has a sock in the toe.' Passive listening during release of the correction reveals a vector that is anterior, outside the thorax and of medium length. Passive listening during correction and release of the shoulder girdle (scapula) reveals the same vector of pull (see Miyuki's story in Chapter 5). Two techniques will be described for this muscle. These are release with awareness for an overactive fascicle of the right serratus anterior attaching to the 4th rib and dry needling for an overactive fascicle of the right serratus anterior attaching to the 2nd rib.

Release with awareness: The patient is left side lying with the head supported and the therapist stands in front of the patient. With the fingers of the left hand, palpate the overactive fascicle of the serratus anterior attaching to the 4th rib (Fig. 6.29A). It is often extremely tender, so palpation should be light but firm enough to control the rib. With the right hand, hold the patient's right arm in approximately 90 degrees of shoulder flexion. Protract the scapula over your right hand ensuring that the 4th thoracic ring does not rotate and follow the protraction (Fig. 6.29B). As your right hand slides beneath the scapula and the scapula protracts, the specific fibers of the fascicle of the serratus anterior attached to the 4th rib will approximate. Hold this position for 10 to 15 seconds and monitor the change in activation of the serratus anterior. Cue the patient to: 'allow the shoulder blade to float off the rib cage.' If this cue is successful, another level of release of the serratus anterior will occur. Hold the scapula in the same position and rotate the 4th thoracic ring beneath the scapula to the next barrier. Hold and repeat the cue three to four times.

Myofascial stretch component of the release with awareness technique: Hold the 4th thoracic ring corrected through the 4th rib and retract the scapula with your right hand and arm (Fig. 6.29C). Once the myofascial barrier is reached (it can be exquisitely tender), hold the

scapula retracted and with the fingertips of the right hand 'fan the tissue' in a craniocaudal manner to release any myofascial restrictions between the scapula and the rib cage. Following this release, reassess the alignment, biomechanics, and control of the 4th thoracic ring during the relevant screening task.

Dry needling: The patient is in side lying with the head supported and the therapist stands in front of the patient. Elevate and medially rotate the scapula so that the medial border is not approximated to the thorax. Overactivation of the fibers of the serratus anterior from the 2nd rib will make this difficult but it is an important step for lung safety when dry needling. See Figure 1.35B for the location on the scapula into which the upper fascicle of serratus anterior from the 2nd rib inserts, inside of the superior angle of the scapula. This is the point to aim for with your needle (Fig. 6.29D). The depth of insertion is to the bone. Either a muscle-grab or twitch response is desired. Wait for the grab to let go before removing the needle. Following this release, reassess the alignment, biomechanics and control of the thoracic ring during the relevant screening task.

The release can be maintained with the following home practice in side lying, four-point kneeling or standing weight bearing through the elevated arm on a wall (Fig. 6.29E) (see shoulder girdle mobility dissociated from interthoracic ring mobility, Stage 3, Level 2 in Chapter 7). Instruct the patient to self-correct the 4th thoracic ring through the right rib (gently lift the anterior aspect of the rib and push it back toward the right axilla) using the left hand. Hold this correction and protract the right scapula with the glenohumeral joint in 90 degrees of flexion. Slowly retract the scapula only as far as optimal alignment of the 4th thoracic ring can be maintained. Repeat three to four times and retest the screening task. There should be a notable change in the experience of performing the task.

Pectoralis major

The two parts of the pectoralis major (clavicular and sternal) (Fig. 1.36) impact different parts of the thorax and the shoulder. The clavicular fibers impact the upper thoracic rings (1st and 2nd) and the clavicle while the sternal fibers impact the middle thoracic rings (3rd to 7th) and humerus. Overactivation can be specific to one thoracic ring.

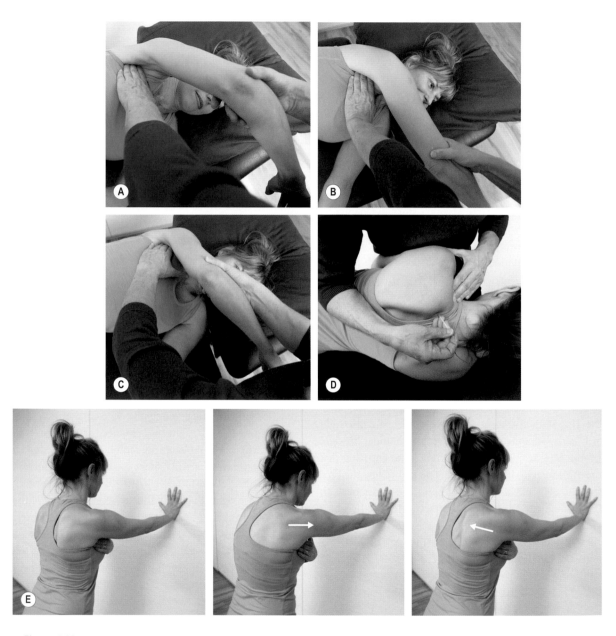

Figure 6.29

Release with awareness for a fascicle of serratus anterior attaching to the right 4th rib. (A) The overactive fascicle of serratus anterior is palpated along the body of the 4th rib. (B) Hold the 4th rib still and protract the scapula over your hand, thereby shortening the fibers of serratus anterior. This is the first part of a release with awareness technique. (C) After verbal cuing for more release, hold the 4th rib and retract the scapula to stretch the myofascial component of the serratus anterior. (D) Dry needling location for the fascicle of serratus anterior that attaches to the superior angle of the scapula from the 2nd rib. (E) Home practice to maintain the release of the serratus anterior.

Overactivation of the clavicular fibers of pectoralis major results in medial compression of the clavicle and while the lateral sternoclavicular joint (between the clavicle and disc) remains mobile, the medial part of the joint (between the disc and the manubrium) often does not. Consequently, the clavicle has limited osteokinematic rotation during all tasks. The 2nd thoracic ring tends to be rotated to the opposite side and passive listening on correction and release of both the clavicle and the 2nd thoracic ring reveals a horizontal vector of pull from the anterior thorax that is subclavicular.

The sternal fibers of pectoralis major do not impact the clavicle; however, they can impact the alignment and biomechanics of the glenohumeral joint. The humeral head is often anterior to the glenoid, the shoulder girdle protracted, and the scapula anteriorly tilted. The relevant thoracic ring or rings is or are translated to the same side and rotated to the opposite side. Passive listening on correction and release of the humerus, shoulder girdle, or middle thoracic rings (3rd to 7th) reveals an oblique anterior and inferior vector of pull that remains outside the thorax. The lower the thoracic ring, the more obliquely inferior the vector of pull.

Release with awareness for the right pectoralis major clavicular fibers: The patient is left side lying with the head supported and the therapist stands behind the patient. With the fingers of the right hand palpate the overactive fascicle of the clavicular part of the pectoralis major. With the other hand, support the scapula (Fig. 6.30A). Protract the shoulder girdle and shorten the overactive fascicle (with fingers of the right hand (Fig. 6.30B). Hold this position for 10 to 15 seconds and monitor the change in activation of the clavicular pectoralis major muscle. Cue the patient to: 'let this muscle soften and imagine the chest is broadening.' If this cue is successful, another level of release of the muscle will occur.

Myofascial stretch component of the release with awareness technique: With the right hand correct the 2nd thoracic ring. With the left hand decompress the clavicle at the sternoclavicular joint and retract the shoulder girdle to stretch the clavicular part of the pectoralis major (Fig. 6.30C). Following this release, reassess the alignment, biomechanics, and control of the clavicle and upper thoracic rings during the relevant screening task.

Release with awareness for the right pectoralis major sternal fibers: The patient is left side lying with the head supported and the therapist stands behind the patient. With the fingers of the right hand, palpate the overactive fascicle of the sternal part of the pectoralis major. With the other hand, support the scapula and shoulder (Fig. 6.31A).

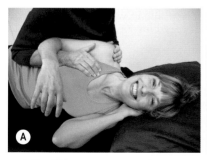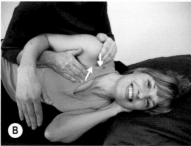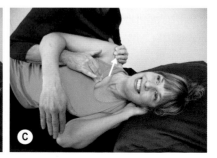

Figure 6.30

Release with awareness for the clavicular fibers of pectoralis major. (A) One hand monitors the overactive fascicle within the muscle while the other positions the shoulder girdle. (B) Shorten the fascicle by protracting the shoulder girdle with one hand and draw the fascicle toward the humerus (point of insertion) with the other. (C) Hold the 2nd thoracic ring corrected and stretch the myofascial component of the clavicular fibers of the pectoralis major by retracting the shoulder girdle.

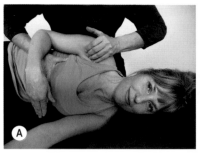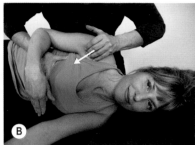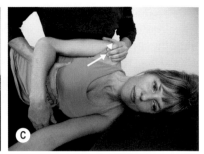

Figure 6.31

Release with awareness for the sternal fibers of the pectoralis major. (A) One hand stabilizes the rib to which the overactive fascicle of the sternal fibers of the pectoralis major attaches. The other hand controls the shoulder girdle. (B) Shorten the origin and insertion by protracting and anteriorly tilting the shoulder girdle. (C) This muscle often pulls the humeral head forward when overactive. Center the humeral head and then retract and posteriorly tilt the shoulder girdle while stabilizing the relevant thoracic ring anteriorly.

Protract and anteriorly tilt the shoulder girdle to shorten the overactive fascicle and stabilize the rib that this fascicle attaches to (Fig. 6.31B). Hold this position for 10 to 15 seconds and monitor the change in activation of the sternal pectoralis major. Cue the patient to: 'let this muscle soften and imagine the chest is broadening.' If this cue is successful, another level of release of the muscle will occur.

Myofascial stretch component of the release with awareness technique: With one hand correct the relevant middle thoracic ring. Hold this correction and with the other hand center the humeral head and retract and posteriorly tilt the shoulder girdle to stretch the sternal part of the pectoralis major (Fig. 6.31C). Following this release, reassess the alignment, biomechanics and control of the humerus and middle thoracic rings during the relevant screening task.

Pectoralis minor

When the position of the scapula is more resistant to change than the thorax, overactivation of pectoralis minor (Fig. 1.36) will posteriorly rotate ribs 3 to 5. More often, the position of the scapula is less resistant to change than the thorax and overactivation of the pectoralis minor results in elevation and an anterior tilt of the scapula associated with anterior rotation of the relevant rib. The impacted thoracic ring commonly translates to the same side and rotates to the opposite side as the scapula elevates

and anteriorly tilts. Like serratus anterior, overactivation of pectoralis minor often produces a co-driver between the scapula and the thoracic ring. Passive listening during correction and release of the shoulder girdle reveals a vector of pull that is anterior and inferior outside the thorax. Passive listening during correction and release of the 3rd to 5th thoracic rings is interesting in that the rib merely floats into anterior rotation (does not feel pulled into anterior rotation) and then the scapula elevates and anteriorly tilts strongly. Two techniques will be described for this muscle. These are release with awareness for an overactive fascicle of the right pectoralis minor attaching to the 5rd rib and dry needling for a fascicle attaching to the 3rd rib.

Release with awareness: The patient is left side lying with the head supported and the therapist stands behind the patient. Monitor the overactive fascicle of the right pectoralis minor to the 5th rib with the right hand and shorten this fascicle by elevating and anteriorly tilting the scapula with the left hand (Fig. 6.32A). Hold this position for 10 to 15 seconds and monitor the change in activation of the pectoralis minor muscle. Cue the patient to: 'soften the muscle under my fingers,' to 'relax the shoulder girdle and let me totally support it.' If this cue is successful, another level of release of the pectoralis minor will occur. Hold and repeat the cue a few times.

Myofascial stretch component of the release with awareness technique: Correct the 5th thoracic ring, hold this correction, and take the shoulder girdle into a posterior tilt and depression (Fig. 6.32B). An exhale breath can facilitate this stretch.

Dry needling: The patient is supine with the head supported and the right arm slightly abducted. With the thumb of the one hand, palpate the costal surface of the pectoralis minor and lift the muscle ventrally off the rib cage (Fig. 6.32C). The overactive fascicle will feel like a 'pepperoni stick in the middle of a salami' between your thumb and fingers. Localize this fascicle and aim the needle toward your thumb to prevent it going through an intercostal space into the lung (Fig. 6.32D). Either a muscle-grab or twitch response is desired. Wait for the grab to let go before removing the needle. Following this release, reassess the alignment, biomechanics and control of the thoracic ring during the relevant screening task.

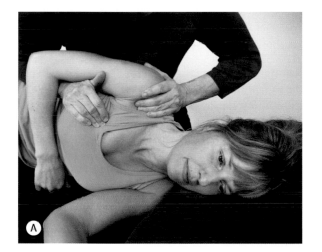
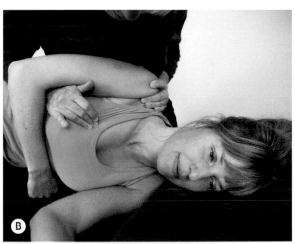
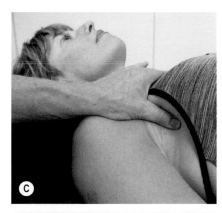
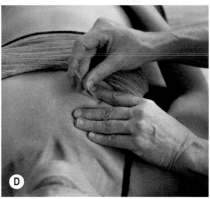

Figure 6.32

Release with awareness for the pectoralis minor. (A) Monitor the overactive fascicle and shorten it by approximating the coracoid process toward the rib to which the overactive fascicle attaches. (B) After the neural component of the release has occurred, the myofascia is stretched by stabilizing the rib and taking the coracoid away from it. The exhale breath anteriorly rotates the rib and when the coracoid is stabilized and this can facilitate more myofascial stretching. (C, D) Dry needling for the pectoralis minor.

The release for both pectoralis major and minor can be maintained with the following home practice. Instruct the patient to lie supine with their head supported on a small pillow. Palpate the rib that the overactive fascicle attaches to with the opposite hand. Hold the rib into anterior rotation and 'circle the shoulder girdle onto the back' (elevate, retract, then depress) (Fig. 6.33A). Abduct and externally rotate the glenohumeral joint (cactus arm) (Fig. 6.33B). Do not let the rib posteriorly rotate with this shoulder girdle and shoulder motion. Actively maintain the retraction and depression of the shoulder girdle, hold the rib in anterior rotation, and then take a small breath in and a long breath out. On the exhale increase the shoulder girdle retraction and depression and gently pull the rib into anterior rotation.

Subclavius

The subclavius (Fig. 1.37) is a compressor of the clavicle and thus important for control of the sternoclavicular joint. When it is overactive, and fails to eccentrically lengthen, the clavicle is compressed medially and 'rides up' the concave facet on the manubrium. This compresses the medial sternoclavicular joint and limits the ability of the clavicle to rotate anteroposteriorly. The result is increased fascial tension in both the superficial and deep fascia of the neck and multiple possible consequences follow. Overactivation of the subclavius is often associated with overactivation of the clavicular fibers of the pectoralis major and this creates mobility restrictions of the upper thorax and manubrium. Active listening to the clavicle during head and neck rotation reveals a motion of the clavicle that should not occur – medial translation. Passive listening during correction and release of the clavicle reveals a vector of pull that is anterior, horizontal, and subclavicular.

Release with awareness: To release the right subclavius, the patient is left side lying with the head supported and the therapist stands behind the patient. Monitor the overactive subclavius with one hand while shortening the two ends of the muscle. Hold the clavicle compressed medially with the other hand (Fig. 6.34A). Hold this position for 10 to 15 seconds and monitor the change in activation of the subclavius. Cue the patient to: 'soften the muscle under

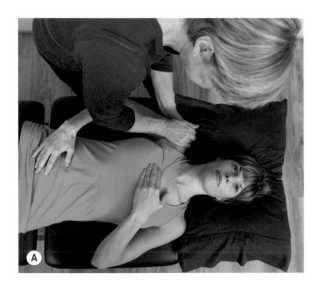
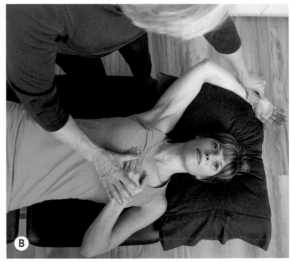

Figure 6.33

Home practice for maintaining release of both the pectoralis major and pectoralis minor. (A) Stabilize the rib to which the overactive fascicle attaches, circle the shoulder onto the back. (B) For further stretch, abduct and externally rotate the shoulder (cactus arm) taking care to not allow the rib to posteriorly rotate. On the exhale breath, gently pull the rib into more anterior rotation.

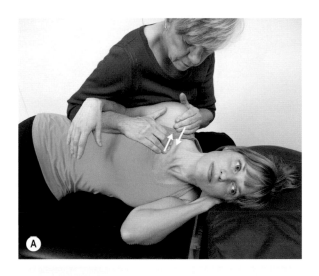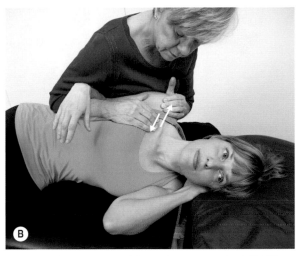

Figure 6.34

Release with awareness for the subclavius. (A) To shorten the muscle, the clavicle is compressed medially toward the manubrium and the subclavius muscle is drawn laterally toward the shoulder. (B) After release of the neural component, the muscle is stretched by distracting the clavicle from the manubrium and drawing the subclavius medially.

my fingers; relax the collar bone and imagine the collar bone floating away from the midline.' If this cue is successful, another level of release of the subclavius will occur. Hold and repeat the cue a few times.

Myofascial stretch component of the release with awareness technique: Decompress the sternoclavicular joint by distracting the clavicle as the subclavius is manually stretched (Fig. 6.34B). Following this release, reassess the alignment, biomechanics, and control of the clavicle and 1st thoracic ring during the relevant screening task.

External oblique

The external oblique (EO) (Fig. 1.24, 1.38) is a strong compressor of the thorax and abdomen. It is common to find this muscle overactive when it is used as part of a suboptimal strategy for transferring loads between the thorax and pelvis. It is often overactive in women with low back and pelvic girdle pain, urinary incontinence, pelvic organ prolapse or diastasis rectus abdominis (DRA). It is also common to find *specific fascicles* of the EO overactive and limiting motion of just one or two thoracic rings. This has significant

implications for tasks requiring rotation of the thorax, as well as for breathing. Lower thoracic rings that are translated and rotated are often related to dyssynergistic recruitment strategies of the abdominal wall (Lee D 2016, 2017a, Lee L-J 2016). The thoracic ring or rings will be translated to the same side, and rotated to the opposite side, as the overactive fascicle or fascicles of the EO when this muscle produces the dominant vector perturbing the alignment and biomechanics. Passive listening during correction and release of the impaired thoracic ring or rings reveals a vector of pull that is anterior, obliquely inferior and long (Fig. 6.24A). The vector of pull remains outside the thorax and abdomen. Release with awareness and dry needling are both useful release techniques; however, one must be very accurate when landmarking the thorax to avoid inadvertently inserting the needle through the intercostals and into the lung.

Release with awareness: The patient is supine, with hips and knees flexed, and the therapist stands at the patient's side. Palpate the specific overactive fascicle of the EO over the body of the relevant rib. Shorten the fascicle by approximating the rib obliquely toward the linea alba and contralateral side of the pelvis (Fig. 6.35A). Hold this position

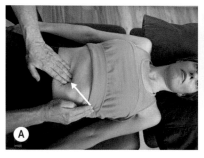 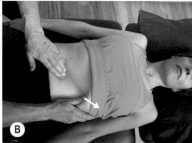 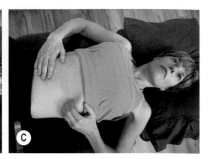

Figure 6.35

Release with awareness for external oblique. (A) Approximate the rib to which the overactive fascicle of EO attaches towards the linea alba to shorten the muscle. (B) After the neural component is released, the external oblique is stretched by posteriorly rotating the relevant rib on the inhale breath. (C) Home practice to maintain release of the EO.

for 10 to 15 seconds and monitor the change in activation of the EO. Cue the patient to: 'let my fingers sink into the abdomen; let the rib cage relax and widen.'

Myofascial stretch component of the release with awareness technique: Lengthen the fascicle manually between the relevant rib and the linea alba by lifting the anterior part of the rib up toward the ipsilateral shoulder (posteriorly rotate the rib) and then cue a lateral costal inhale breath (Fig. 6.35B). If the overactive fascicle cannot eccentrically lengthen and relax, it will try to anteriorly rotate the rib. Hold the rib against the vector of force on inspiration and release and relax on expiration. Repeat three to four times.

The release can be maintained by instructing the patient how to use a manual self-correction of the thoracic ring while anchoring the linea alba combined with an inhale lateral costal breath to release the specific fascicle of the EO (Fig. 6.35C). Repeat three to four times and retest the screening task (usually thoracic rotation). There should be a notable change in the experience of performing the task. Supine wipers (see the home release practice for the internal oblique below) can also be used to maintain release of the EO.

Internal oblique

Overactivation of the intermediate fibers of the internal oblique (IO) (Figs 1.24, 1.39) impact the function of the 10th thoracic ring, and by the aponeurotic expansion of

the IO, the 9th to 7th thoracic rings. The vector of force pulls the rib into anterior rotation and when these fibers produce the dominant vector the thoracic ring will be held translated to the same side as the vector and contralaterally rotated. When the IO is recruited more than the EO and upper fibers of the transversus abdominis, the rib cage and infrasternal angle will widen during a short head and neck curl-up task. Passive listening during correction and release of the relevant lower thoracic ring reveals a vector that is anterior, obliquely lateral and inferior, outside the abdomen. Two techniques will be described to release the intermediate fibers of the IO: release with awareness and dry needling.

Release with awareness: It is common to find a tender trigger point in the intermediate fibers halfway between the iliac crest and the 10th rib in the midaxillary line when this part of the muscle is overactive. The patient is side lying with the muscle to be released on the uppermost side and the therapist stands in front of the patient. Support, and control, the thorax by winding the cranial arm through the patient's upper arm. Palpate the overactive fascicle of the IO with one hand and the 10th rib with the other. Shorten the specific fascicle with ipsilateral side bending and rotation of the thorax and specifically the 10th thoracic ring (Fig. 6.36A). Hold this position for 10 to 15 seconds and monitor the change in the activation of the IO. Cue the patient to: 'let the muscle in the waist soften; let the pelvis roll backwards; let my fingers sink into the waist; let the

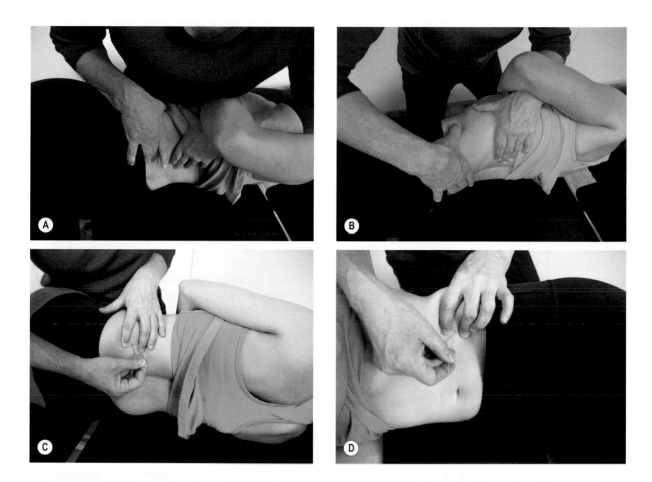

Figure 6.36

Release with awareness and dry needling for the internal oblique. (A) The intermediate fibers of the internal oblique are shortened with ipsilateral side bending and rotation of the thorax. (B) After the neural component is released, the internal oblique is stretched with contralateral side bending and rotation of the thorax. (C) Dry needling the origin of the internal oblique at the posterior iliac crest. (D) Dry needling the intermediate fibers midway between the iliac crest and the 10th rib.

ribs relax into my hand.' If this cue is successful, another level of release of the IO will occur.

Myofascial stretch component of the release with awareness technique: Lengthen the fascicle by bringing the lower thorax into contralateral rotation and side-bending in a direction that lengthens the overactive IO (Fig. 6.36B). Continue to use words to encourage relaxation and release and monitor the fascicle for any recurrence of overactivation. Following this release, reassess the alignment,

biomechanics, and control of the relevant thoracic ring during the screening task.

Dry needling: For the left IO, the patient is in right side lying with the head supported and the therapist stands in front of the patient. Palpate the overactive fascicle of the IO and trace the origin of this fascicle to the iliac crest. The depth of insertion of the needle is to the iliac crest (Fig. 6.36C). Alternately, the middle part of this fascicle can be dry needled by squeezing the anterior and posterior part of the muscle together, lifting the muscle away from the abdomen and ensuring that the colon is not between your fingers. The needle is then inserted horizontally from anterior to posterior (not directly into the abdomen) (Fig. 6.36D).

The release of both the EO and IO can be maintained with the following home practice called 'supine wipers' (Lee D 2017a, 2017b). The patient is supine with the head supported and the hips and knees flexed. Have them take a few breaths here and visualize the thighs sinking into the hips like telephone poles in mud. Let the sitting bones widen and the thighs be heavy so that they sink deep into the back of the acetabulum (center the femoral heads). These are cues to release and relax any overactivation of the deep hip and pelvic floor muscles that may be reacting to increased intra-abdominal pressure from thoracic ring impairments. Gently activate the deep muscles responsible for lumbopelvic control with the appropriate connect cue (see intrapelvic ring motor control training in Chapter 7) and do not allow the pelvis to tilt.

1. On the exhale breath, slowly take both knees to the left only as far as they can go without the thorax leaving the floor (Fig. 6.37A). Inhale to hold this position for three to four seconds and on the next exhale increase the recruitment of the deep muscles and derotate the pelvis to neutral. Notice if it is easier or harder to go to the right or left. Work on the side that is more difficult until they are the same.

2. Progression: With one hand, hold the relevant thoracic ring to the floor (do not let it lift) and recruit the deep muscles and exhale as the knees move to the left. Inhale to hold and then exhale, increase the recruitment and rotate the pelvis to the right to return the knees to neutral (i.e., do not lead the movement with the knees). Repeat to the right.

3. Progression: Take the arms into 'cactus arms' (elbows bent with the back of the palms on (or near) the floor by the head), and take three to four deep breaths expanding the rib cage sideways (lateral costal breath) to release any overactivation of the abdominal wall. Activate the deep muscles as you exhale and take the knees to the right (Fig. 6.37B). Use the superficial muscles (abdominals and back muscles) to keep the thorax on the floor. Try to keep the arms relaxed and not engaged in this movement practice. Inhale and hold, and lengthen the thigh by 'reaching the femur away from the pelvis.' This cue is used to relax the superficial long muscles of the thigh that are compressing the hip joint. Exhale, increase the recruitment to the deep system and derotate using the pelvis, not the knees. Repeat three to four times each side. Focused attention to each part is important for building these recruitment strategies.

4. Further progression: Repeat this sequence and reverse the breathing pattern.

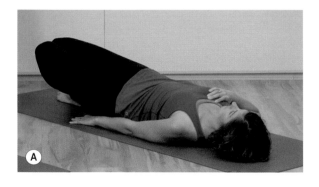
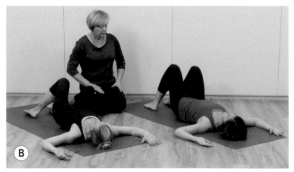

Figure 6.37

Supine wipers. (A) Manually maintaining the alignment of the 3rd thoracic ring. (B) Progressing to using imagery for alignment of the thoracic rings (in cactus arms).

Rectus abdominis

Overactivation of the upper compartment of the rectus abdominis (Figs 1.24, 1.40) can impact function of the 5th to 7th thoracic rings. If bilaterally overactive, the rectus abdominis will hold the left and right ribs in anterior rotation and limit posterior tilting of thoracic rings 5 to 7, a required motion for extension of the thorax in, for example, backward bending of the trunk. Unilateral overactivation will hold one rib in anterior rotation and cause the thoracic ring to rotate to the ipsilateral side. In this instance, rotation of the thorax is the main motion impaired.

Passive listening during correction and release reveals a vector of pull that is anterior and inferior with minimal obliquity, and outside of the thorax and abdomen. A release with awareness technique to facilitate elongation of this muscle is described.

Release with awareness: The patient is supine with the hips and knees flexed. Palpate the cranial and caudal extent of the overactive fascicle within the rectus abdominis. Approximate the two ends and hold the fascicle in this shortened position (Fig. 6.38A). Hold this position for 10 to 15 seconds and monitor the change in the fascicle's activation. Cue the patient to: 'allow the belly to soften; let my fingers sink into the abdominal wall; open the space between the pelvis and the ribcage.' If this cue is successful, another level of release will occur.

Myofascial stretch component of the release with awareness technique: Lengthen the fascicle by taking the two ends of the overactive fascicle apart. Continue to use words to encourage relaxation and release and monitor the fascicle for any recurrence of overactivation. Following this release, reassess the alignment, biomechanics, and control of the 5th to 7th thoracic rings during the relevant screening task.

The release can be maintained by any exercise that extends the thorax relative to the pelvis (supported back bridge over a gym ball, cobra pose in yoga (Fig. 6.38B), passive prone push-up, etc.).

Back extensors and rotators

This group of muscles includes the semispinalis thoracis (part of the transversospinalus group) and the erector spinae (spinalus thoracis, longissimus thoracis pars thoracis, iliocostalis thoracis, and iliocostalis lumborum [Fig. 1.47], serratus posterior superior or serratus posterior inferior [Fig. 1.49]). Bilateral overactivation of these muscles compresses the posterior aspect of the rib cage and spine preventing anterior tilt of the thorax and flexion of the thoracic spine. Unilateral overactivation of multiple fascicles creates a side bending compressive force, often with contralateral translation of multiple thoracic rings. More common is the 'subtle redistribution of activation' (Hodges & Smeets 2015) of specific fascicles that then impact mobility and control of one thoracic ring. This may occur as a dominant vector causing the

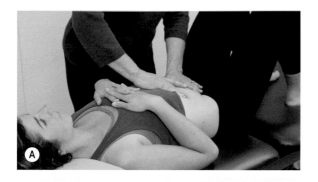
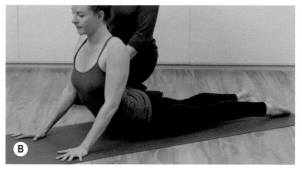

Figure 6.38

(A) Release with awareness for rectus abdominis. This is an intramuscular release technique. (B) Cobra pose for home practice to lengthen the released fascicle of rectus abdominis.

thoracic ring to translate and rotate or in reaction to another vector to prevent further translation and rotation of the thoracic ring. Iliocostalis lumborum attaches to the posterior aspect of a rib and the iliac crest (Fig. 1.48) and when overactive will posteriorly rotate that rib and create a contralateral translation and ipsilateral rotation of the entire thoracic ring if unopposed. It can potentially create a superior pull on the posterior ipsilateral innominate. If this force is beyond that which the force closure mechanism of the pelvis can oppose, loss of SIJ control can occur. Longissimus thoracis pars thoracis inserts via long tendinous slips into the thoracolumbar fascia and sacrum and when overactive, nutates the sacrum. This increases the force closure mechanism for the pelvis (see Leah's story in Chapter 5); however, it is not an ideal strategy since thoracolumbar mobility is lost. Passive listening during correction and release reveals a vector of pull that is posterior and inferior with minimal obliquity, and outside the thorax and abdomen. A release with awareness technique and a muscle recoil technique are described.

Iliocostalis cervicis has the opposite biomechanical impact on the rib than iliocostalis thoracis and iliocostalis lumborum when overactive. Arising from the neck and inserting into the posterior aspect of the rib (Fig. 1.47), when overactive iliocostalis cervicis can anteriorly rotate the rib and cause an ipsilateral translation and contralateral rotation of the relevant thoracic ring. Passive listening during correction and release of a cervical vertebra reveals a vector of pull that is posterior and inferior with minimal obliquity, and outside the thorax. When the relevant thoracic ring is corrected, passive listening reveals a vector of pull that is posterior and superior with minimal obliquity. A release with awareness technique is described.

Release with awareness: The patient is prone with the head neutral and the arms by the sides. Palpate the cranial and caudal extent of the overactive fascicle within the relevant back extensor muscle. Approximate the two ends and hold the fascicle in this shortened position (Fig. 6.39A) for 10 to 15 seconds and monitor the change in the fascicle's activation. Cue the patient to: 'let the muscle soften; let my fingers sink into the back; relax and allow the spine to lengthen.' If this cue is successful, another level of release will occur.

Myofascial stretch component of the release with awareness technique: Lengthen the fascicle by taking the two ends of the overactive fascicle apart (Fig. 6.39B). Continue to use words to encourage relaxation and release and monitor the fascicle for any recurrence of overactivation. Following this release, reassess the alignment, biomechanics and control of the thoracic ring or rings and cervical vertebrae during the relevant screening task.

Muscle recoil or muscle manipulation technique: The patient is prone with the head neutral and the arms by the sides. With the heels of the hands, palpate the cranial and caudal extent of the overactive fascicle (thorax, not neck). Approximate the two ends and hold the fascicle in this shortened position for 10 to 15 seconds (Fig. 6.39C). Then, apply a high-velocity, low-amplitude thrust of the hands toward each other (staying within the muscle layer and not

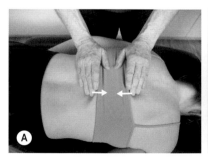 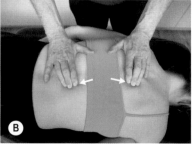 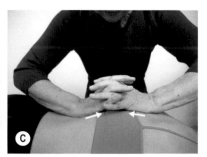

Figure 6.39

Release for the back extensors. (A) Release with awareness for a fascicle of the right erector spinae. Begin by approximating either end of the overactive fascicle and hold for 10 to 15 seconds. (B) Take the muscle into passive stretch. (C) Muscle 'recoil' or manipulation technique. First, approximate either end of the over-active fascicle for 10 seconds.

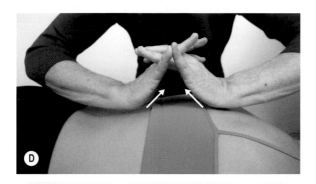 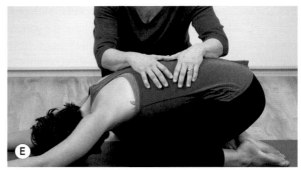

Figure 6.39 *continued*

(D) Then, a high velocity, low amplitude approximation of the heels of the hands is followed by immediate release of the tissue. (E) Balasana (Child's Pose) and breath are excellent practices to maintain reduced activation of the back extensors.

compressing into the skeletal thorax) followed by immediate release of the muscle (Fig. 6.39D). This technique activates the golgi tendon organs and results in relaxation of the extrafusal muscle fibers. If this technique is successful, another level of release will occur.

The release can be maintained with any exercise that facilitates flexion of the neck and thorax (prone over a gym ball, Child's Pose (Balasana) and interthoracic ring mobility and control with sagittal plane movement training (see Chapter 7)). Instruct the patient to breathe into the areas of the thorax that require release (Fig. 6.39E).

General, non-structure-specific technique for multiple system impairments

This is a general, non-structure-specific, precise technique aimed to release multiple system vectors and restore alignment and biomechanics of a thoracic ring. Thoracic ring stack and breathe (Lee L-J 2016) combined with hold–relax and vector-specific articular mobilization for relevant zygapophyseal and costotransverse joint restrictions are all integrated into this technique. It can be used for multiple directions of restriction for any thoracic ring. Simply modify the landmarking according to the restricted ring and apply the biomechanics from Chapter 2 into the technique. One example follows below; innovate others as needed.

In this example, the 7th thoracic ring is translated right and rotated left (right 7th rib anteriorly rotated, left 7th rib posteriorly rotated, T6–T7 left rotated and left side-bent, entire thoracic ring translated right and rotated left) with neural and visceral vectors. The patient is sitting with their arms crossed to opposite shoulders. Ensure that the pelvis is in neutral rotation and that the SIJs are not unlocked. If the pelvis is rotated (transverse plane rotation or intrapelvic torsion) or one SIJ is unlocked in a vertically loaded position, neuromuscular vectors connecting the pelvis and thorax for control will not relax since they are needed to provide control for the pelvis. The therapist stands behind the patient. With both hands, palpate the left and right 7th ribs. Remember that the ribs will not be on the same horizontal level (see Chapter 1 for how to landmark ribs in the vertebrochondral region). Correct the 7th thoracic ring and ensure that the 6th and 8th thoracic rings are capable of independent motion relative to the 7th and that their alignment does not worsen with this correction. If they do, then either a two or three thoracic ring correction is required. If the vectors impairing optimal alignment and biomechanics of the 7th thoracic ring are neural or visceral or both, it will be possible to correct the thoracic ring or rings. Hold the 7th thoracic ring corrected and instruct the patient to:

1. Breathe diaphragmatically (belly breath);

2. Breathe with lateral costal expansion in the low thorax, then with middle thorax expansion;

3. Breathe apically.

Pick the breathing pattern that attempts to pull the 7th thoracic ring out of alignment the most and have the patient repeat the inhale and exhale three to four times (Fig. 6.40A). If inhalation pulls more, have them take a short breath out and a long breath in. If exhalation pulls more, have them take a short breath in and a long breath out. Then, instruct the patient to rotate to the right only until the first resistance to this motion is felt. Repeat the breathing pattern three more times in this position (Fig. 6.40B). Be sure to keep the thorax stacked vertically over the pelvis; do not allow the thorax to excessively translate laterally or sidebend as they rotate. After three more breaths, apply a gentle resistance to further right rotation and instruct the patient to 'meet your resistance' (hold–relax) (Fig. 6.40C). See if this provides more release and mobility into right rotation. Repeat two to three times.

If a complete correction of the 7th thoracic ring is not possible, there may be a combination of neural, visceral, and articular system vectors restricting mobility. For this situation, begin with thoracic ring stack and breathe, followed by hold–relax and then add a specific arthrokinematic glide that is appropriate for the direction of rotation being treated. For this example, apply an inferior glide to the right T6–T7 zygapophyseal joint, an anterolateroinferior glide to the right 7th costotransverse joint, a superior glide to the left T6–T7 zygapophyseal joint, and a posteromediosuperior glide to the left 7th costotransverse joint. One or more of these joints may require a vector-specific mobilization technique, which can be integrated into this combined technique for neural, visceral, and articular system impairments that restrict mobility of the 7th thoracic ring.

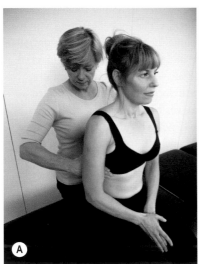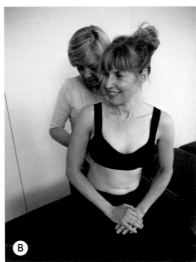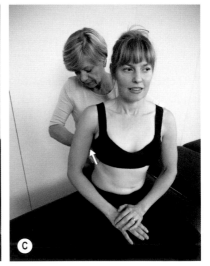

Figure 6.40

Thoracic ring stack and breathe (Lee L-J 2016) and hold–relax. (A) Correct the thoracic rings of interest and find the breathing pattern (abdominal, lateral costal, apical) that attempts to pull the thoracic rings out of alignment. Have the patient breathe this way three to four times and do not release the correction. (B) Rotate the thorax and facilitate the optimal biomechanics of the individual thoracic rings until the first resistance is felt. Repeat the breathing pattern previously found to perturb the alignment of the thoracic rings being treated three to four times. (C) Rotate the thorax to the next barrier. Ask the patient to 'meet your resistance' as you try to rotate them further (arrow) (hold–relax). Repeat two to three times. Maintain the alignment of the thoracic rings as they rotate back to neutral and release the thoracic rings slowly. Recheck seated thoracic rotation with no manual correction and note any change in amplitude and the patient's experience of the task.

Dural and perineural system impairments

When the alignment of the body is the cause for insufficient dural or perineural mobility, correcting the alignment will improve the ability of the dural or perineural system to elongate and move, and more range of motion will be gained (Figs 3.82A–F, 3.83A–C). Vector analysis of the driver or drivers subsequently determines the underlying system impairment and the required treatment intervention (Fig. 6.41A–C).

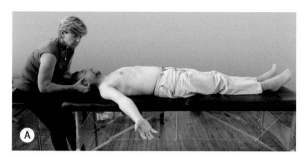

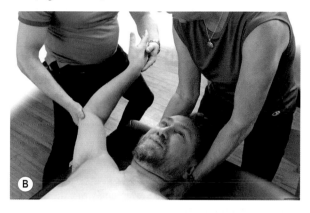

Figure 6.41

These figures continue the story first introduced in Figure 3.83A–C in Chapter 3. This man's meaningful complaint was neuralgic-type symptoms in the right arm with elevation or abduction of his right arm, particularly movements that stretched the right ulnar nerve. He presented with a left intracranial torsion (ICT) and a congruently left rotated sphenoid, C7 translated right and rotated left, the 2nd thoracic ring alternating between left and right rotation, and the 4th thoracic ring translated right and rotated left. His primary driver for abduction of the right arm was his cranium. Correcting his cranium restored the alignment of C7 and the 2nd and 4th thoracic rings.

(A) In supine, the patient was only able to abduct his right arm to 45 degrees before neuralgic symptoms started in his hand and his cranium was felt to twist more into a left ICT. (B) The intracranial vectors (cerebellar tentorium, transverse and sigmoid sinuses) were released and he was surprised to note that he could elevate his right arm completely even when the forearm was pronated. (C) Repeat analysis of his meaningful task revealed more amplitude of elevation of the right arm with no consequences to the alignment of his 2nd or 4th thoracic rings, C7 or the cranium.

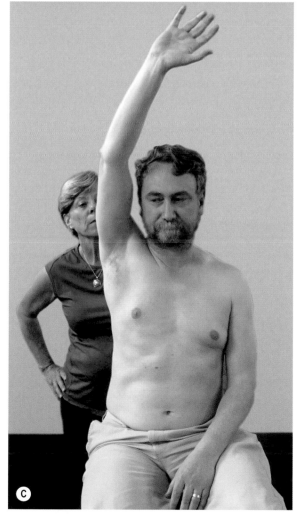

When the dura, or its peripheral extension into the perineural tissue, is the primary system impairment, and the dural or perineural system has exhausted its capacity to elongate, a correction in alignment of one body region will worsen the alignment in another, as well as the performance of the task (Fig. 3.81A–C). The entire length of the dural and perineural vector then requires release before suboptimal alignment, biomechanics, and control of the skeleton can be addressed. If only one part of the restriction is addressed (e.g., upper or lower limb, spinal column, cranium) the other end of the vector will shorten and no absolute release, or length, will be gained. On occasion, two or more therapists will be required to 'capture' the entire extent of the vector (cranium to sacrum, cranium to two feet, cranium to two hands) for complete release. Since most of us do not have ISM personal assistants the patient becomes the additional therapist and is guided through various active movements while the primary therapist retains the alignment of the cranium.

Cranium to sacrum

The patient is in hook lying, with their arms by the sides. The therapist is seated at the head. Begin by correcting the cranium (see the sections on intracranial torsion (ICT) and the sphenoid in Chapter 3) and ask the patient to contract their pelvic floor muscles. When the dura in the cranium and spinal canal does not permit elongation, a contraction of the pelvic floor muscles often pulls the cranium caudally. If the pelvic floor contraction is asymmetric, the cranium often twists (ICT) and becomes compressed into the upper neck (C1, C2). Release any suboccipital neuromuscular vectors using a release with awareness technique. Maintain a complete cranial correction (cranium, C1, C2) and slide your middle and ring fingers onto

the occipitoatlantal (OA) membrane; the spinal dura attaches here (Fig. 6.42A). Instruct the patient to posteriorly tilt the pelvis just until you feel the response in the OA membrane or cranium. If a second therapist is available, they can provide more specific stabilization of the sacrum and coccyx with the palm of their hand (Fig. 6.42B). Apply a steady, moderately strong, distraction force to the spinal dura while maintaining the correction of the cranial region (cranium, C1 and C2). The second therapist stabilizing the sacrum and coccyx should feel the pull on the sacrum and coccyx and applies a gentle counterforce. Hold the distraction until a release between the cranial region and sacrum is felt. Add more posterior pelvic tilt (caudal pull on the sacrum and coccyx) and wait for further release. Have the patient return their pelvis to a neutral position, retain the correction of the cranial region, and ask the patient to contract their pelvic floor muscles. If the release has been successful, you should not feel this contraction pull on the upper neck or cranium.

The next step depends on the patient's story and whether the restriction continues into the lower or upper extremities.

Cranium to lower extremity

Posterior lower extremity perineural mobilization: Maintain the correction of the cranium and moderately strong spinal dura traction and ask the patient to flex one hip and knee to 90 degrees and then dorsiflex and evert the foot as they straighten the knee. Stop the motion of the lower extremity when any pull or twist on the cranium is felt (Fig. 6.43A & B). The leg and foot can be supported on a wall in this position or held by a second therapist. Wait until this part of the dural and perineural system releases;

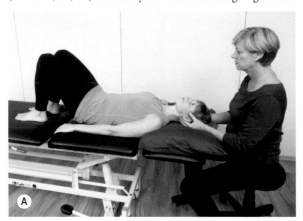

Figure 6.42

Release of the dura from the cranium to sacrum. (A) Correct the cranial region and then distract the cranium from the spine. Maintain this distraction as the patient either contracts their pelvic floor muscles or posteriorly tilts their pelvis. Do not let the cranium twist.

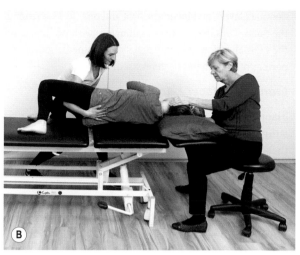
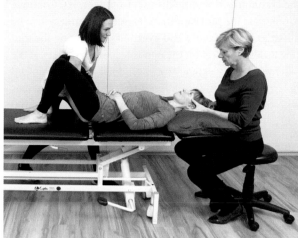

Figure 6.42 *continued*

(B) When a second therapist is available to stabilize the sacrum and coccyx distally the long vector in the dura between the cranium and sacrum and coccyx is more easily localized and released.

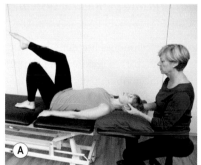
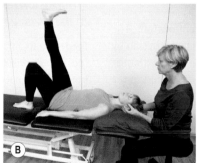
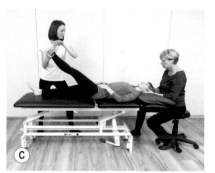

Figure 6.43

Release of the dura and perineurium from the cranium to the posterior lower extremity. (A) While maintaining the cranium corrected and a moderately strong distraction force to the spinal dura, ask the patient to flex one hip to 90 degrees and then begin to straighten the knee. Stop when any compression or torsion is felt in the cranium, hold and wait for the dura and perineurium to release. (B) Progress by adding extension of the knee, dorsiflexion of the ankle and inversion or eversion of the foot. (C) A second therapist is a useful assist for this release technique. The therapist at the cranium guides the movements of the lower extremity and instructs when to hold a position and when to progress further.

the cranium will slightly distract from the atlas. Continue to lengthen the posterior lower extremity neural system by dorsiflexing the ankle and everting or inverting the foot (Fig. 6.43C). Repeat on the opposite lower extremity. If the patient can fully extend the knee, dorsiflex and evert and invert the foot, and only feel a stretch in the hamstrings with no impact on the cranium, then the posterior dural and perineural system has been released.

Anterior lower extremity perineural mobilization:
Maintain the correction of the cranium and moderately strong spinal dura traction and ask the patient to extend one hip and flex the knee over the side of the table. Vary the plantarflexion and dorsiflexion of the ankle, inversion and eversion of the foot and assess the response in the cranium. Stop the lower extremity motion when any pull on the cranium is felt. The leg and foot can be supported on a footstool or held by a second therapist (Fig. 6.44A). Wait until this part of the dural and perineural system releases; the cranium will slightly distract from the atlas. Continue to lengthen the anterior neural system by extending the hip and flexing the knee (Fig. 6.44B).

Medial lower extremity perineural mobilization: The medial perineural system of the thigh can be addressed by adding abduction of the hip to the anterior lower extremity mobilization. Repeat on the opposite lower extremity. If the patient can fully extend and abduct the hip, flex the knee, dorsiflex, evert, and invert the foot and only feel a stretch in the quadriceps, hip flexors or adductors with no impact on the cranial region, then the anterior and medial dural and perineural system has been released.

Cranium to upper extremity

Maintain the correction of the cranial region and moderately strong spinal dura traction and ask the patient to supinate the forearm and abduct the glenohumeral joint (Fig. 6.45A). Stop the upper extremity motion when any pull on the cranium is felt. Wait until this part of the dural and perineural system releases; the cranium will slightly distract from the atlas. Continue to lengthen the upper extremity perineural system with further abduction to 90 degrees (Fig. 6.45B). Once the perineural system can tolerate this with no impact on the cranium, add elbow flexion, wrist extension and pronation of the forearm (Fig. 6.45C). If the patient can reach this position with no neural symptoms and no impact on the cranium, then the upper extremity perineural system has been released. Repeat on the opposite side.

Progression for the dural and perineural system to the lower extremity

Progressions for the above techniques are done in sitting (posterior), or side lying (anterior) to restore more elongation of the spinal dura and the peripheral perineurium that is influenced by the position of the hip.

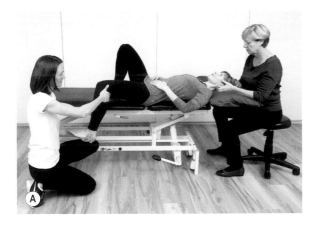
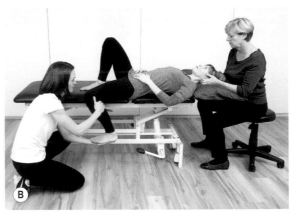

Figure 6.44 A & B

Release of the dura and perineurium from the cranium to the anterior and medial lower extremity.

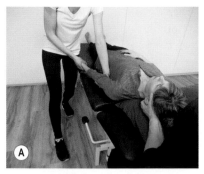
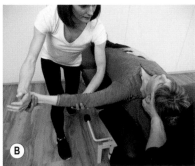
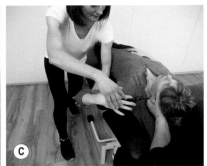

Figure 6.45 A–C

Release of the dura and perineurium from the cranium to the upper extremity.

Dural and posterior perineural system to the lower extremity

The patient is sitting on a well-controlled, neutral pelvis (neither SIJ is unlocked and there is no TPR or IPT or tilt) with the knees flexed and feet initially unsupported. Maintain correction of the cranial region and instruct the patient to posteriorly tilt the pelvis only until a pull or twist is felt in the cranium (Fig. 6.46A & B). The thoracic rings will attempt to translate and rotate if the spinal flexion is taken too far. This defeats the intention of the technique so watch for this compensatory pattern. Instruct the patient to dorsiflex one ankle and evert that foot. Repeat on the other side. Often the perineural system in one lower extremity has less ability to elongate than the other; start with the more restricted side. Gradually add more spinal flexion and knee extension while maintaining the correction of the cranium and position of the ankle and foot (Fig. 6.46C). A second therapist is very useful in this technique to control the foot and knee positioning. A dural and perineural system that permits full elongation will allow the patient to completely slump, flex the head and neck, and extend the knee with the ankle dorsiflexed and the foot everted. Forward bending of the trunk at the hip (hip flexion) depends on the ability to elongate the dural and perineural system, the posterior myofascial system in the neck, the trunk (erector spinae and its fascial connections) and the lower extremity (hamstrings, gastrocnemius, tibialis posterior, peroneus longus, flexor digitorum).

Dural and anterior perineural system to the lower extremity

The patient is side lying on a table, with the lower extremity to be treated uppermost. Maintain correction of the cranial region and instruct the patient to extend the upper leg in line with the pelvis until a pull or twist is felt in the cranium (Fig. 6.47A). Instruct the patient to dorsiflex the ankle and evert the foot. Have the patient anteriorly tilt the pelvis taking care to avoid any increase in low back pain. Gradually add more hip extension with the knee extended while maintaining the correction of the cranium and position of the ankle and foot. A second therapist is very useful in this technique to control the foot and hip positioning. Progress by adding knee flexion or hip rotation to this mobilization (Fig. 6.47B & C). A dural and perineural system that permits full elongation will allow the patient to completely extend the spinal column and hip with the knee fully flexed, the ankle dorsiflexed or plantarflexed, and the foot everted or inverted. Backward bending of the trunk at the hip depends on the ability to elongate the dural and perineural system, the anterior myofascial system in the trunk (psoas, iliacus), all hip flexors in the thigh, extensors of the knee and anterior tibial muscles. Abduction of the thigh in the extended hip position will require more elongation of the medial neural system of the thigh as well as the short and long adductors.

Complete mobilization of the dural and perineural system may take four to six treatment sessions. If there are strong intraspinal adhesions from previous inflammation

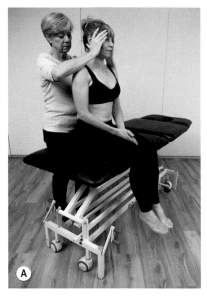
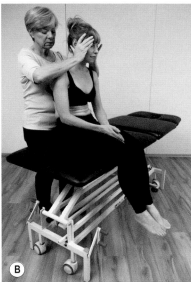
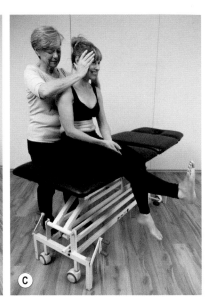

Figure 6.46

Progressions for dural and perineural mobilization into the lower extremity. (A) Begin with the patient in neutral sitting and correct any torsion of the cranium. (B) Have the patient posteriorly tilt the pelvis only until you feel an increase in the intracranial torsion. Progressively increase the degree of spinal flexion, stopping each time you feel the cranium twist and wait for the dura to 'release' and the pull on the cranium to soften. (C) Further progressions into the posterior perineural system involve adding extension of the knee, dorsiflexion of the ankle, and eversion or inversion of the foot.

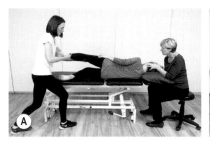
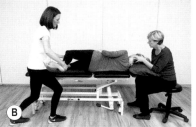
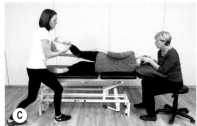

Figure 6.47 A–C

Progressions for releasing the dura and perineurium into the lower extremity.

or infection or congenital disorders (spina bifida), full mobility may not be achieved. Mobilization of the peripheral myofascial interfaces of the peripheral nerves are often added to the treatment session.

Once full, or the best possible, dural or perineural mobility has been achieved, attention can be directed to skeletal alignment, drivers found for meaningful tasks, and

posture, motor control and movement training can begin (see Chapter 7).

Myofascial system impairments

The myofascial system includes muscles, and their tendinous and fascial and aponeurotic connections, as well as the regular dense and loose connective tissue. Surgical

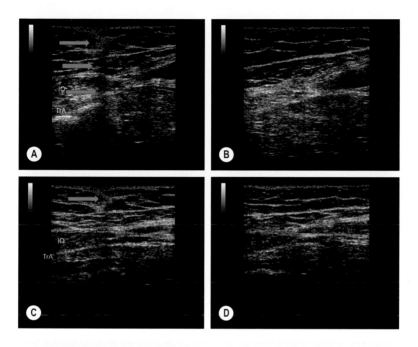

Figure 6.48

Impact of minimally invasive surgery on the fascial compartments of the abdominal wall. (A) Ultrasound image of the abdominal wall directly over one of four portals used to enter the abdomen, 17 days postsurgery. Fascial disruption can be seen along the vertical line indicated by the arrows. (B) Ultrasound image of the abdominal wall one inch lower than the portal imaged in (A) for comparison. Note that there is no vertical echogenic line. (C) Ultrasound image of the abdominal wall over the same portal at four weeks postsurgery. The fascial compartments of the internal oblique and transversus abdominis appear healed and the adhesion in the superficial layers has persisted (arrow). (D) Ultrasound image of the abdominal wall one inch lower than the portal imaged in (C) for comparison. Note that there is no vertical echogenic line. IO = internal oblique, TrA = transversus abdominis.

or traumatic scars can adhere tissue and prevent the necessary intermyofascial sliding and tissue elongation and shortening required for function (Fig. 6.48A–D). Passive listening on both correction and release of the driver reveals vectors that are of variable length and usually firmer than the neuromuscular system and less firm than the articular system. The location (left and right, front and back), direction (up and down), and quality of the vector on passive listening (correction and release of the driver) direct where to palpate for possible adhesions or dehydration of the loose connective tissue preventing myofascial mobility. Several textbooks, authored by various clinicians of different disciplines have been published by Handspring Publishing and are useful resources for

techniques on how to mobilize the myofascial system. The ISM principles for when and how to treat this system are:

1. Vector analysis of the driver for any screening task that pertains to the patient's movement goals (meaningful task) reveals the first vector to be a specific structure in the myofascial chain or system;

2. Release any overactivation of the muscles pertaining to the restricted myofascia first (release with awareness); and then

3. Complete the release technique by directly lengthening the myofascia (take into stretch) and hold until release is obtained.

Myofascial release techniques in an ISM approach are often integrated with other system release techniques. Dry needling can also be used to release 'stubborn' connective tissue bonds and ultrasound guidance is preferred for accuracy (Fig. 6.49A & B).

Visceral system impairments

It is beyond the scope of this text to describe release techniques for specific visceral structures. The reader is referred to the extensive curriculum developed by Dr. Jean-Pierre Barral (www.barralinstitute.com) for more information on how to acquire the skills and clinical reasoning to treat this system. While specificity is always preferred, general techniques are a useful start. Many intrathoracic visceral vectors from the lungs and mediastinum can be addressed with the general, non-structure-specific release technique described in this chapter (thoracic ring stack and breathe [Lee L-J 2016]). When the vector revealed on passive listening is the pericardium of the heart (Fig. 3.71A), it

is not uncommon to see an S-curve posture in the sagittal plane between C6 and T5 with excessive extension at C6–C7, flexion between C7–T2, and extension between T2 and T5 (Fig. 3.71B). If the posture changes in an inverted position (Fig. 3.71C), the hypothesis is that the central tendon of the diaphragm is too low and that the pericardium is the victim of its descent. Because of the strong attachments of the pericardium to the ventral aspect of C6, T2 and T4, this posture is the result. Further assessment to determine why the central tendon of the diaphragm is too low should follow. The motor supply to the diaphragm is via the phrenic (C3, C4, and C5) and vagal (exits via the jugular foramen) nerves and parts of the diaphragm may be overactive in response to changes in neural drive from drivers in the cranium or upper thorax or both that tense, or change the vascularity of, these nerves. If correcting the cranium or upper thorax or both changes the posture from C6–T5, then treatment is focused on whatever vector analysis of the cranium or upper thorax reveals. The diaphragm

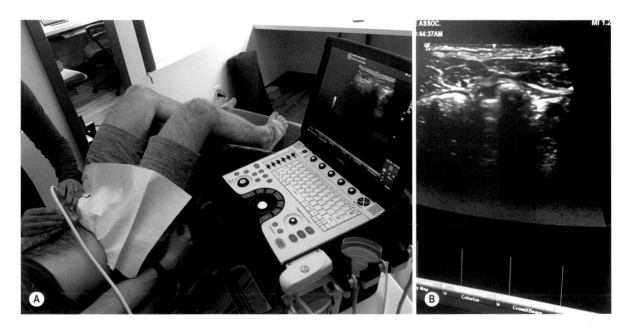

Figure 6.49

(A) This young man had a prior history of an intramuscular abdominal hernia. His persistent complaint of a local 'tug' in the abdominal wall was not relieved with local soft tissue mobilization techniques. Dry needling was used to release the 'stubborn' connective tissue bonds. (B) Ultrasound guidance enhances safety with this dry needling technique.

can also be too low because of poor abdominal or pelvic-floor muscle function; multiple conditions can lead to this state. The goal here is to restore optimal abdominal canister function with an ISM approach that ultimately results in elevation of the central tendon of the diaphragm and reduction of the pericardial vector on the neck and thorax. Finding the driver is critical since a low diaphragm can have whole body implications. If the diaphragm is weak, hypopressive training (Low Pressure Fitness™, www.lowpressurefitness.com) appears to be an effective way to restore its strength and conditioning. Alignment and breath training precedes diaphragm strengthening (see the section on hypopressive exercise and Low Pressure Fitness™ in Chapter 7).

Summary

The Integrated Systems Model approach for treatment contains two components (see Fig. 4.1):

1. Addressing the cognitive, emotional, and sensorial (physical) barriers that are creating suboptimal strategies for function, in conjunction with

2. Teaching optimal strategies for function that relate to the patient's goals and meaningful tasks.

Physical barriers that perpetuate suboptimal strategies for function can be addressed with a wide variety of release techniques. The release of specific system impairments helps to change sensory input to the cortical body matrix from these sources, and potentially reduce threat and an output of pain. Treatment is directed initially to the primary system impairment noted on vector analysis of the driver.

Following release of the primary and secondary system vectors, postural instruction combined with taping (if necessary) and motor learning and movement training are used to reinforce improved alignment and biomechanics for the meaningful task (see Chapter 7). This instruction also facilitates a change in the sensory input to the cortical body matrix from multiple tissues of the body (articular, myofascial, neural, visceral), as well as the mind (cognitive beliefs and emotional states) and thus potentially changes the motor output and strategies for function. Release techniques are initially applied to the driver or drivers, which may change after release. All drivers are addressed and released in conjunction with motor control and movement training and they should change both within and in between treatment sessions unless a major myofascial or articular system impairment is present.

Introduction and principles for motor learning and movement training

The final and critical part of each treatment session is to train better strategies for function and performance, which requires motor learning and movement training. The aim is to build and use new and better 'brain maps' and movement strategies that share loads and control excessive canister pressures (cranial, thoracic, abdominal, pelvic) in a way that sustains tissue structure, blood flow and drainage, function, and overall health. The principles of this approach are derived from those presented in 1999 by Richardson et al. for low back pain, a model which has continued to evolve with new evidence (Falla & Hodges 2017, Hodges et al. 2016, van Dieën et al. 2017). The approach is prescriptive and individual:

'... management of spinal pain should be considered within a biopsychosocial framework which embraces biological, psychological and social features and their interactions, all of which may contribute to the disorder and to recovery. Yet the relevant contribution of each component will vary for each individual. The large variability in underlying pain mechanism (relevance of nociceptive input or central sensitization processes) and variability of motor adaptations noted between individuals with neck or low back pain likely contributes to the variable symptomatic benefit experienced by patients following standardized exercise programs. It is not surprising when some studies show little or no effect of exercise interventions in people with spinal pain considering that the people included in the trial may have psychological or social features contributing to their disorder which outweigh physical features that were not addressed with the applied exercise program. Because of this heterogeneity, there can be no recipe approaches and it is likely that better outcomes will be achieved if each patient is regarded as an individual and management programs are designed and tailored to individual's needs.' (Falla & Hodges 2017)

The training suggested in this chapter is not a recipe, nor is it protocol driven.

'Motor control training for low back and pelvic pain aims to restore optimal control of the spine and pelvis, with consideration of posture/postural alignment, muscle activation and movement. Sensation and the multiple functions of the trunk are also key considerations. The objective of this approach is to optimize load on the structures of the spine and pelvis (that may be a source of ongoing nociceptor discharge), in a manner that is matched to the changes in motor control that are specific to the individual and matched to his or her functional demands. This requires consideration of the role of biology (e.g., role of ongoing nociceptor discharge in the maintenance of pain and/or the role of exposure to healthy movement to recovery) within the biopsychosocial presentation of the patient.' (Hodges et al. 2016)

Postural alignment, muscle activation and movement are known to be important considerations in the management of spinal pain. Treatment should be matched to the individual and their functional demands, and therefore meaningful.

'Optimal control is generally thought to be the outcome of reinforcement learning. Efference copies [internal copy of an outflowing, movement-producing signal generated by the motor system] of the motor commands and feedback on the consequences of the motor actions provide the individual with information on performance and associated costs, allowing adaptation of motor commands to achieve the task goal with minimal costs in terms of neural drive (control effort) or metabolic or mechanical costs of muscle force production. It has been suggested that movement planning occurs sequentially at two hierarchical levels: initially to plan the kinematic trajectory and subsequently to plan a muscle recruitment pattern that fits the planned kinematic trajectory.' (van Dieën et al. 2017)

'Motor learning involves the acquisition and refinement of movement and coordination that leads to permanent change in movement performance.' (Hodges et al. 2016)

There are three phases of motor learning (Fitts & Posner 1967):

1. Cognitive phase: Tasks are organized cognitively with attention to feedback, movement sequence, and quality of performance. Parts of the movement are practiced and feedback is critical on both the quality of performance (self-check) and the result of the task (retest the screening test and/or meaningful task).

2. Associative phase: The focus shifts to emphasize the consistency of performance and the cognitive demands are reduced.

3. Automatic phase: Requires considerable practice; the focus shifts to transferring the task between environments.

For the purposes of this text, these three phases have been categorized as 'Stages of motor learning and movement training' and the principles and specifics of each stage are outlined in Table 7.1.

When the thorax is the primary driver, intrathoracic ring alignment and control is trained first (Stage 1), if necessary. This is followed by training for alignment and control of multiple thoracic rings (interthoracic ring or rings) (Stage 1). Capacity training for the new strategy (increasing load tolerance and endurance – Stage 2) follows. At this phase of motor learning, Stage 1 followed by Stage 2 training can be added for alignment and control of any secondary driver (pelvis and hip, cranium, neck and shoulder girdle). Once all drivers can be statically controlled with both upper and lower limb loading, Stage 3 inter-regional movement training of more complex whole-body tasks can then begin.

There are three levels of progression in Stage 3 training. Stage 3, Level 1 tasks require aligned and controlled interthoracic ring movements in a variety of planes (sagittal, coronal, transverse, combination of planes) with a focus on those that pertain to the meaningful task. Once interthoracic ring mobility and control is restored, Stage 3, Level 2 tasks can be introduced. These require the thorax to be controlled during movement while simultaneously controlling a secondary driver, or region, and then moving both regions in congruent and incongruent directions in multiple planes. Stage 3, Level 3 tasks add a further level

of challenge by reducing the base of support and creating unpredictable situations.

The principles of motor learning and neuroplasticity guide all stages of training. What is neuroplasticity?

'The ability of the nervous system to respond to intrinsic and extrinsic stimuli by reorganizing its structure, function and connections.' (Snodgrass et al. 2014)

'Neurons that wire together, fire together.' (Hebb 1949)

The key principles required for neuroplastic change are:

- Focused attention: Training should occur with minimal distraction (i.e., no music or noise). The therapist must have skills to teach the patient how to 'feel with awareness' the differences in the experiences of the body when recruitment strategies are different (what works and feels better, the same, or worse). This is part of the cognitive phase of motor learning.

- Training tasks that have meaning or purpose: For any movement training prescribed, the patient must understand the purpose of the training. Ask them 'Why do you think this exercise is important?' Often it is important to break down complicated meaningful tasks into component parts and rebuild the movement pattern. The component part may look nothing like the final movement pattern, yet it may be essential for building a better strategy. This is also part of the cognitive phase of motor learning.

- Massed practice of high-quality performance: Tsao and Hodges (2007, 2008) and Tsao et al. (2010) showed that the timing of transversus abdominis (TrA) recruitment in response to perturbations of the trunk through rapid arm movement could be improved within 30 repetitions of high quality contractions with focused attention. The initial dosage for training the TrA was three sets of 10 10-second holds with a two-minute rest in between sets. If this practice was done at least twice per day (preferably three to four times per day) Tsao et al. (2010) found that by two weeks, the recruitment pattern of the TrA to perturbations of the trunk with rapid arm loading was restored (i.e., within 50 ms anticipatory timelines).

Table 7.1
Stages of motor learning and movement training

STAGE	PRINCIPLES	INTRATHORACIC RING CONTROL SPECIFICS	INTERTHORACIC RING MOTOR CONTROL AND MOVEMENT TRAINING SPECIFICS	INTRAPELVIC RING CONTROL SPECIFICS	CERVICAL SEGMENTAL CONTROL SPECIFICS	LUMBAR SEGMENTAL CONTROL SPECIFICS
Stage 1	Posture and alignment training with ability to produce independent contraction of deep segmental muscles responsible for control without overactivation of superficial muscles (static alignment control)	Release all restrictive vectors Find the best release and connect cue for the specific intrathoracic ring impairment Taping for intrathoracic ring alignment and control	Release all restrictive vectors Find the best release and connect cue for the specific interthoracic ring alignment and control Motor control training for upper fibers of the TrA and diaphragm for the vertebrochondral region Taping for interthoracic ring control and appropriate sensory input to cortical body matrix	Release all vectors impacting alignment of pelvis and hips Training for deep muscles responsible for pelvic control (low fibers of TrA, sacral deep multifidus, diaphragm, pelvic floor) Minimize superficial muscle recruitment Taping or belts for intrapelvic ring control	Release all vectors impacting alignment of head, neck, shoulder girdle, and upper thorax Training for deep muscles responsible for cervical segmental control Minimize superficial muscle recruitment	Release all vectors impacting alignment of thorax, pelvis and lumbar spine Training for deep muscles responsible for lumbar control (middle fibers of TrA, lumbar deep multifidus, diaphragm) Minimize superficial muscle recruitment
Stage 2	Strategy capacity training Add load and movement of distal segments while maintaining static position and alignment of region being trained	Progress to interthoracic ring motor control and movement training	Release and connect cues with home self-check tasks Strategy capacity training for static interthoracic ring control Add motor control training of any secondary driver (pelvis, cervical, lumbar, etc.)	Release and connect cues with self-check tasks Strategy capacity training for static intrapelvic ring control Progress to Stage 3 inter-regional movement training	Release and connect cues with self-check tasks Strategy capacity training for static cervical segmental control Progress to Stage 3 inter-regional movement training	Release and connect cues with self-check tasks Strategy capacity training for static lumbar segmental control Progress to Stage 3 inter-regional movement training
Stage 3	Add controlled movement of region being trained in multiple planes Progress to controlled movement of region with either static control or controlled movement of other regions Further progression to add wide variety of equilibrium and predictability challenges					

Continued

Table 7.1 continued

STAGE	PRINCIPLES	INTRATHORACIC RING CONTROL SPECIFICS	INTERTHORACIC RING MOTOR CONTROL AND MOVEMENT TRAINING SPECIFICS	INTRAPELVIC RING CONTROL SPECIFICS	CERVICAL SEGMENTAL CONTROL SPECIFICS	LUMBAR SEGMENTAL CONTROL SPECIFICS
Stage 3 Level 1	Move just the region, i.e., the thorax, and not the arms, legs or head		Thorax mobility and control in the sagittal and transverse planes to maintain center of gravity (COG) over base of support (BOS) without arm movement			
Stage 3 Level 2	Move the thorax with either static control or controlled movement of another region Congruent and incongruent directions of motion of two regions in any plane – sagittal, coronal or transverse Shoulder girdle and arm and thorax Head and neck and thorax Pelvis and lower extremity and thorax		Progressions to mid- and high-load strength training for interthoracic ring mobility and control integrated with shoulder and arm, head and neck, pelvis and lower extremity			
Stage 3 Level 3	Add complex movement tasks involving the whole body Progress training to higher equilibrium challenges or unpredictable situations		Progressions into whole-body tasks with mobility and control of all drivers and all body regions			

TrA = transversus abdominis.

Similar principles have been applied clinically to other muscles for intrathoracic and interthoracic ring control. Over time this meets the 2nd and 3rd phases of motor learning, which are the associative and automatic phases.

- Normalizing the sensory input: This is essential if change in the motor output is to occur. The sensory input should be nonthreatening.

- Positive feedback.

- Specificity.

The rest of this chapter will focus on the description and illustration of specific training practice at each Stage and Level for intrathoracic and interthoracic ring alignment, biomechanics, and control. Examples include motor control and movement training with:

- weights and resistance bands,

- Reformer and Cadillac Pilates, and

- intermediate and advanced yoga sequences (provided by Chelsea Lee [Lee D 2017b]).

Intrathoracic ring motor control training

Intrathoracic ring function requires optimal alignment, biomechanics and control of the bones and joints that comprise one thoracic ring (Fig. 1.2). Intrathoracic ring training is applicable for the individual with an articular system impairment that has compromised the form closure mechanism, or passive control, of the joint or joints of the thoracic ring. The story reveals past, or recent, trauma with or without episodic joint fixation (i.e., fixation of the costotransverse joint or lateral translation and rotation fixation of the entire thoracic ring; see Chapter 6).

The active osteokinematic mobility findings are variable and depend on the individual's motor adaptation to pain. Depending on the specific impairment, the passive control tests may reveal:

1. Excessive anterior or posterior translation of the costocartilage or rib at the sternocostal or costochondral joint. This is often associated with a palpable step or 'bump' at the relative joint (Fig. 7.1A).

2. Excessive anterior, posterior or mediolateral translation within the thoracic ring in the close-packed position (either flexion or extension).

3. Excessive superior or inferior glide of the costotransverse joint of one rib.

When the strategy for alignment and control within the thoracic ring is suboptimal, the active control tests reveal loss of static alignment combined with suboptimal intrathoracic ring biomechanics when the load exceeds the capacity of the thoracic ring in question (Fig. 7.1B). Prolotherapy may be required to completely restore intrathoracic ring control, which should be restored before training progresses to interthoracic ring training (between two thoracic rings).

Stage 1 release and connect cues for intrathoracic ring impairments

All vectors preventing optimal alignment and mobility of any part of the thoracic ring should be released prior to motor control training (see Chapter 6). This includes restoring articular mobility when there is a specific joint fixation (i.e., costotransverse joint fixation, lateral translation and rotation fixation of the thoracic ring). As mobility is restored, Stage 1 intrathoracic ring motor control training begins.

Sternocostal or costochondral joint impairment

The anterior or middle intercostals and transversus thoracis are often overactive when there is a form closure deficit of the costochondral or sternocostal joint. Release cues with or without manual assistance include:

1. Create space between the adjacent ribs (vertical dimension); and

2. Think about broadening the front of the chest (lateral dimension) and allowing the rib to 'float' laterally (Fig. 7.1C).

A manual assist can be applied by correcting the alignment of the relative rib. The step deformity of the costochondral or sternocostal joint should reduce if the release cue is effective. Taping the rib to distract the costochondral and/or sternochondral joint and then compressing the rib

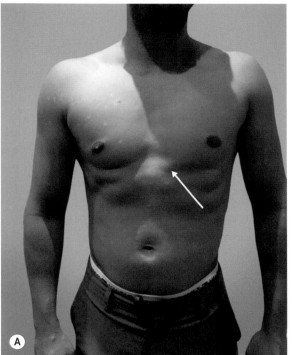

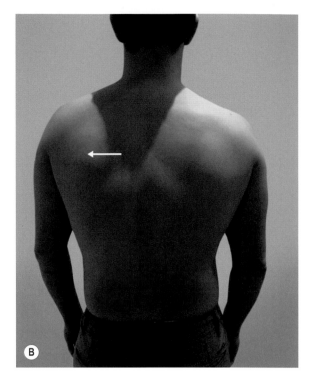

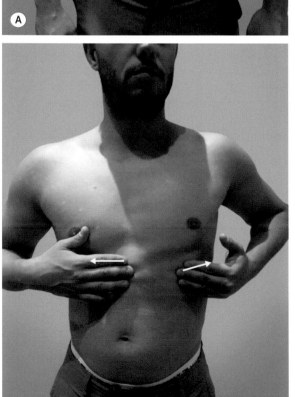

Figure 7.1

This man sustained a compression injury to his rib cage eight years ago while wrestling and felt a 'pop in his left 6th rib adjacent to the lower sternum,' which was subsequently 'manipulated back in with another pop.' He experiences intermittent shortness of breath, midthoracic pain, and difficulty rotating his thorax to the left. He gets relief when he 'pushes the bump at the junction of his sternum and rib flat.' (A) There is a notable step deformity between the sternum and the costocartilage of the left 6th rib (arrow). The 6th thoracic ring is translated left and rotated right with an intrathoracic ring buckle at the sternocostal joint. All other thoracic rings in the vertebrosternal region are translated left and rotated right. (B) Note the regional left translation of the middle thorax. The 6th thoracic ring is translated left and rotated right (arrow) further than the thoracic rings above and below (suboptimal alignment and loss of control). (C) A manual assist (arrows), combined with a release cue (think about creating space between the ribs and then letting the left 6th rib slowly float laterally) to decompress and restore alignment to the 6th thoracic ring. A connect cue from the midaxillary line up to the midthoracic spine (J-hook image, see text) was added for interthoracic ring alignment and control.

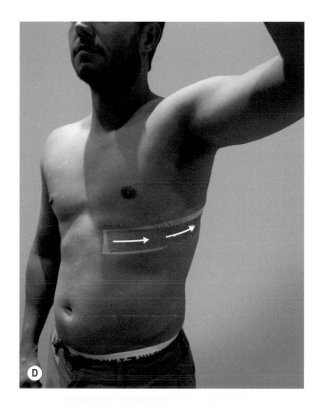

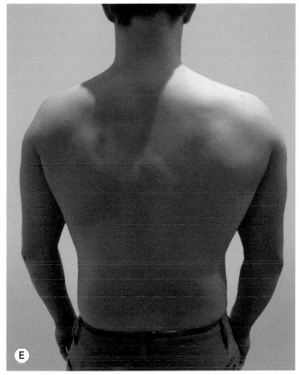

Figure 7.1 *continued*

The intent of this manual correction, combined with the release and connect cues, is to facilitate a better recruitment strategy of the intercostals and other segmental muscles for both intrathoracic ring alignment and interthoracic ring alignment and control. (D) Tape is used to reinforce the motor learning for both what to release and what to connect to. For this sternocostal joint impairment, the tape is anchored to the 6th costocartilage, which is then distracted laterally from the sternum. This lateral distraction force then continues around the thorax to compress the 6th rib medially into the costovertebral joints at T5–T6 (cross the tape across the spine in the midline). (E) The intrathoracic ring release and connect cues should result in improved interthoracic ring alignment as well. Note the improvement in alignment of the midthorax here compared to Figure 7.1B.

posteriorly into the relevant costovertebral joints can assist with both the release cue for alignment and motor control training for better biomechanics and control (Fig. 7.1D).

The goal of Stage 1 motor control training for a sterno-costal or costochondral joint impairment is to maintain optimal alignment *within* the thoracic ring using mental cuing (imagery) and over time lessen the need for manual assistance and tape. Cues for training the deep segmental muscles responsible for intra- and inter-thoracic ring alignment and control (intercostals, multifidus and rotatores) are collectively called 'connect cues.' Appropriate connect cues for this impairment include the following:

1. Imagine a guy wire from the body of the rib in the midaxillary line to the vertebra of the same number (e.g., 6th rib to T6) and gently connect the rib to the vertebra (J-hook cue).

2. As the rib connects posteriorly, create space between it and the ribs above and below. The intent of this cue is to prevent over-activation of the superficial back extensors.

Once intrathoracic ring alignment can be achieved with mental imagery, Stage 1 interthoracic ring motor control training can begin.

Thoracic ring lateral translation and rotation impairment

This intrathoracic ring impairment is released with a high-velocity, low-amplitude thrust technique (see Chapter 6). After release, the lateral translation passive control test is often positive (excessive amplitude of motion) in the direction of the lateral translation impairment with associated inhibition of the deep segmental muscles responsible for interthoracic ring control (intercostals, multifidus and rotatores). Taping the rib *above* the impaired thoracic ring into medial translation can help to prevent translation of the superior vertebra of the impaired thoracic ring and thus translation of the entire thoracic ring (Fig. 7.2A–C).

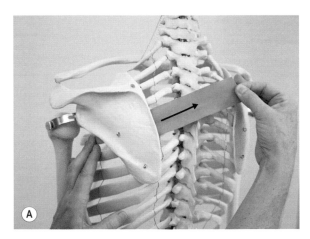

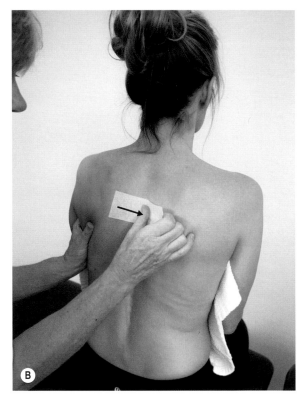

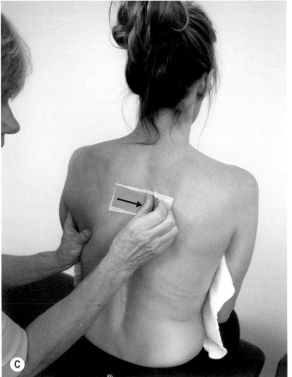

Figure 7.2

Taping for a lateral translation and rotation fixation of the thoracic ring after release. (A) The thoracic ring above the impaired one is taped into medial translation. Here, the 5th rib is being taped to control left lateral translation of the 6th thoracic ring. (B) Attach the Fixomull® over the back of the left 5th rib just lateral to the costotransverse joint. Compress the 5th rib medially in the midaxillary line (left hand) to control the T6 vertebra. Pull the Fimomull® across the spine (arrow) and attach to the opposite 5th rib. (C) Repeat the process with the Leukotape®.

For example, if the 6th thoracic ring was fixated in left lateral translation and right rotation, T5 and the left and right 6th ribs have translated to the left relative to T6. After reduction of this fixation, the left 5th rib is compressed into T5 with taping such that left lateral translation of T5 and the left and right 6th ribs is prevented. Stage 1 motor control training for the 6th thoracic ring can then begin.

The goal of Stage 1 motor control training for a lateral translation and rotation impairment is to maintain optimal alignment *within* the thoracic ring using mental cuing (imagery) and over time lessen the need for manual assistance and tape. Appropriate connect cues for this impairment include the following:

1. Imagine a guy wire from the body of the 6th rib in the midaxillary line to the spinous process of the superior vertebra of the thoracic ring (e.g., 6th rib to T5) and connect the rib to the superior vertebra along this line (Fig. 7.3A); then

2. Imagine a second guy wire attached to the spinous process of the superior vertebra (T5 in this example) that extends toward the ceiling. Think about gently suspending, or lifting, this vertebra (along with the connected rib) 1 mm above the one below (T6) (Fig. 7.3B).

Collectively, these two connect cues should align the bones of the 6th thoracic ring. Once intrathoracic ring alignment can be achieved with mental imagery, Stage 1 interthoracic ring motor control training can begin.

Posterior translation impairment of a thoracic spinal segment

This intrathoracic ring impairment is often associated with overactivation of the superficial spinal extensors (spinalis thoracis and longissimus thoracis, iliocostalis) (Fig. 7.4). After release, the posterior translation passive control test is often positive (excessive amplitude of motion) and associated with inhibition of the deep segmental muscles responsible for control (intercostals, multifidus and rotatores). Taping this impairment is not often helpful.

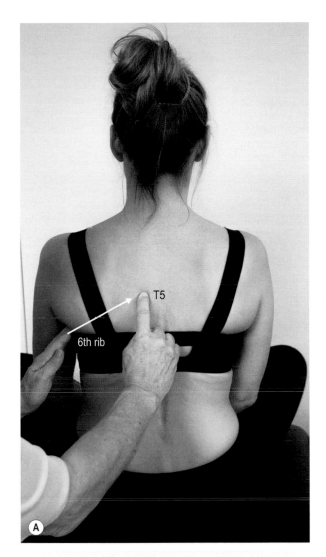

Figure 7.3

Connect cues for alignment and control of a 6th thoracic ring lateral translation and rotation impairment: Stage 1 motor learning after release. (A) Palpate the left 6th rib in the midaxillary line and the paraspinal muscles lateral to the spinous process of T5. The connect cue (imagine a guy wire from the body of the 6th rib to T5) should result in correction of the alignment (palpable in the midaxillary line) and activation of the segmental muscles at T5–T6 (multifidus and rotatores) without overactivation of the long spinal extensors. *Continued*

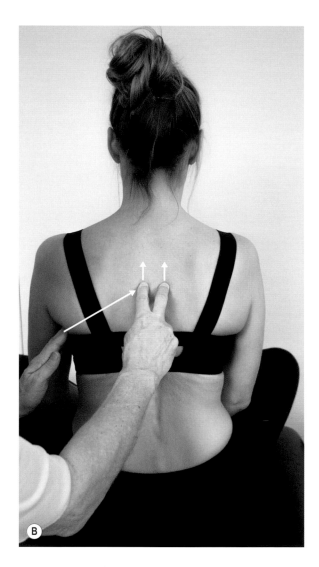

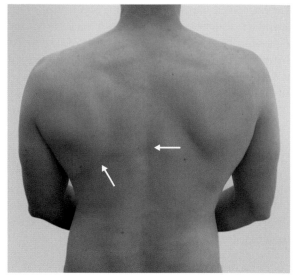

Figure 7.4

This man presented with a posterior translation impairment at T7–T8 (right arrow). Note the posterior step deformity and overactivation of the spinal extensors, which is associated with inhibition of the related intercostals on the left (left arrow).

Figure 7.3 *continued*

(B) Palpate the paraspinal muscles on the left and right sides of T5. The 2nd connect cue (suspend T5 1 mm above T6 – 'think about lifting this vertebra just a little') should result in more recruitment of the multifidus and rotatores and less recruitment of the long spinal extensors. Hold the isometric contraction for 10 seconds and repeat 10 times, or as many times as can be managed accurately.

The goal of Stage 1 motor control training for a posterior translation impairment is to maintain optimal alignment *within* the thoracic ring using cuing (imagery) and over time lessen the need for manual release. Appropriate release and connect cues for this impairment include the following:

1. If the thorax is overly extended: Imagine the sternum softly settling toward the abdomen and the long back extensors relaxing such that the individual thoracic rings float apart in your back (release cue) (Fig. 7.5); then

2. Imagine a guy wire attached to the spinous process of the superior vertebra of the segment that is posteriorly translated and continue the image of the guy wire to the ceiling. Think about gently suspending, or lifting, this vertebra 1 mm above the one below.

Collectively, these two cues should improve the alignment of the bones of the impaired thoracic ring.

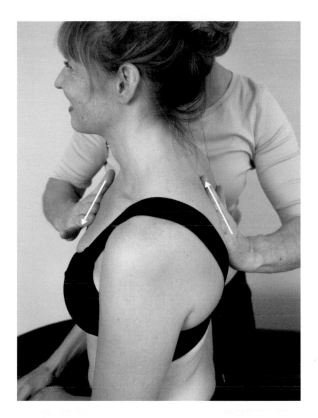

Figure 7.5

Release and connect cues for Stage 1 motor control training for a posterior translation impairment. Instruct the patient to 'soften the sternum into flexion, don't collapse, and think about suspending the superior vertebra of the impaired segment toward the ceiling.'

Once intrathoracic ring alignment can be achieved with mental imagery, Stage 1 interthoracic ring motor control training can begin.

Costotransverse joint fixation

This intrathoracic ring impairment is specific to the costotransverse joint and is released with a high-velocity, low-amplitude thrust technique (see Chapter 6). After release, the passive control test for anterior distraction of the costotransverse joint is positive (excessive amplitude of motion). If the costotransverse joint was fixated in superior glide, then taping the rib into posterior rotation (inferior glide) is indicated (Fig. 7.6A & B). If the joint was fixated in inferior

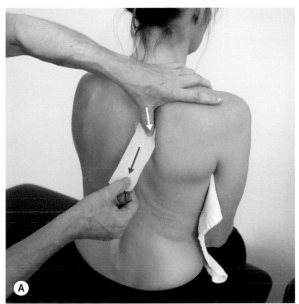

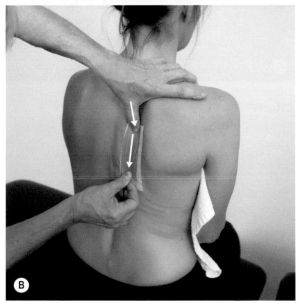

Figure 7.6

Taping for a fixation of the costotransverse joint after release. (A) Superior fixation: Attach the Fixomull® in the intercostal space above the rib to be controlled. Glide the rib inferiorly at the costotransverse joint (short arrow) (posteriorly rotate the rib) and pull the tape directly inferior (long arrow). (B) Repeat the process with the Leukotape®. *Continued*

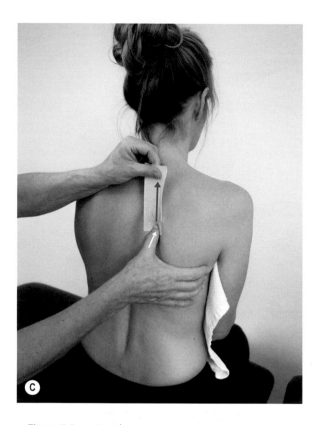

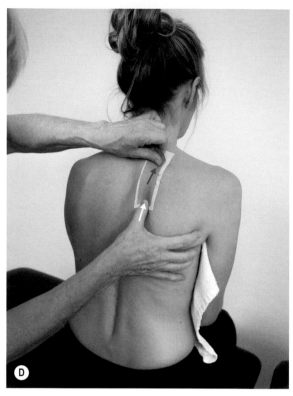

Figure 7.6 *continued*

(C) Inferior fixation: attach the Fixomull® in the intercostal space below the rib to be controlled. Glide the rib superiorly at the costotransverse joint (short arrow) (anteriorly rotate the rib) and pull the tape directly superior (long arrow). (B) Repeat the process with the Leukotape®.

glide, then taping the rib into anterior rotation (superior glide) is indicated (Fig. 7.6C & D). Stage 1 intrathoracic ring motor control training then follows.

The goal of Stage 1 motor control training for this impairment is to maintain optimal alignment within the thoracic ring using mental connect cues and over time lessen the need for tape. Appropriate connect cues include the following:

1. Superior laxity (tendency for the rib to fixate in anterior rotation, or superior glide, at the costotransverse joint): Activate the intercostals between the affected rib and the one *below* by 'closing the space' between the two ribs without recruiting the superficial spinal extensors.

2. Inferior laxity (tendency for the rib to fixate in posterior rotation, or inferior glide, at the costotransverse joint): Activate the intercostals between the affected rib and the one *above* by 'closing the space' between the two ribs without recruiting the superficial spinal extensors.

3. Hold the connect cue and breathe. The strategy should not completely brace the costotransverse joint and the superior and inferior glide should still occur during inhalation and exhalation.

It is not uncommon for the intrathoracic ring release and connect cues to result in improved interthoracic ring alignment as well (Fig. 7.1E).

Interthoracic ring motor control training

Interthoracic ring function requires optimal alignment, biomechanics and control between the 10 thoracic rings, 1 to 10. This training is applicable after intrathoracic ring alignment and control has been restored (articular system impairment), or when the interthoracic ring strategy for alignment, biomechanics, and control is suboptimal for the task being evaluated in the absence of an intrathoracic ring impairment. Trauma to the thorax is not always part of the story; poor posture and movement habits can, over time, lead to suboptimal strategies for interthoracic ring alignment, biomechanics, and control.

The active osteokinematic mobility findings are often reduced prior to release of the vectors contributing to the suboptimal strategies. The thoracic ring position (alignment) and biomechanics are commonly incongruent with the required alignment and biomechanics for the task when restricting vectors are present. A 6th thoracic ring that is held translated left and rotated right will restrict left rotation of the thorax and any task that requires left rotation of the thorax.

After releasing the restricting vectors, the impaired thoracic ring or rings may demonstrate optimal alignment, biomechanics, and control for a few repetitions of the screening task and then lose control and alignment, which then impacts the osteokinematic mobility findings. The 6th thoracic ring noted above may appear aligned and able to translate right and rotate left during left rotation of the thorax for a few repetitions, and then it may:

- Translate left and rotate right and restrict left rotation on the subsequent repetition (incongruent thoracic ring biomechanics for the task); or

- Translate too far right and rotate too far left during left rotation of the thorax. This is called a suboptimal congruent thoracic ring translation and rotation.

- Alignment and control may be optimal for left rotation; however, the 6th thoracic ring may lose neutral alignment and control when load is added (e.g., during elevation of the arm).

Inconsistency of findings between tasks and between repetitions of the same task is the consistent feature of this interthoracic motor control impairment. The tests for passive control of the articular system of the thoracic ring are normal.

Motor control and movement training for interthoracic ring control begins with:

1. Stage 1: Release all restricting vectors and build a new strategy for static interthoracic ring control.

2. Stage 2: Increase capacity of the strategy for interthoracic ring control by adding load to the thorax without allowing any movement of the thorax to occur.

Stage 3 training (inter-regional movement and control) then follows, but first the secondary drivers may need attention and training.

Stage 1 release and connect cues for interthoracic ring impairments

All vectors preventing optimal alignment and mobility of any part of the thoracic ring should be released prior to motor control training (see Chapter 6). If releasing the thoracic ring or rings automatically restores a better strategy for controlled interthoracic ring alignment and biomechanics, then specific motor control training is not required and training can progress to Stage 2 strategy capacity training. The thoracic rings should be monitored in the early stages of Stage 2 training to determine if there is any loss of interthoracic ring alignment, biomechanics, and control as loading is increased and movements prescribed become more complex. If releasing the thoracic ring or rings does not result in restoration of better strategies for interthoracic ring function then specific motor control training is required.

Stage 1: Release and connect cues are combined while monitoring the alignment, and then control of the thoracic ring during loading. The seated patient is taught initially how to monitor the primary thoracic ring shift (glued thoracic rings should have been released at this stage) and the impact on any compensatory thoracic ring shift in another region of the thorax. It is common to find a primary thoracic ring impairment in the vertebrosternal region (4th thoracic ring translated left and rotated right) and a compensatory one in the vertebrochondral region (8th thoracic ring translated right and rotated left). If the 4th thoracic ring is the primary impairment, manual correction of the 4th ring will either fully or partially correct the incongruent 8th thoracic ring. Let's continue with the assumption that the 4th thoracic ring correction fully corrects the 8th thoracic ring. The patient will then monitor the 4th thoracic ring in the midaxillary line and note the impact of the following release and connect cues on the alignment:

1. Release cue: Think about creating space between the adjacent ribs (vertical dimension) at the side, front, and back of the thorax. Let the thoracic rings 'float apart.'

2. Release cue: Think about broadening the front (or back depending on what they need) of the chest (lateral dimension), and note what happens to the 'bumpy rib in the axilla.'

If it automatically corrects, then no connect cues are required. If the thoracic ring only partially corrects, add one of the following connect cues:

1. Connect cue: Imagine a guy wire from the body of the 4th rib in the midaxillary line to the vertebra of the same number (e.g., 4th rib to T4) and gently connect the rib to the vertebra (J-hook cue). As the 4th rib connects posteriorly, keep creating space between it and the ribs above and below. The intent of this cue is to prevent overactivation of the superficial back extensors and retractors of the scapula.

2. Connect cue: Imagine a second guy wire attached just to the right of the spinous process of the superior vertebra (T3 in this example) that extends toward the ceiling. Think about gently suspending, or lifting, this vertebra (along with the connected rib) 1 mm above the one below (T4). When the 4th thoracic ring is translated left and rotated right, T3–T4 will be right side-bent and right rotated (see Chapter 2 for biomechanics of the thorax). Thinking about suspending the right side of T3 a little more

than the left will facilitate a reduction in the right side bending and assist in restoring neutral alignment of the entire 4th thoracic ring.

If the thorax is overly extended, add a release cue that results in flexion of the thorax (e.g., soften the sternum and gently allow the back extensors to lengthen (Fig. 7.5)). If the thorax is overly flexed, add a release cue that results in extension of the thorax (e.g., lift the sternum and gently allow the abdominals to lengthen). If the thorax is overly side-bent, add a release cue that results in lengthening of the lateral side of the body (e.g., create more space between the ribs and then the lower thorax and the pelvis on the same side). Both the release and connect cues should be independent of the respiratory cycle. Some patients will attempt to 'move the thoracic ring' using their breath. While this may be helpful initially, it is not a sustainable strategy. Brain maps for alignment and control should be independent of breathing, which is another loading task. Have the patient maintain the release and connect cue for three to five complete breaths and note if any part of the breathing cycle is more challenging for maintaining alignment and control of the thoracic ring.

Once the patient can completely correct the 4th thoracic ring (which in turn will fully correct the 8th ring in this clinical scenario), as well as the entire thorax over the pelvis, ask them to stop 'thinking' about their cues and note what happens to the 4th thoracic ring. If the cues have been successful, the 4th thoracic ring will translate left and rotate right when the mental images are released, and this is clearly felt in the axilla. The intention of this stage of training is to build a new 'brain map,' or strategy, for interthoracic ring alignment and control; therefore, the patient must have a way of knowing if their training is being effective and how to test the response of their mental cuing. This is a home self-check for their release and connect cues. As their ability to automatically maintain better alignment of the 4th thoracic ring improves, the difference in alignment of the 4th thoracic ring will lessen when they 'turn on and shut off' their cuing. They often report 'I can't find the bumpy rib anymore.' This is progress.

Another home self-check is to add a light load to the thorax by elevating the arm to 30 degrees and noting the difference in effort required to initiate the task without, and then with their cues. When the thorax is optimally aligned and control maintained during loading, the effort required to initiate arm elevation should be less. As the strategy moves through the three phases of motor learning (cognitive, associative, automatic) the differences in effort between the two strategies (i.e., thinking prior to movement versus not thinking and just moving) should decrease.

If the patient is unable to restore better alignment of the 4th thoracic ring in sitting, and all restrictive vectors have been released, then this thoracic ring should still be taped and Stage 1 training for interthoracic ring alignment should begin in the hook-lying position.

Stage 1 motor control training for the upper fibers of the transversus abdominis and diaphragm

The upper fibers of the TrA (Fig. 1.28) interdigitate with the sternal and anterior costal portion of the diaphragm (Fig. 1.31) and connect the left and right common cartilaginous bar of the vertebrochondral region. Suboptimal motor control strategies of the upper fibers of the TrA and this region of the diaphragm impact function of the vertebrochondral thoracic rings. Often correcting the alignment of the thoracic rings results in automatic improved recruitment of the TrA and diaphragm.

In this author's experience, in thorax-driven abdominal wall dysfunction, a symmetric bilateral transversus abdominis muscle contraction is often restored in response to both abdominal wall and pelvic floor cues when the thoracic ring driver is corrected (Fig. 3.74). A similar change in the abdominal wall recruitment response with a thoracic ring correction has also been noted during a short head and neck curl-up task (Fig. 3.75A & B) (Lee D 2017b).

Sometimes, the recruitment response of the TrA does not change with correction and release of the thoracic ring driver. In this situation, another body region may be driving the suboptimal behavior of the abdominal wall (pelvis, hip, neck or cranium) or, alternately, specific motor control training for the individual muscle is required. Widening of the infrasternal angle, combined with bulging of the upper abdomen during a short head and neck curl-up

task, with or without associated doming of the upper linea alba (Fig. 7.7), that cannot be changed with correction of any body region, suggests that specific training of the upper fibers of the TrA and diaphragm is indicated.

Stage 1 training: With the patient in hook lying, palpate the left and right TrA just lateral to the rectus abdominis between the 10th ribs and the xyphoid. Ensure the depth of palpation is accurate to reach the TrA layer (Fig. 3.76C).

Connect cues for upper fibers of the TrA: There is no research to guide cuing for recruitment of the upper fibers of the TrA. The current evidence provides information about the middle fibers and suggests that a 10 to 15 per cent contraction of the pelvic floor muscles should result in an automatic contraction of the middle fibers of the TrA

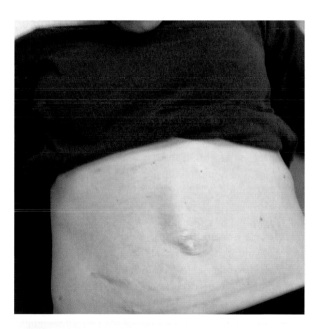

Figure 7.7

This woman has a suboptimal automatic recruitment strategy for a short head and neck curl-up task. She is not recruiting the upper fibers of her left or right TrA. Note the doming of the linea alba, which suggests insufficient tension has been generated by her automatic strategy for this task. The internal oblique is also dominating the external oblique since the infrasternal angle has widened during this task.

that is isolated from the superficial abdominals (Hodges et al. 2003). Clinically, contracting the pelvic floor does not always result in an automatic contraction of the upper fibers of the TrA. If a gentle contraction of the pelvic floor does not change the behavior of the upper abdomen during a single leg lift (active bent leg raise), or during a short head and neck curl-up task, try the following local upper abdominal connect cue. First, palpate the upper fibers of the TrA at the appropriate depth with the left and right thumb and gently pull your thumbs laterally to take up any laxity in the linea alba and rectus sheaths. Then:

1. Ask the patient to bring their attention to your left and right thumb and to imagine a guy wire connecting them.

2. Ask them to gently find a way to connect along this guy wire to draw the left and right infrasternal angle narrower. Watch for the external oblique (EO) to activate instead of the upper fibers of TrA. The EO contraction will be more superficial than the TrA contraction and will render the rib cage more rigid. A deep, gentle increase in tension is the optimal response.

This contraction is easily seen on ultrasound imaging and its impact on tension in the linea alba for those with diastasis rectus abdominis can clearly be seen (see Amanda's story in Chapter 5).

The following is a useful home self-check to ensure the recruitment strategy for Stage 1 training of the upper abdomen for control of the vertebrochondral thoracic rings is optimal. Have the patient lie in hook lying and, without imagining a connection to anything, lift the right leg and then the left leg 5 cm off the floor. Does one leg seem harder or heavier to lift than the other? Palpate the upper abdomen, have them think of nothing, and repeat the single leg lift. Did any bulging of the upper abdomen occur (Fig. 7.8)? If there is a DRA did the midline of the abdomen dome when the leg was lifted? Instruct the patient to activate the upper fibers of TrA and the diaphragm with the previously found connect cue and repeat the single-leg-lift task. Is there any difference in the effort it took to lift the leg with this new strategy? Is there any difference in the

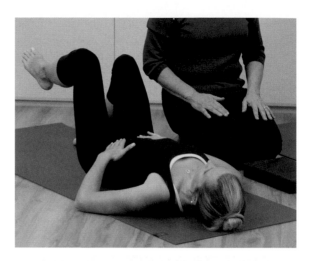

Figure 7.8

The active bent leg raise, with and without activating the deep muscles responsible for thoraco-lumbopelvic control (transversus abdominis, pelvic floor, multifidus), is useful for determining the difference various recruitment strategies have on the effort it takes to lift one leg.

upper abdominal bulging or midline doming with the use of the connect cue?

Stage 1 motor control training prescription dosage

The goal for this stage of motor learning (cognitive stage) is to achieve three sets of 10 10-second holds with a two-minute rest in between (Tsao & Hodges 2007, 2008; Tsao et al. 2010). If there is fatigue prior to reaching this dosage, the home self-check test will reveal more effort to lift the arm or leg. When monitoring the behavior of the upper abdomen, the abdomen will bulge or the linea alba will dome, or become less tense, when the strategy is less optimal. Stop, reconnect, and try once more. If there is no improvement in the quality of the contraction, stop.

Taping for interthoracic ring control

The following taping techniques were developed by Linda-Joy Lee (2003a) and provide biomechanical support and proprioceptive feedback during Stage 1 and early Stage 2 motor control training for interthoracic ring control.

Single thoracic ring translated and rotated in the vertebrochondral region

All restrictive vectors should be released prior to taping a thoracic ring. In the vertebrochondral region of the thorax (thoracic rings 7 to 10), the thoracic ring is corrected and then tape is applied to the thoracic ring to prevent the lateral translation component. For example, if the 8th thoracic ring is persistently translated right and rotated left and is the primary driver for the meaningful task, the 8th thoracic ring is manually corrected and taped into left lateral translation (Fig. 7.9A). The direction of the translation is not in the pure transverse plane of the body, it follows the plane of the body of the rib.

1. Apply hypoallergenic tape, such as Fixomull®, from the midaxillary line of the 8th rib, along the body of the rib posteriorly, and then cross the T8 vertebra ending the tape just lateral to the spinal column (Fig. 7.9B & C). Do not correct the 8th thoracic ring during the application of the Fixomull®; it is the 'landing strip' for the next tape application.

2. Anchor a strong, nonelastic tape, such as Leukotape®, over the Fixomull® in the midaxillary line ensuring that none of this tape contacts the patient's skin (Fig. 7.9D).

3. With one hand, correct the 8th thoracic ring, maintain this correction, and apply the Leukotape® along the body of the 8th rib with gentle medial and superior translation (over the Fixomull®). End the Leukotape® across the spinal column, avoiding contact with the patient's skin (Fig. 7.9E). Recheck the alignment of the 8th thoracic ring and note the impact of the connect cue, combined with taping, to retain control and alignment of the 8th thoracic ring during a static loading task such as arm elevation, as well as the relevant screening task. This is an essential requirement prior to progressing to Stage 2 motor learning and movement training.

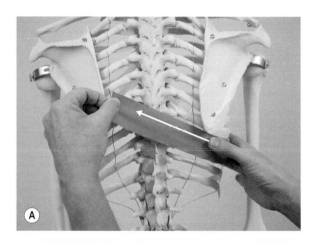

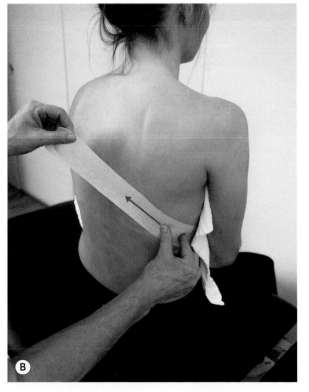

Figure 7.9

Taping a single thoracic ring in the vertebrochondral region for interthoracic ring alignment and control (Lee L-J 2003a). (A) In the vertebrochondral region the vector of force for taping the thoracic rings can be lateromedial translation since the scapula does not overlap the ribs and direct access to the rib is possible. (B) Attach the Fixomull® over the body of the rib in the midaxillary line. *Continued*

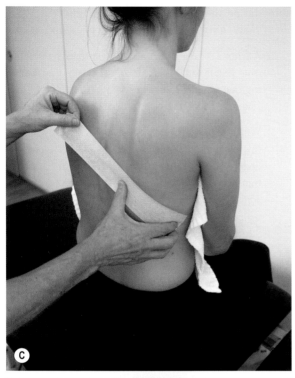

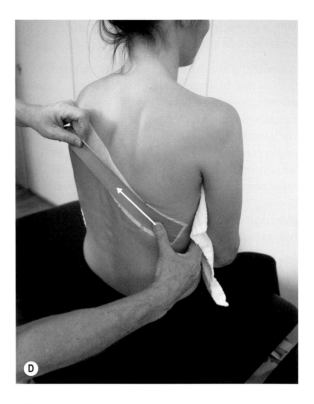

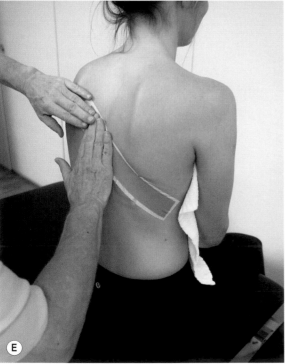

Figure 7.9 *continued*

(C) Do not guess; landmark the rib accurately by moving your thumb along the back of the rib as the Fixomull® is applied. (D) Attach the Leukotape® over the Fixomull® in the midaxillary line, correct the thoracic ring, and pull the tape along the line of the rib (medial and superior translation). (E) End the tape across the spine medial to the scapula.

Single thoracic ring translated and rotated in the vertebrosternal region

All restrictive vectors should be released prior to taping a thoracic ring. In the vertebrosternal region of the thorax (thoracic rings 3 to 6), the scapula prevents taping the thoracic ring from the midaxillary line. In this region, the thoracic ring is corrected and then tape is applied to the thoracic ring to control anterior rotation of the relevant rib. For example, if the 4th thoracic ring is persistently translated left and rotated right and is the primary driver for the meaningful task, the 4th thoracic ring is manually corrected and the left 4th rib is taped into posterior rotation (Fig. 7.10A) to control the entire thoracic ring. The thoracic ring should still be able to move when taped.

1. Apply hypoallergenic tape, such as Fixomull®, in the posterior intercostal space between the left 3rd and 4th ribs with the tape oriented inferiorly and to the right (Fig. 7.10B). Monitor the 4th thoracic ring in the left axilla, pull on the Fixomull® in a variety of inferior/medial planes until the line of pull that corrects the 4th thoracic ring is found (Fig. 7.10C). Lay the Fixomull® across the spinal column making sure to cross over the right 5th rib.

2. Anchor a strong, nonelastic tape, such as Leukotape®, over the Fixomull® in the intercostal space between the left 3rd and 4th ribs ensuring that none of this tape contacts the patient's skin.

3. With one hand, correct the 4th thoracic ring, maintain this correction and apply the Leukotape® along the line of the Fixomull®. As you pull the tape inferiorly and to the right, the 4th thoracic ring should correct (note in the axilla) (Fig. 7.10D). End the Leukotape® across the spinal column crossing the right 5th rib, avoiding contact with the patient's skin.

Recheck the alignment of the 4th thoracic ring and note the impact of the connect cue, combined with taping, to retain control and alignment of the 4th thoracic ring during a static loading task such as arm elevation, as well as the relevant screening task. This is an essential requirement prior to progressing to Stage 2 motor learning and movement training.

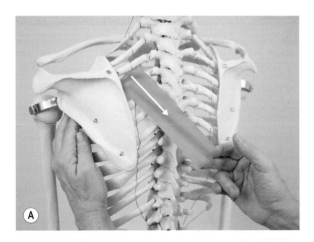

Figure 7.10

Taping a single thoracic ring in the vertebrosternal region for interthoracic ring alignment and control (Lee L-J 2003a). (A) In the vertebrosternal region posterior rotation of the relevant rib in the thoracic ring is used since the scapula overlaps the ribs and direct access for taping from the midaxillary line is not possible. (B) Attach the Fixomull® in the intercostal space above the thoracic ring of interest. *Continued*

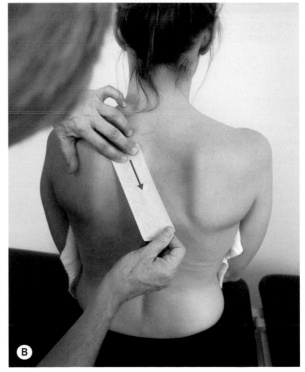

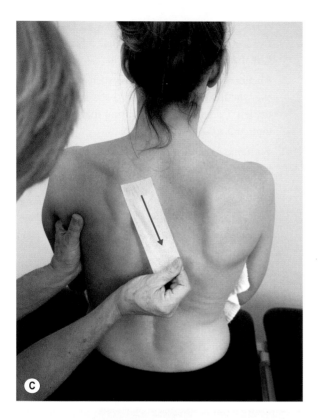

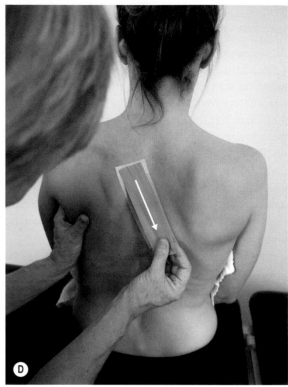

Figure 7.10 *continued*

(C) As you pull the tape inferiorly and medially, monitor the reaction of the thoracic ring in the axilla; it should begin to correct.

(D) Attach the Leukotape® over the Fixomull®, correct the thoracic ring, and pull the tape inferiorly and medially ending across the spinal column.

Multiple adjacent thoracic rings translated and rotated

The principles for taping multiple adjacent or nonadjacent thoracic rings are the same as for taping one. Begin by taping the thoracic ring that has the biggest impact on the other thoracic rings. For example, if there are three adjacent thoracic rings translated and rotated in alternate directions (3rd translated right and rotated left, 4th translated left and rotated right and 5th translated right and rotated left), note the thoracic ring that when corrected results in the best correction of the other two. Tape this thoracic ring first then tape the other two. Remember to release all restrictive vectors prior to taping multiple rings. Glued thoracic rings

should be released prior to taping. If taping a thoracic ring in the vertebrosternal region results in only partial correction of a thoracic ring in the vertebrochondral region, and all restrictive vectors have been released, tape the vertebrosternal thoracic ring first and then the vertebrochondral thoracic ring.

Taping should facilitate better alignment, biomechanics, and control and remind the patient of when their thoracic rings are losing alignment and control. If the tape is used to augment motor learning, strategies appear to improve more quickly than if the patient ignores the pulling of the tape and reverts to old, poor strategies.

Taping the scapula

When the shoulder girdle is either a primary driver or a co-driver and poor control of the thoracic rings is secondary to, or in conjunction with, poor function of the shoulder girdle, taping the scapula can assist both Stage 1 and Stage 2 motor control training of the thorax, neck, and shoulder girdle. The axillary sling taping technique for the scapula was developed by Lyn Watson (Watson & Dalziel 1996). The goal is to create a hammock of support for the inferior angle of the scapula such that the shoulder girdle is slightly elevated (Fig. 7.11A). This reduces the compression force on the thorax, and the downward pull on the head and neck, from the shoulder girdle. All restrictive vectors to the shoulder girdle (clavicle, scapula), head, neck and thorax should be released prior to taping the scapula. Correct the scapula (align the spine of the scapula to the 3rd thoracic ring) and mark with a pen where the inferior angle rests on the rib cage; it should be close to the 7th rib.

1. Attach hypoallergenic tape, such as Fixomull®, in the midaxillary line at approximately the 7th rib.

2. Elevate and correct the scapula and then apply the Fixomull® along the posterior aspect of the thorax crossing the X where the inferior angle of the scapula will rest when the scapula is released (Fig. 7.11B). Extend the Fixomull® across the opposite side of the posterior thorax up to the 2nd thoracic ring. Avoid applying the tape over the contralateral scapula.

3. Release the scapula, note its resultant position and impact on the alignment of the thoracic rings, cervical segments, and cranium.

4. The inferior angle of the scapula should be supported in the Fixomull® like a person in a hammock (Fig. 7.11C).

5. Reinforce the Fixomull® with Leukotape® Fig. 7.11D & E.

6. Additional taping to correct protraction of the scapula can be added. If the scapula continues to anteriorly tilt, it is likely that an anterior restrictive vector remains and should first be released.

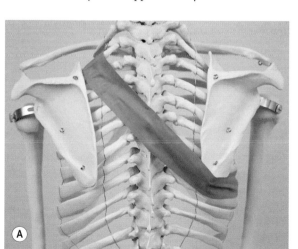

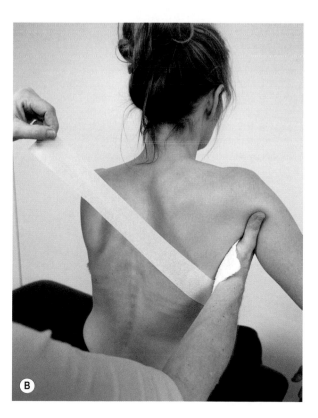

Figure 7.11

(A) A hammock taping technique for the scapula to unload the cervical segments and thoracic rings (Watson & Dalziel 1996) (B) After marking where the inferior angle of the scapula rests on the posterior thorax, attach the Fixomull® in the midaxillary line, elevate and correct the scapula, and cross the mark with the tape. Ensure that the tape crosses the spine but does not contact the contralateral scapula. *Continued*

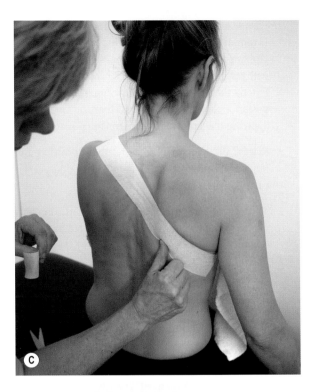

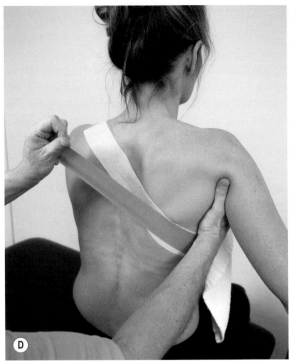

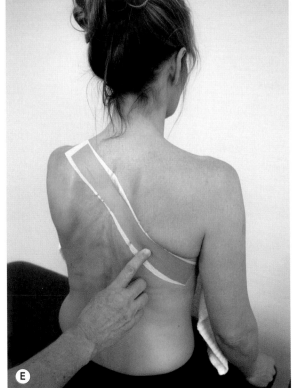

Figure 7.11 *continued*

(C) Release the scapula and check to ensure the inferior angle is resting and supported in the tape. (D) Repeat the process with the Leukotape®. (E) When applied correctly, and for the right condition, the alignment of the thoracic rings and cervical segments will improve. This taping facilitates the motor learning and movement training for the neck and thorax by reducing the vertical load.

Stage 2 strategy capacity training for interthoracic ring control

Once the patient can recruit a better strategy for static interthoracic ring alignment and control, training can progress to improve the capacity of the strategy to tolerate more load applied through distal body regions.

Stage 2 training examples using body weight, free weights, and light equipment

Instruct the patient on how to monitor interthoracic ring alignment and control, as well as the recruitment strategy for the upper fibers of the TrA and diaphragm, for any training given. Ensure they understand how to dose their training (e.g., three sets of 10 repetitions per side three to four times per day) ensuring that every repetition occurs with the better motor control strategy. Stage 1 release and connect cues recruit the strategy; breathing and arm and leg movements add further challenge and load to the task. The goal is to maintain static alignment of the thoracic rings during all loading. At this stage of training, a symmetric recruitment response of the upper fibers of the TrA with a connect cue will have been restored without further manual correction of any driver.

1. Arm loading progressions (hook lying, side lying where appropriate, prone, then progress to sitting):

    a. Single and double arm elevation to 90 degrees, then progress to adding weights (Fig. 7.12A–D);

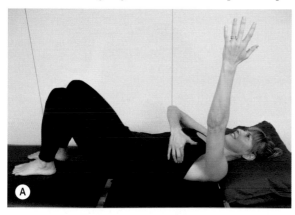
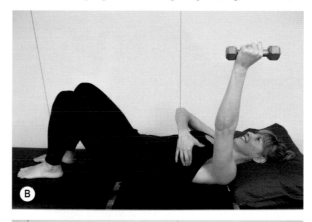
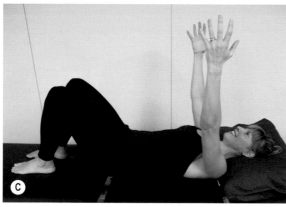
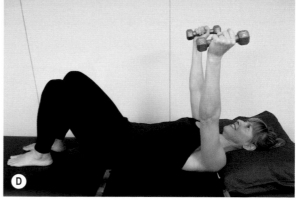

Figure 7.12

Stage 2 strategy capacity training in hook lying. The principles of this stage of training are to maintain optimal alignment of the target region (thorax) while adding load through distal segments (arms, legs) in a variety of positions. (A–D) Arm loading: Single and double arm elevation to 90 degrees initially monitoring alignment of the relevant thoracic ring, progressing to adding light weights.

b. Protraction and retraction of the scapula (dissociated movement of shoulder girdle) Fig. 7.13A–D);

c. As capacity for controlling interthoracic ring alignment and control improves, light weights or resistance bands can be added in more challenging positions (sitting, standing, squat, lunge) (Fig. 7.14A–D).

2. Leg loading progressions (supine, side lying, prone):

   a. Single leg lift, progress to single leg extension, abduction, and circles (Fig. 7.15A–C).

   b. Prone knee flexion, hip rotation (Fig. 7.15D & E).

3. Wall planks: This task requires control of multiple body regions and dissociated, independent movement of the shoulder girdles and upper extremities (Fig. 7.16A & B).

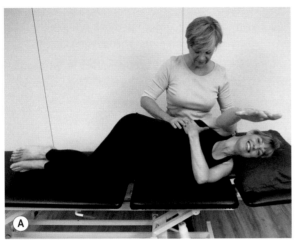
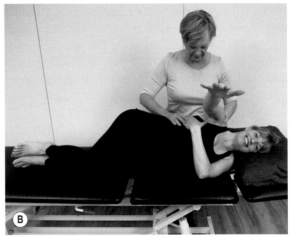
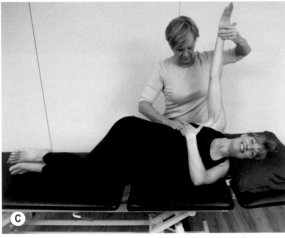
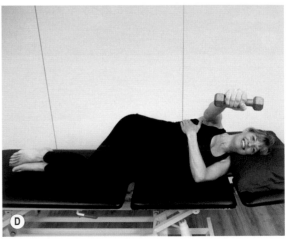

Figure 7.13

Stage 2 strategy capacity training in side lying. (A–D) Arm loading: Protraction and retraction of the scapula while maintaining alignment and control of the thoracic rings (i.e., training independent movement between the scapula and the vertebrosternal thoracic rings) progressing to adding light weights.

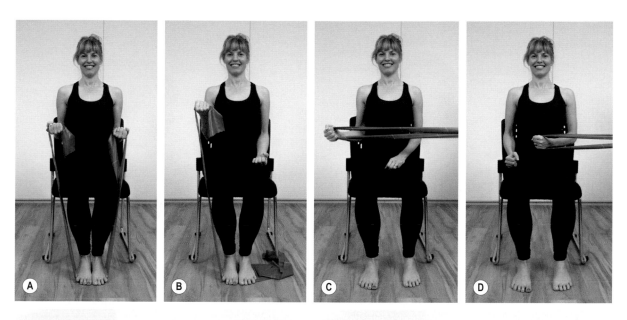

Figure 7.14

Stage 2 strategy capacity training in sitting: Arm loading. (A) Bilateral biceps curls without losing thoracic ring alignment or control add further sagittal plane challenge. (B) Unilateral biceps curls add a side bending and rotation challenge for the thorax. (C & D) Elastic band resistance for additional rotation control challenge for the thorax. In Stage 2 training, the goal is to maintain static thoracic ring alignment and control under increasing loads.

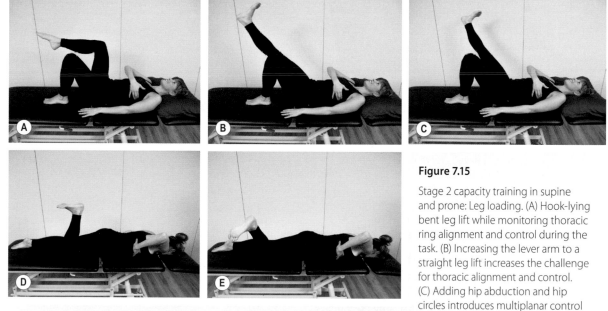

Figure 7.15

Stage 2 capacity training in supine and prone: Leg loading. (A) Hook-lying bent leg lift while monitoring thoracic ring alignment and control during the task. (B) Increasing the lever arm to a straight leg lift increases the challenge for thoracic alignment and control. (C) Adding hip abduction and hip circles introduces multiplanar control challenges for the thorax. (D) Prone knee bend while monitoring thoracic ring alignment and control during the task. (E) Adding hip rotation to the prone knee bend task for further multiplanar challenge.

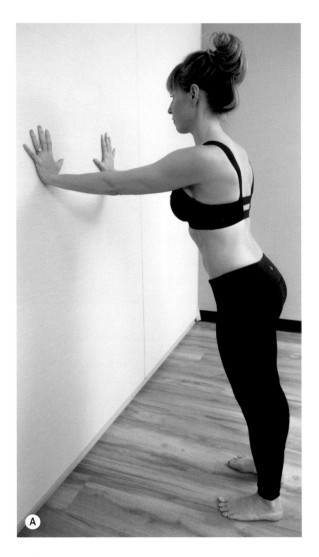

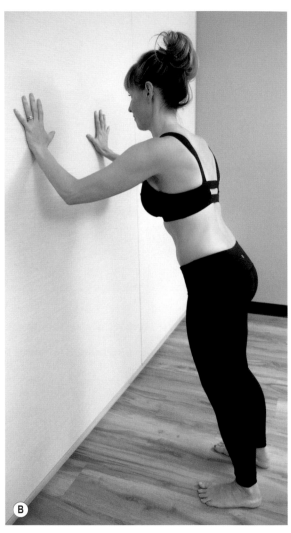

Figure 7.16

Stage 2 strategy capacity training for multiple body region control and independent movement of the shoulder girdle and upper extremity. (A & B) Wall planks. The thorax does not move when this task is performed well; therefore, this is still a Stage 2 strategy capacity training task.

Stage 2 training examples using Pilates equipment

The goal at this stage of motor learning is to maintain static alignment of the thoracic rings during all loading through the upper extremity. Lower extremity training on Pilates equipment requires confirmation that any secondary pelvis or hip driver can be controlled with loading (see the next section). Using load through the upper extremity to build capacity for interthoracic ring control also requires that the shoulder girdle is not a driver for the training task. The assumption for all training presented here is that the thorax is the primary driver and that interthoracic ring control is the main impairment for the task being trained:

1. Seated box work on the Pilates Reformer (variety of arm loading in multiple planes) (Fig. 7.17A–C);

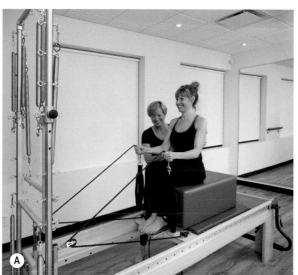
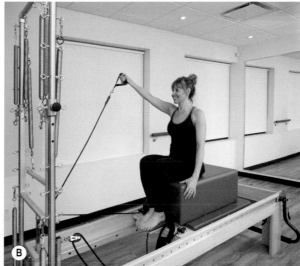
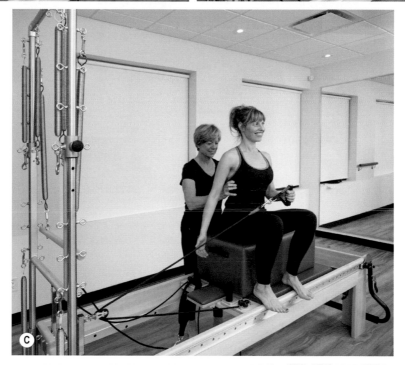

Figure 7.17

Stage 2 strategy capacity training using the Pilates Reformer. (A) Biceps curls seated on a box. No loss of thoracic ring alignment or control should occur during this task. (B) One-arm fly seated on a box. This is a much harder challenge for the thorax. (C) Resisted external rotation of the shoulder while maintaining optimal thoracic ring alignment and control.

2. Prone box work on the Pilates Reformer;

3. Four-point kneeling arm and leg movements with thoracopelvic control on the Pilates Reformer (Fig. 7.18A–E).

Before progressing to Stage 3 training for the thorax (interregional movement), control of any secondary driver should be addressed.

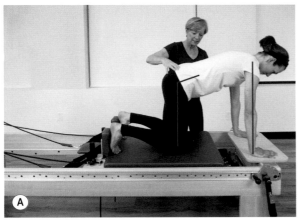

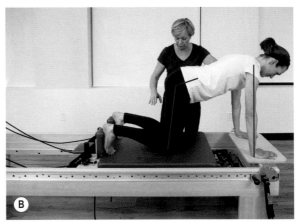

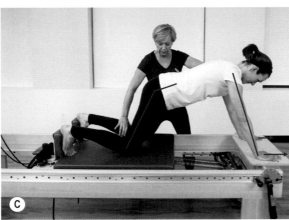

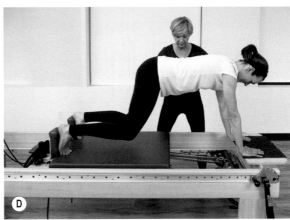

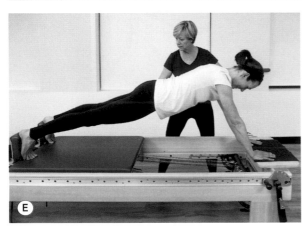

Figure 7.18

Stage 2 strategy capacity training using the Pilates Reformer with progressions. Instruct the patient as follows. (A) In four-point kneeling, begin with the wrists directly beneath the shoulders and knees beneath the hips with the spine in neutral. (B) Push the carriage back by extending only the hips, keep the wrists directly beneath the shoulders and the spine in neutral. (C) Push the platform forward using the arms and keep the thorax, lumbar spine, and pelvis in neutral. (D) Hover the knees off the carriage. (E) Push the carriage back by extending the hips and knees into a full plank position. Reverse to return to neutral four-point kneeling.

Intrapelvic ring motor control training

If intrapelvic ring control is not completely restored with treatment of the thorax, the pelvis is a secondary driver and specific motor control training for the pelvis is indicated before tasks are given that require control of both the thorax and pelvis, with or without mobility of either region. It is not the intention of this text to describe motor control and movement training for the pelvis in detail; the reader is referred to *The Pelvic Girdle* (Lee D 2011) for more information on this topic. The principles for motor control and movement training to restore intrapelvic ring control are the same as those presented in this text for the thorax.

Stage 1: Release all restricting vectors and build a new strategy for static intrapelvic ring control (low fibers of the TrA and IO, sacral fibers of the multifidus, pelvic floor muscles, diaphragm). If there is a form closure deficit with loss of passive articular integrity, prolotherapy may be required before motor control training begins. Taping, or a sacroiliac belt (www.babybellypelvicsupport.com), may be required at this stage of training for both biomechanical support (increased force closure) and for providing non-threatening proprioceptive input.

Stage 2: Increase strategy capacity for intrapelvic ring control by adding load to the pelvis through the lower extremity without allowing any intrapelvic motion to occur.

Stage 3: Inter-regional control and movement then follows.

Lumbar and cervical segmental control

If segmental lumbar or cervical control is not completely restored with treatment of the thorax, specific motor control training for the relevant segment is indicated before tasks are given that require inter-regional movement and control. The principles for motor control and movement training to restore segmental lumbar and cervical control (secondary driver) are the same as those presented in this text for the thorax.

Stage 1: Release all restricting vectors and build a new strategy for static lumbar and cervical segmental control.

Stage 2: Increase strategy capacity for segmental lumbar and cervical control by adding load without allowing any lumbar and cervical motion to occur.

Stage 3: Inter-regional control and movement then follows.

Inter-regional movement and control – moving into function

Stage 3 movement training

Stage 3 movement training is based on the patient's meaningful tasks such that training is specific to their functional goals. The goal is broken down into component tasks and training is initially focused on improving the alignment, biomechanics and control of the primary and secondary drivers for that task. Eventually, the whole body is trained and integrated. Stage 3 training can be divided into three levels:

1. Level 1: Movement training for the thorax in multiple planes with the thorax centered over a controlled base of support – the pelvis. Arm or leg movements are not part of this level of movement training for the thorax.

2. Level 2: Progress and add:

   a. lumbopelvic control in the sagittal plane

   b. the shoulder girdle and arm (closed and open kinetic chain training), with interthoracic ring movements and lumbopelvic or cervical segmental control (sagittal and transverse planes),

   c. the lower extremity (closed and open kinetic chain training) added to (a) above (sagittal and transverse planes), and

   d. incongruent head and neck movements in the direction of movement of the thorax (sagittal and transverse planes).

3. Level 3: Whole-body complex tasks with varying levels of task predictability and perturbation.

Table 7.2 provides examples of Stage 3, Levels 1 to 3 training goals and tasks and it is followed by illustrations of each movement training practice with key features explained in the captions. Select appropriate movement training that is matched to the task demands of the patient's goals.

Table 7.2
Stage 3 Movement training

LEVEL	TRAINING GOALS	TRAINING TASK	FIGURE
1	Interthoracic ring mobility and control – sagittal plane	Seated thorax flexion and extension	7.19A and B
1	Interthoracic ring mobility and control – transverse plane	Seated thorax rotation integrated with breathing	7.20
1	Interthoracic ring mobility and control – sagittal plane	Upper abdominal curls with a Pilates Spine Corrector Barrel or mat	7.21A and B
2	Interthoracic ring mobility and lumbopelvic control – sagittal plane	Seated lumbopelvic–hip and thorax roll-back (curls)	7.22
2	Interthoracic ring mobility, lumbopelvic control, and shoulder girdle control – sagittal plane	Seated lumbopelvic and thorax roll-back with spring-resistance assistance on the Pilates Cadillac	7.23A–E
2	Interthoracic ring mobility, lumbopelvic control, and shoulder girdle control – sagittal plane	Four-point-kneeling cat-cow with the addition of incongruent head and neck movements, knee hover, and Downward Facing Dog	7.24A–D
2	Interthoracic ring mobility, hip mobility, and lumbopelvic control – sagittal plane	Supine bridge roll-up and roll-down	7.25
2	Interthoracic ring mobility, hip mobility, and lumbopelvic control – sagittal plane	Pilates Reformer supine bridge roll-up, leg press, and roll-down	7.26A–I
2	Interthoracic ring mobility, hip mobility, and lumbopelvic control – sagittal plane	Pilates Reformer short spine	7.27A–F
2	Interthoracic ring mobility, shoulder mobility and control, hip mobility, and lumbopelvic control – sagittal plane	Pilates Cadillac teaser and progressions	7.28A–G
2	Interthoracic ring mobility and lumbopelvic–hip mobility – transverse plane	Supine wipers	7.29
2	Interthoracic ring mobility, shoulder girdle dissociation, head and neck congruent rotation – transverse plane	Side-lying protraction–retraction of shoulder girdle and arm with congruent thoracic rotation with a Pilates Spine Corrector	7.30
2	Interthoracic ring mobility, shoulder girdle dissociation, head and neck rotation, and lumbopelvic control – transverse plane	Four-point kneeling Thread the Needle	7.31
2	Interthoracic ring mobility, hip mobility, and lumbopelvic control - transverse plane	Supine bridge roll-up, rotate pelvis, and roll-down	7.32
2	Interthoracic ring mobility, hip mobility and lumbopelvic control – transverse plane	Supine bridge roll-up, lift and extend one leg, replace, and roll-down	7.33
2	Interthoracic ring mobility, lumbopelvic control, and shoulder girdle control – transverse plane	Seated thorax rotation with arm weights or resistance bands with congruent and incongruent head and neck rotation	7.34
2	Interthoracic ring mobility, lumbopelvic control, shoulder girdle control – transverse plane	Pilates Reformer Box trunk rotation	7.35
2	Interthoracic ring mobility, lumbopelvic control, and shoulder girdle mobility and control – transverse plane	Pilates Cadillac porte de bras exercises	7.36A–F
3	Integration of regional movement and control, inter-regional movement and control with varying levels of task predictability and perturbation	High kneeling, thorax rotation with resistance bands. Progress to lifting the back knee into a lunge	7.37
3	Integration of regional movement and control and inter-regional movement and control with varying levels of task predictability and perturbation	Squats, with thorax rotation, resistance, and different head and neck positions	7.38
3	Integration of regional movement and control and inter-regional movement and control with varying levels of task predictability and perturbation	Pilates Reformer – standing leg abduction press with contralateral thorax rotation with the head and neck in neutral position	7.39A–C

Table 7.2 *continued*

LEVEL	TRAINING GOALS	TRAINING TASK	FIGURE
3	Integration of regional movement and control and inter-regional movement and control with varying levels of task predictability and perturbation	Lunges with congruent or incongruent rotation of the thorax, with the head and neck in neutral position	7.40A–C
3	Integration of regional movement and control and inter-regional movement and control with varying levels of task predictability and perturbation	Pilates Cadillac waterwheel	7.41A–H
3	Yoga flow sequences	Ardha Bhujangasana to Bhujangasana to Urdhva Mukha Svanasana	7.42A–C
		Baby Cobra to Cobra to Updog	
3	Yoga flow sequences	Phalankasana to three-legged Adho Mukha Svanasana to Knee to Nose (triceps) to Camatkarasana to Vasisthasana	7.43A–E
		Plank to three-legged Downward Dog to Knee to Nose (triceps) to Fallen Triangle to Side Plank	
3	Yoga flow sequences	Virabhadrasana II to Viparita Virabhadrasana to Utthita Parsvakonasana	7.44A–C
		Warrior II to Reverse Warrior to Extended Side Angle	
3	Yoga flow sequences	Utthita Hasta Padangusthasana to Parivrtta Hasta Padangusthasana to Virabhadrasana III	7.45A and B
		Extended Hand-to-Big Toe to Revolved Hand-to-Big Toe to Warrior III	
3	Yoga flow sequences	Virabhadrasana II to Trikonasana to Ardha Chandrasana	7.46A–D
		Warrior II to Triangle to Half Moon	
3	Yoga flow sequences	Utkatasana to Parivrtta Utkatasana to Parivrtta Anjaneyasana	7.47A–C
		Chair to Revolved Chair to Revolved High Lunge	
3	Yoga flow sequences	Setu Bandha Sarvangasana to Urdhva Dhanurasana. Bridge to Wheel	7.48A and B
3	Yoga flow sequences	Virasana to Supta Virasana to Ustrasana	7.49A–C
		Hero to Reclined Hero to Camel	
3	Dynamic training – equilibrium challenge, agility, and speed	Jumping, agility ladders, skipping, Bosu jumps, ball toss on two SITFIT® pads	—

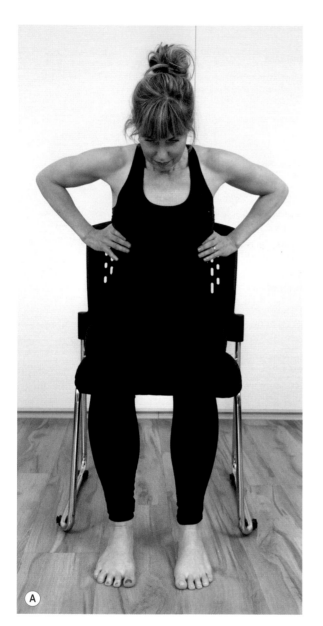
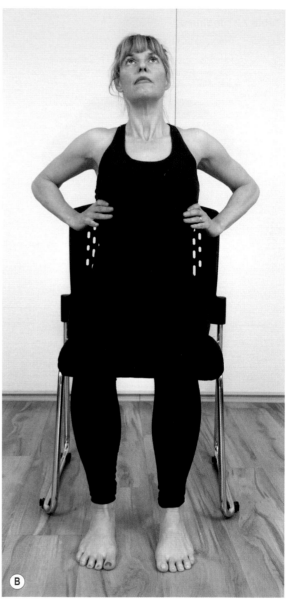

Figure 7.19

Stage 3, Level 1 movement training for the thorax in the sagittal plane. The individual release and connect cues for the thoracic ring driver, as well as any secondary drivers, precede any movement of the thorax in the sagittal plane. (A) Forward bending with sequenced flexion and anterior tilt of each thoracic ring while monitoring the alignment and control of the thoracic ring being trained. (B) Backward bending with sequenced extension and posterior tilt of each thoracic ring while monitoring the alignment and control of the thoracic ring being trained.

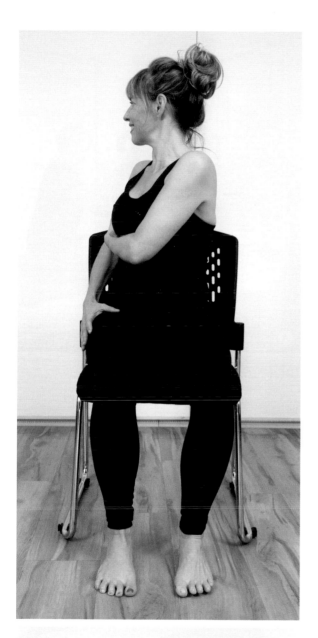

Figure 7.20

Stage 3, Level 1 movement training for the thorax in the transverse plane. The individual release and connect cues for the thoracic ring driver, as well as any secondary drivers, precede any movement of the thorax in the transverse plane. This image shows rotation while monitoring the alignment and control of the thoracic ring being trained.

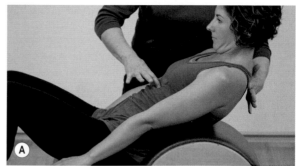

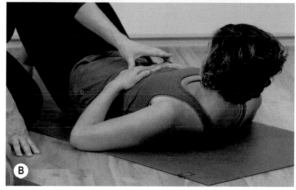

Figure 7.21

Stage 3, Level 1 movement training for the thorax in the sagittal plane. (A) The Pilates Spine Corrector Barrel supports the lower back and pelvis so that attention can be focused on interthoracic ring alignment, biomechanics, and control during sagittal plane motion (forward and backward bending). The individual release and connect cues for the thoracic ring driver, as well as any secondary drivers, precede any movement of the thorax in the sagittal plane. Here the therapist is cuing activation of the upper fibers of the TrA and palpating to ensure no bulging of the upper abdomen or widening of the infrasternal angle occurs during the forward and backward bending task. (B) The same movement practice can be performed on a mat. The curl-up should only be as far as the thorax can be maintained in optimal alignment with a correct abdominal strategy (i.e., no bulging of the abdomen or doming of the linea alba). No widening or narrowing of the rib cage should occur when the superficial abdominals are co-activating.

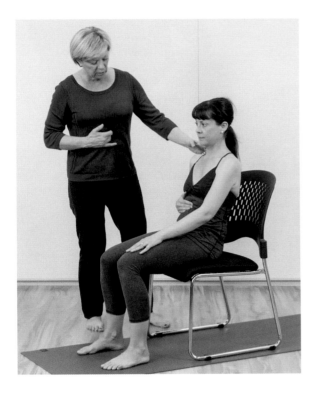

Figure 7.22

Stage 3, Level 2 movement training for sagittal plane interthoracic ring mobility and control in sitting. This task requires controlled mobility of the lumbopelvic and hip region as well as interthoracic ring mobility and control in the sagittal plane. The individual release and connect cues for the thoracic ring driver, as well as any secondary drivers (lumbopelvis or neck), precede any movement of the thorax in the sagittal plane. On the exhale breath, instruct the patient to posteriorly tilt the pelvis keeping the shoulders directly over the base of support (without leaning back). This should be a 'lengthening curve' and not a collapse into flexion. Monitor the abdominal wall for bulging and the midline for doming of the linea alba. Ask the patient to inhale and hold this position for two to three seconds and then curl back up to neutral sitting.

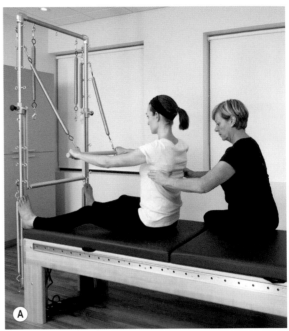

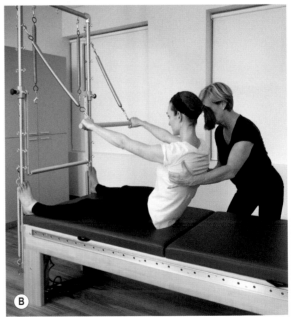

Figure 7.23

Stage 3, Level 2 movement training for sagittal plane interthoracic ring mobility and control in sitting with spring-bar assistance using the Pilates Cadillac.

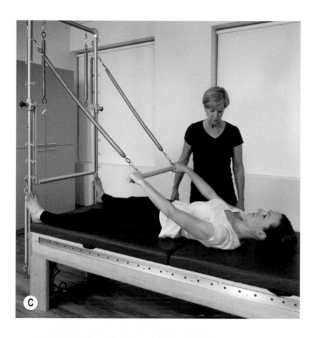

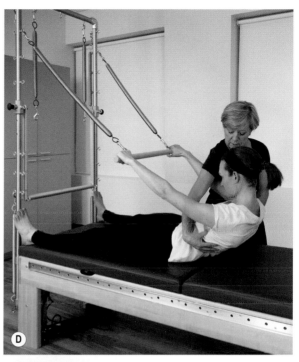

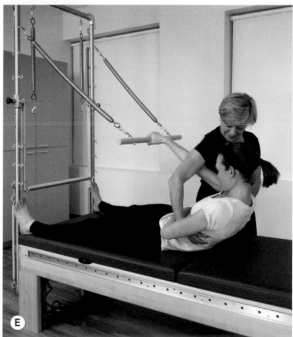

Figure 7.23 *continued*

(A–D) This task requires controlled mobility of the lumbopelvic and hip region as well as interthoracic ring mobility and control in the sagittal plane. (E) A further challenge to rotation control can be added by doing the same exercise with one arm on the spring-loaded bar. Only sagittal plane motion of the thorax is allowed.

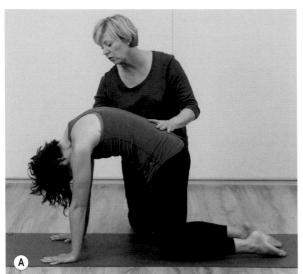 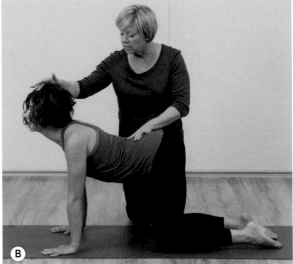

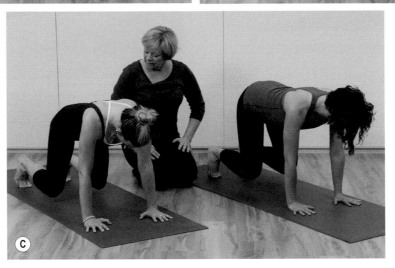

Figure 7.24

Stage 3, Level 2 movement training for sagittal plane interthoracic ring mobility and lumbopelvic and shoulder girdle control.
(A) Four-point kneeling cat with congruent head and neck flexion. The individual release and connect cues for the thoracic ring driver, as well as any secondary drivers, precede any movement of the thorax in the sagittal plane. Instruct the patient as follows. Posteriorly tilt the pelvis, flex the lumbar spine, then each individual thoracic ring, and finally the neck and head. Hold this position and extend the head and neck only (incongruent direction of motion to the thorax and low back). (B) Four-point kneeling cow with congruent head and neck extension. Maintain the individual release and connect cues for all drivers, then extend the head and neck (avoid compressing the back of the neck by looking up too far), soften the chest toward the floor, and allow the scapulae to gently retract (dissociated movement of the shoulder girdles on the thorax). Extend the lumbar spine with control and finally anteriorly tilt the pelvis by flexing the hips. Maintain this position and flex the head and neck (incongruent motion). (C) Find the neutral spine position in four-point kneeling, then further challenge alignment and control by shifting the weight to one side and lifting one hand or leg, then the other hand or leg, or by hovering both knees off the floor.

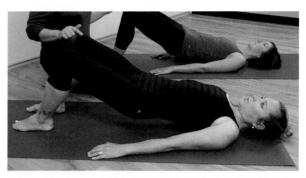

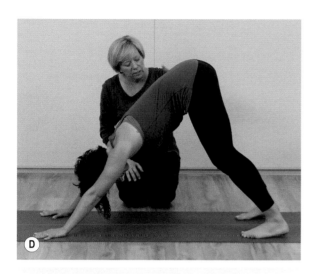

Figure 7.24 *continued*

(D) From the four-point kneeling position, tuck the toes under, spread all fingers and thumbs, and gently activate the muscles of the hands by 'clawing' the floor without bending the knuckles (lumbrical grip) until you feel a slight lift through the center of the palm. Feel the deep muscles of the hands 'wake up' and the wrists lift slightly. Lift the hips up and back and keep the arms straight until you are in an inverted 'V' position. Keep the scapular muscles engaged without overly compressing the thoracic rings. Bend the knees as much as necessary to retain an anterior tilt of the pelvis and a gentle curve in the low back. As the hamstrings lengthen, begin to straighten the legs and lower the heels to the floor. Stay here for three to four lateral costal breaths. Feel the weight of the viscera on the diaphragm and try to expand the rib cage in all directions (lateral costal, or umbrella, breath) with each inhale. This is an excellent practice progression for those with a 'low diaphragm' and pericardial vectors pulling on the thoracic rings (Figures 3.71B & C).

Figure 7.25

Stage 3, Level 2 sagittal plane interthoracic ring mobility and control, hip mobility, and lumbopelvic control. Supine bridge roll-up and roll-down. The individual release and connect cues for the thoracic ring driver, as well as any secondary drivers, precede any movement of the thorax in the sagittal plane. Instruct the patient as follows. On the next exhale, slowly posteriorly tilt the pelvis to flatten the low back to the mat. Monitor the abdominal wall for bulging, midline doming and sagging and the perineum to ensure no descent. Slowly release the curl and come back to a neutral low back and pelvis position. Once able to perform 10 high-quality repetitions of the low abdominal reverse curl, movement of the thorax is added to the task. This is not a plank 'lever' bridge; it is a roll-up, roll-down bridge. Imagine the spine like a string of pearls. On the exhale breath, connect and roll up into the bridge, flexing each individual lumbar vertebra and then each individual thoracic ring one by one, as if you were slowly lifting a string of pearls off the ground. Continue to roll up as far as possible while still maintaining optimal alignment and control. Inhale and hold this position, and on the exhale breath begin to roll down slowly releasing each thoracic ring and lumbar vertebra segment by segment. Allow the thorax to gently soften and let gravity take each thoracic ring back to neutral one segment at a time. Lengthen the entire trunk by reaching the tailbone toward the feet during the roll-down portion of the task. For this to happen, the spinal extensors and superficial abdominals must eccentrically lengthen.

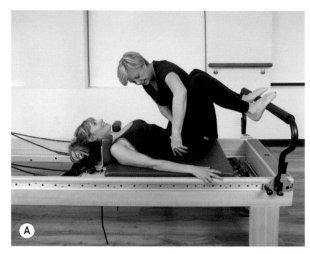

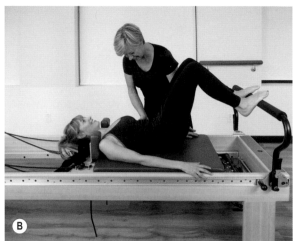

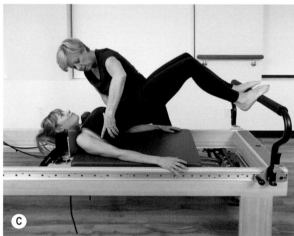

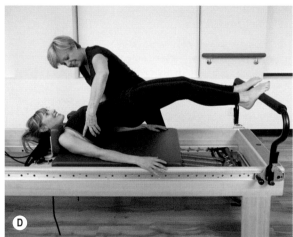

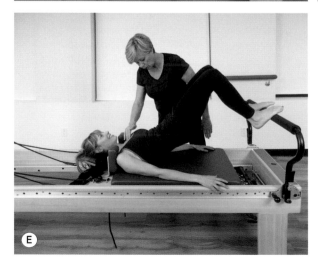

Figure 7.26

Stage 3, Level 2 sagittal plane interthoracic ring mobility and control, hip mobility, and lumbopelvic control using the Pilates Reformer. Supine bridge roll-up, leg press, and roll-down. (A) The individual release and connect cues for the thoracic ring driver, as well as any secondary drivers, precede any movement of the thorax in the sagittal plane. Instruct the patient as follows. On the next exhale, slowly posteriorly tilt the pelvis to flatten the low back to the carriage. (B) Without moving the carriage, continue to flex the low back and then each individual thoracic ring until weight-bearing on the shoulder girdles. (C & D) Maintain the alignment of the thorax, low back and pelvis and extend the hips and knees, the carriage will move and the spring resistance can be increased as capacity increases. (E) Roll-down variation with knees flexed.

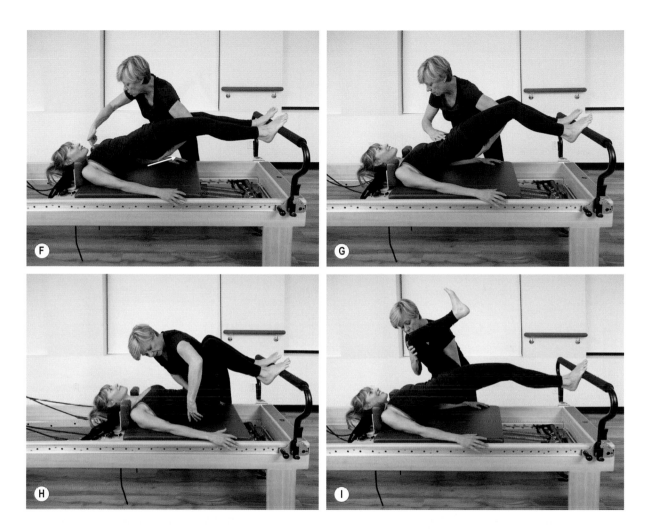

Figure 7.26 *continued*

(F) Roll-down variation with knees extended. Reach the tailbone 'long' (arrow). The therapist's hand is on the sacrum providing gentle longitudinal traction so that the release cue ('reach the tailbone long') makes sense. Begin the roll-down by softening the sternum and flexing the vertebrosternal region first. (G) Ensure the deep muscles responsible for segmental control of the lumbar spine remain engaged (no abdominal bulging). (H) Cue a release of the hips at the end of the roll-down (let your sitting bones go wide and the groin soften). (I) This may be followed by a progression which introduces a rotation control challenge.

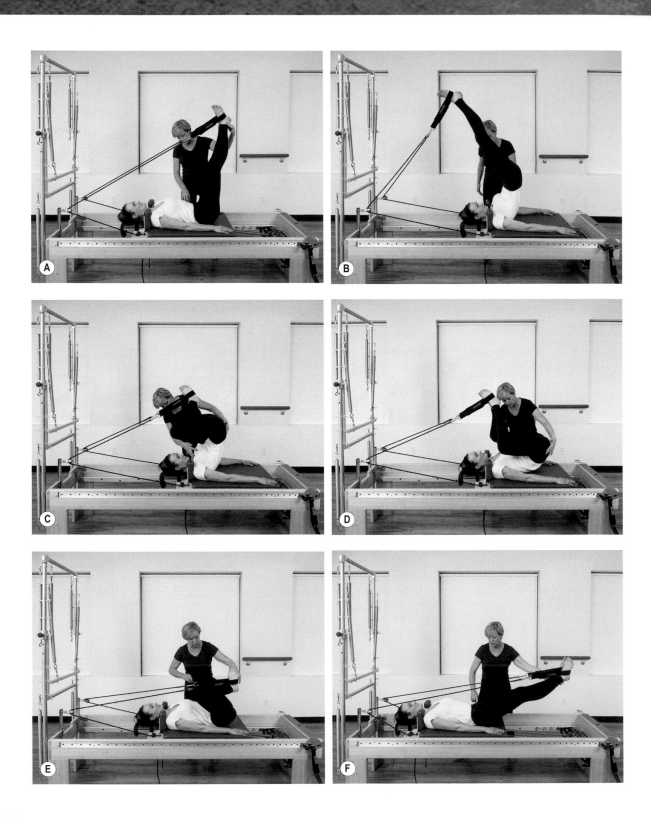

Figure 7.27 *(left)*

Stage 3, Level 2 sagittal plane interthoracic ring mobility and control, hip mobility, and lumbopelvic control using the Pilates Reformer. Short spine. (A) The individual release and connect cues for the thoracic ring driver, as well as any secondary drivers, precede any movement of the thorax in the sagittal plane. Instruct the patient as follows. With the feet in both straps, flex the hips keeping the knees straight. (B) On the next exhale, posteriorly tilt the pelvis, flex the lumbar spine and then each individual thoracic ring until weight-bearing on the shoulder girdles. (C) Inhale, bring the soles of the feet together, flex, abduct, and externally rotate the hips. (D) Keep the feet still in space, exhale and roll down by softening the sternum and flexing the vertebrosternal region first. (E) Once the low back reaches the carriage, pause and inhale, then exhale to bring the heels toward the buttocks. (F) Press the legs into extension.

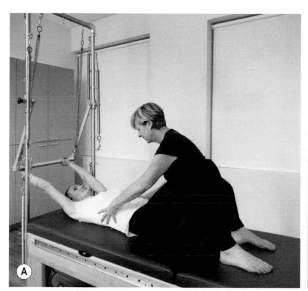

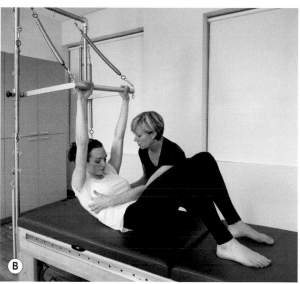

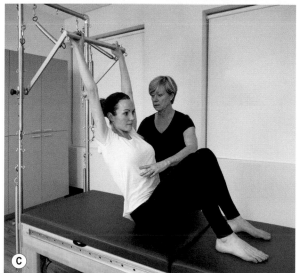

Figure 7.28

Stage 3, Level 2 sagittal plane interthoracic ring mobility and control, hip mobility, and lumbopelvic control using the Pilates Reformer. Teaser. (A) This movement practice begins in hook lying with the arms in full elevation. (B) The spring-loaded bar is pushed through followed by sequential flexion of the head, neck, and thorax. The therapist is using touch to provide sensory input to the nervous system at the level of the thoracic ring that requires attention for alignment and control. (C) The head, neck, and thorax are then extended to neutral. It is common for individuals to overextend at the thoracolumbar junction and to lose engagement of the upper fibers of the TrA and diaphragm at this point. The infrasternal angle then widens and the lower ribs 'pop forward'. Here the therapist is cuing engagement of the upper abdominals and diaphragm. *Continued*

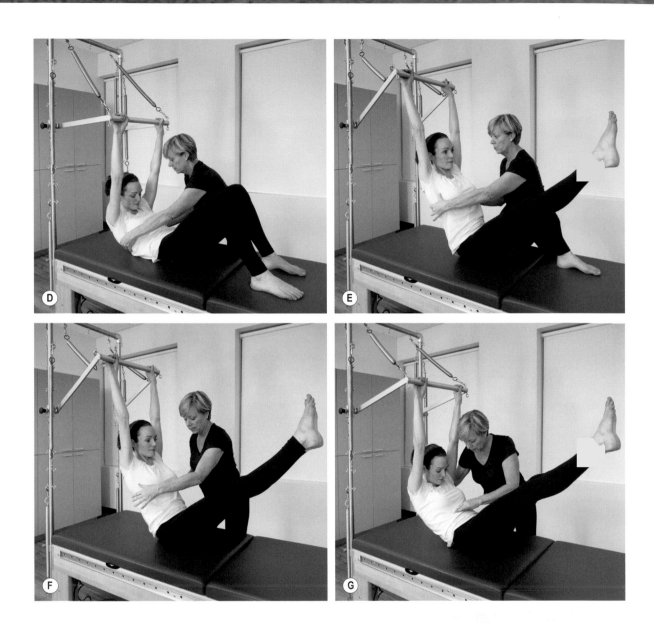

Figure 7.28 *continued*

(D) The return is initiated with a posterior pelvic tilt followed by sequenced flexion of the lumbar spine and thoracic rings, neck and head following which the bar is pushed overhead. (E) Progressions: Unilateral active straight leg raise simultaneous with the extension phase of the trunk. This requires control of the low back and pelvis and recruitment of the muscles responsible for control of these regions. (F) Further progression: Bilateral active straight leg raise. (G) Watch for abdominal bulging, infrasternal angle widening, translation and rotation of the thoracic rings, and chin poking during the return of this highly challenging Stage 3, Level 2 task.

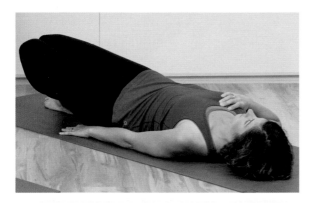

Figure 7.29

Stage 3, Level 2 transverse plane interthoracic ring mobility and lumbopelvic and hip mobility. Supine wipers. The individual release and connect cues for the thoracic ring driver, as well as any secondary drivers, precede any movement of the thorax in the transverse plane. On the exhale breath, the patient slowly takes both knees to the left ensuring all the thoracic rings rotate congruently to the left. Here, the patient is monitoring the 3rd thoracic ring to ensure optimal alignment and biomechanics during this movement practice. She then inhales to hold this position for three to four seconds and on the next exhale reinforces the connect cues and derotates the pelvis, lumbar spine, and thorax to neutral.

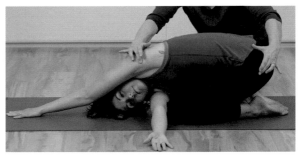

Figure 7.31

Stage 3, Level 2 transverse plane interthoracic ring mobility, shoulder girdle dissociation, head and neck rotation, and lumbopelvic control. Four-point kneeling Thread the Needle. Instruct the patient as follows. Find the neutral spine position in four-point kneeling and engage the individual release and connect cues for all drivers. From this position, thread one arm underneath the other, protract this shoulder girdle ensuring that it can move independently from the thoracic rings. Then, rotate the thorax congruently with the shoulder girdle and rest the shoulder and head on the floor. Hold for three to four breaths then return to neutral and repeat on the other side.

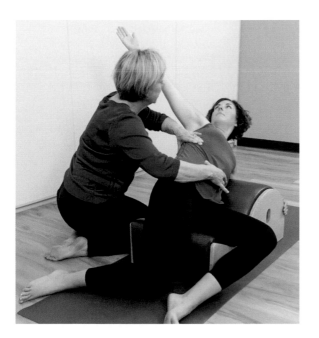

Figure 7.30

Stage 3, Level 2 transverse plane interthoracic ring mobility, shoulder girdle dissociation, and head and neck rotation. The thorax is supported over the Pilates Spine Corrector Barrel and the patient ensures the release and connect cues are engaged. With the upper arm elevated to 90 degrees, the shoulder girdle is retracted then the glenohumeral joint is horizontally abducted. The patient continues to take the arm back rotating the thorax congruently with this motion. Here, the therapist is cuing the upper fibers of the TrA and monitoring the vertebrochondral region for optimal alignment and biomechanics during this task. In this illustration, the head and neck have rotated congruently with the task. For throwing tasks, the head and neck can be trained to maintain a forward gaze as the shoulder girdle and thorax rotates beneath.

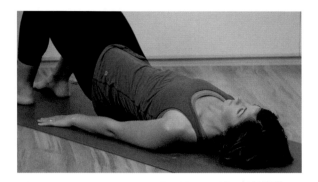

Figure 7.32

Stage 3, Level 2 transverse plane interthoracic ring mobility, hip mobility, and lumbopelvic control. Supine bridge roll-up, rotate pelvis, and roll-down. This is a progression from the supine bridge roll-up and roll-down (see Fig. 7.25). From the roll-up bridge position, the patient lengthens the entire trunk and then rotates the pelvis ensuring the axis about which this rotation occurs is through the spinal column and center of the pelvic floor. All thoracic rings should rotate congruently with the direction of the pelvic rotation. Repeat to the opposite side.

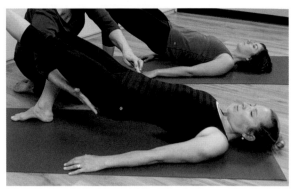

Figure 7.33

Stage 3, Level 2 transverse plane interthoracic ring mobility, hip mobility and lumbopelvic control. In supine bridge roll-up, one leg is lifted, extended, replaced on the floor, and followed by roll-down. This is a more advanced movement practice in that the base of support for transverse plane rotation of the pelvis and low back is reduced.

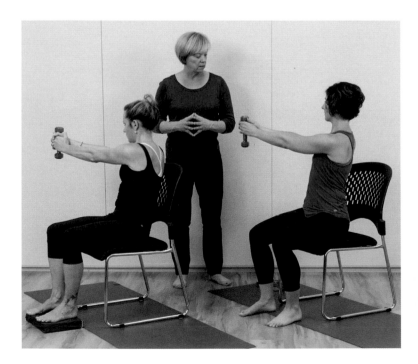

Figure 7.34

Stage 3, Level 2 transverse plane interthoracic ring mobility, lumbopelvic control, and shoulder girdle control. Seated thoracic rotation with arm weights. This is a progression from seated thoracic rotation without arm loading (Fig. 7.20). Once lumbopelvic control and thoracic mobility are well mastered, rotation with arm loading can be added to the task. Instruct the patient as follows. Start in a neutral trunk position, with both arms elevated to 90 degrees, engage the release and connect cues for all drivers, and rotate the thorax initially by maintaining the center of mass over the base of support. Progress by rotating in varying degrees of flexion and extension. Progressively add more weight to the arms with light weights or elastic band resistance. The task can be made more complex and, depending on the meaningful task, more meaningful if the head and neck are rotated to the opposite side or if a forward gaze is maintained.

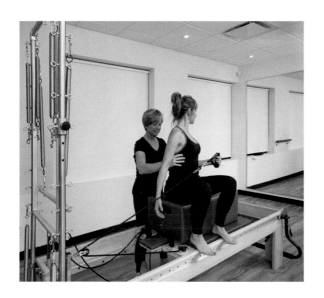

Figure 7.35

Stage 3, Level 2 transverse plane interthoracic ring mobility, lumbopelvic control, and shoulder girdle control. Seated box rotation on the Pilates Reformer. This is a progression from Figure 7.17C. The left shoulder is externally rotated followed by congruent thoracic rotation. The head and neck can be cued to follow the rotation of the thorax, or to remain forward, or to rotate incongruently.

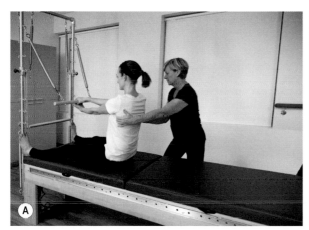

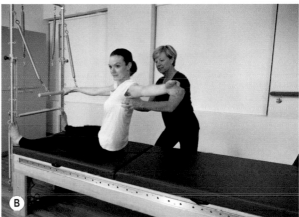

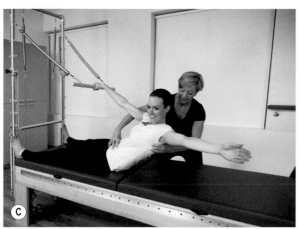

Figure 7.36

Stage 3, Level 2 transverse plane interthoracic ring mobility, lumbopelvic control, and shoulder girdle mobility and control. Porte de bras exercises on the Pilates Cadillac. Instruct the patient as follows. (A) Begin seated in neutral, feet against the tower posts, one hand above, and the other below the spring-loaded bar. (B) Engage the release and connect cues for all drivers, and then horizontally abduct the lower arm, retract the shoulder girdle, then rotate the thorax, head and neck. The therapist is ensuring all thoracic rings are rotating congruent with the requirements of the task. (C) From this position, posteriorly tilt the pelvis and sequentially flex the lumbar spine and thoracic rings. Watch for abdominal bulging, infrasternal angle widening and lower rib cage 'popping'. *Continued*

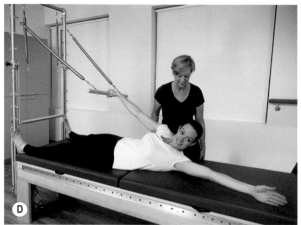

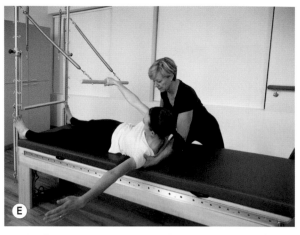

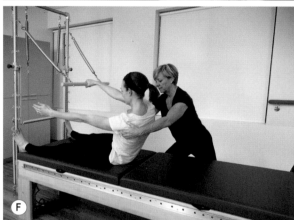

Figure 7.36 *continued*

(D) Press the right foot into the tower post and reach the left arm long to further lengthen the left anterior oblique myofascial sling of the trunk. (E) To return, bring the arm to horizontal abduction and simultaneously left side-bend, derotate, and flex the thoracic rings. Watch for chin poking, abdominal bulging, infrasternal angle widening or loss of contact of the feet with the tower posts. (F) The entire movement practice should flow with both the inhale and exhale breath.

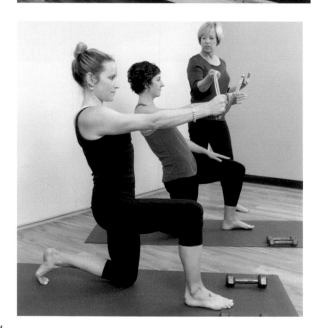

Figure 7.37

Stage 3, Level 3 integration of regional movement and control and inter-regional movement and control with varying levels of task predictability and perturbation. High kneeling, thorax rotation with elastic band resistance in varying trunk postures. Progress the task by lifting the back knee to a lunge position. For all Level 3 training, continue to monitor the alignment, biomechanics, and control of all drivers to ensure appropriateness and dosage for this training.

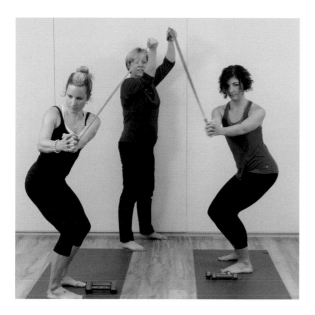

Figure 7.38

Stage 3, Level 3 integration of regional movement and control and inter-regional movement and control with varying levels of task predictability and perturbation. Squats, with thorax rotation, resistance, and different head and neck positions.

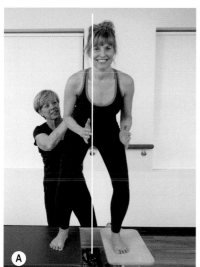

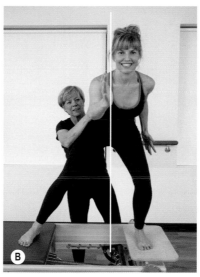

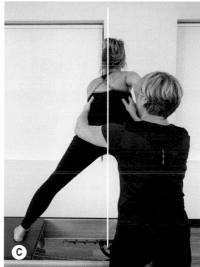

Figure 7.39

Stage 3, Level 3 integration of regional movement and control and inter-regional movement and control with varying levels of task predictability and perturbation. Standing leg abduction and contralateral thorax rotation with head and neck in neutral on a Pilates Reformer. (A) This is a challenging whole-body task and very useful for runners, speed skaters, or anyone training for a task that requires thoracopelvic rotation and leg movement. This task starts in a squat position with the thorax aligned vertically with the pelvis. This individual's thorax is to the left of her pelvis and base of support. (B) The carriage is pushed out with an abduction force from the leg as the thorax is rotated to the left. Her thorax should be centered over her pelvis. There is too much weight on her left leg and she is not rotating her thorax well. (C) On the opposite side, this individual is performing the requirements of the task much better although her upper thorax is left of center and her head and neck right of center.

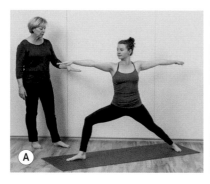
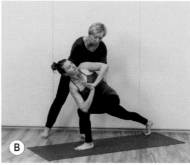
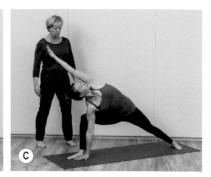

Figure 7.40

Stage 3, Level 3 integration of regional movement and control and inter-regional movement and control with varying levels of task predictability and perturbation. Lunges and variations. (A) Lunge with congruent thorax and pelvis and incongruent head and neck rotation. (B) Lunge with incongruent thorax and pelvis rotation, congruent head and neck, and thorax rotation. (C) Lunge with congruent pelvis, thorax, and head and neck rotation.

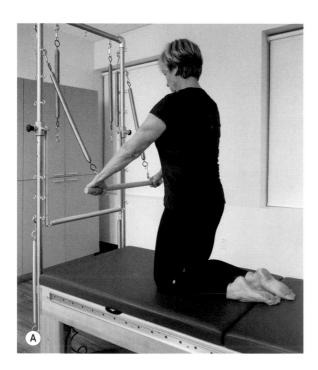
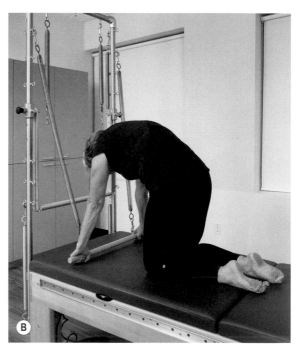

Figure 7.41

Stage 3, Level 3 integration of regional movement and control and inter-regional movement and control with varying levels of task predictability and perturbation. Pilates Cadillac Water Wheel. (A) From a high kneeling starting position, the spring-loaded bar is pressed toward the Cadillac's surface. (B) The head, neck, and thoracic rings sequence through flexion in the preliminary part of the task.

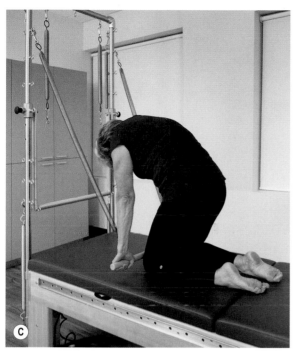

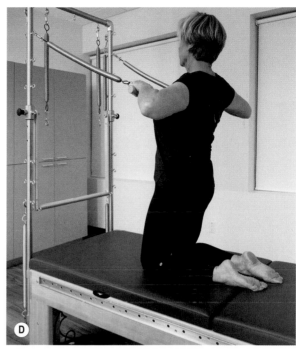

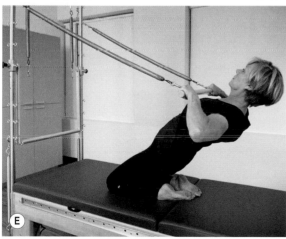

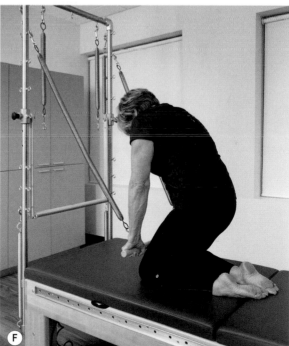

Figure 7.41 *continued*

(C) The bar is then drawn to the knees and up the thighs as the hips, lumbar spine, and thorax return to neutral. (D) The arms are abducted and with the bar held close to the chest (E) the entire trunk is taken posteriorly by flexing the knees. Watch for abdominal bulging or any loss of alignment and control. (F) The goal is now to flex the head, neck, and thorax around the bar and then press the bar down the thighs, back to the Cadillac surface (G, overleaf). *Continued*

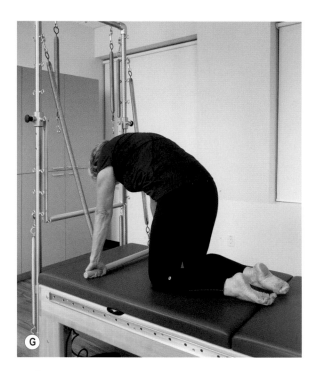
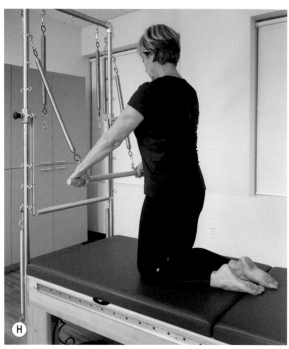

Figure 7.41 *continued*

(H) Return to the starting position is initiated with a posterior pelvic tilt followed by sequential lumbar and thoracic ring extension.

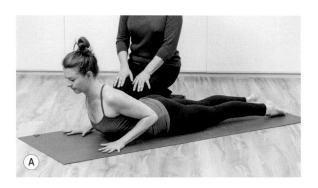
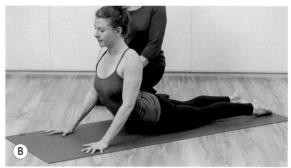

Figure 7.42

Stage 3, Level 3 yoga flow sequences. Ardha Bhujangasana to Bhujangasana to Urdhva Mukha Svanasana. (A) Baby Cobra to (B) Cobra to (C) Updog.

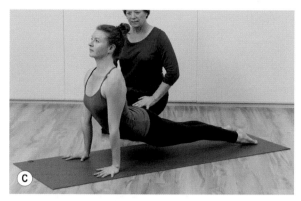

C

Figure 7.42 *continued*

For all these yoga flow sequences ensure optimal alignment, biomechanics, and control of all drivers are maintained and that loads are shared through all body regions.

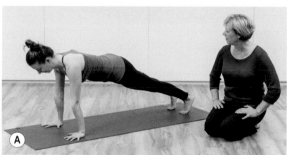

A

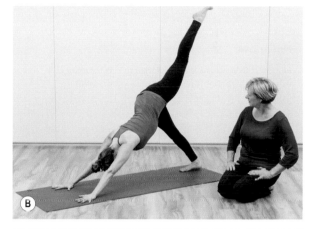

B

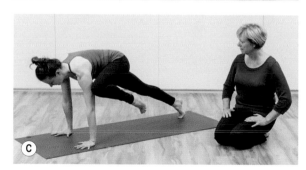

C

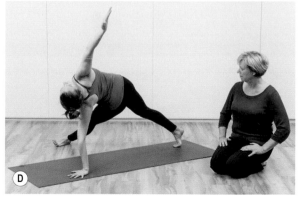

D

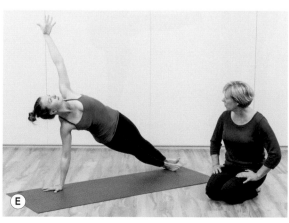

E

Figure 7.43

Stage 3, Level 3 yoga flow sequences. Phalankasana to three-legged Adho Mukha Svanasana to Knee to Nose (triceps) to Camatkarasana to Vasisthasana. (A) Plank to (B) Three-legged Downward Dog to (C) Knee to Nose (triceps) to (D) Fallen Triangle to (E) Side Plank.

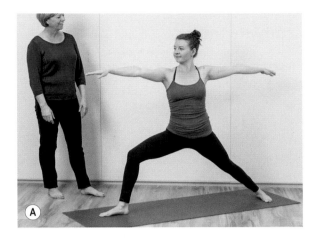

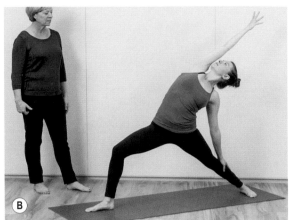

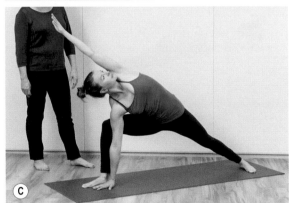

Figure 7.44

Stage 3, Level 3 yoga flow sequences. Virabhadrasana II to Viparita Virabhadrasana to Utthita Parsvakonasana. (A) Warrior II to (B) Reverse Warrior to (C) Extended Side Angle.

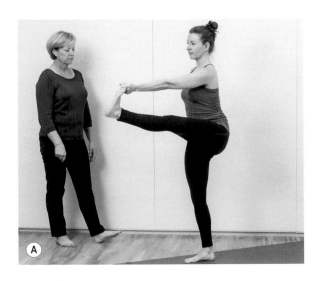

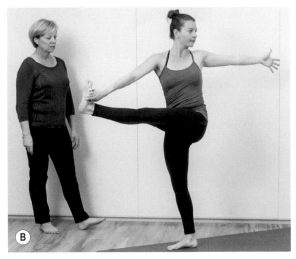

Figure 7.45

Stage 3, Level 3 yoga flow sequences. Utthita Hasta Padangusthasana to Parivrtta Hasta Padangusthasana to Virabhadrasana III. (A) Extended Hand-to-Big Toe to (B) Revolved Hand-to-Big Toe to Warrior III.

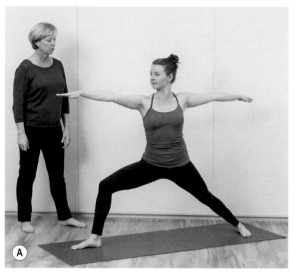

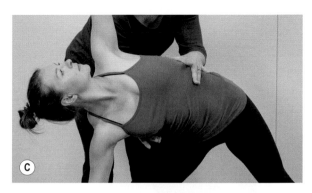

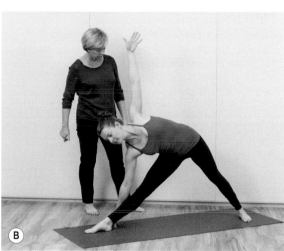

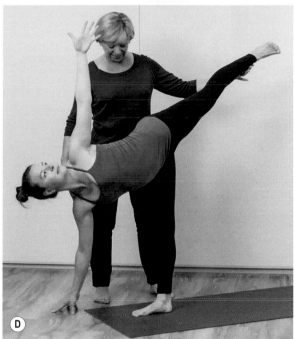

Figure 7.46

Stage 3, Level 3 yoga flow sequences. Virabhadrasana II to Trikonasana to Ardha Chandrasana. (A) Warrior II to (B) Triangle to (C) manual assist to facilitate congruent interthoracic ring rotation to (D) Half Moon.

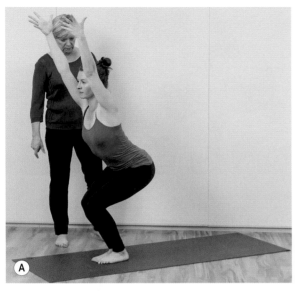

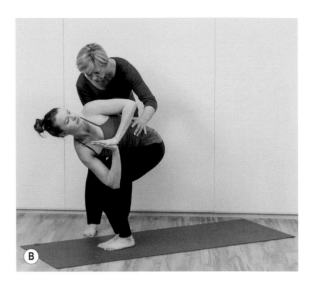

Figure 7.47

Stage 3, Level 3 yoga flow sequences. Utkatasana to Parivrtta Utkatasana to Parivrtta Anjaneyasana. (A) Chair to (B) Revolved Chair to (C) Revolved High Lunge.

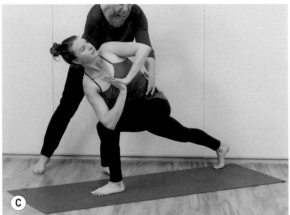

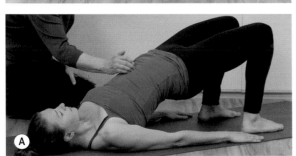

Figure 7.48

Stage 3, Level 3 yoga flow sequences. Setu Bandha Sarvangasana to Urdhva Dhanurasana. (A) Bridge to (B) Wheel.

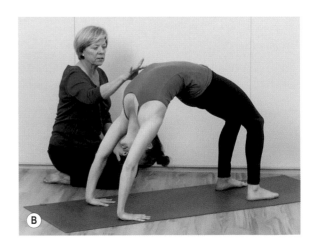

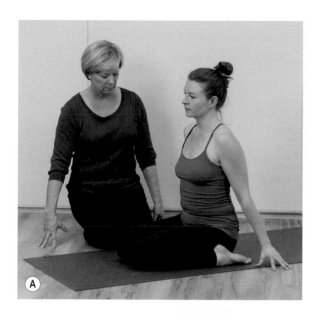

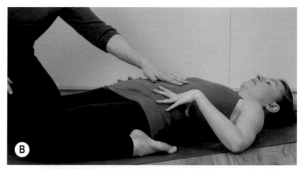

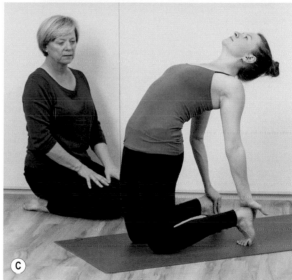

Figure 7.49

Stage 3, Level 3 yoga flow sequences. Virasana to Supta Virasana to Ustrasana. (A) Hero to (B) Reclined Hero to (C) Camel.

Hypopressive exercise and Low Pressure Fitness™

Low Pressure Fitness™, or hypopressive exercise, was originated by Marcel Caufriez, a Belgian physiotherapist, with the goal of helping women prevent or recover from urinary incontinence and pelvic organ prolapse. Low Pressure Fitness™ has evolved with contributions from Tamara Rial and Piti Pinsach from Spain. In Canada, Trista Zinn is the principal trainer for this method (Fig. 7.50A–C). It is an entire program with three component parts that aim to:

1. Restore optimal posture and control of the trunk;

2. Train lateral costal breathing;

3. Use false inhalation, or apnea, combined with the specific postures to decrease intra-abdominal pressure and train the deep muscles responsible for control of the lumbopelvis, including the diaphragm, the transversus abdominis, and the pelvic floor.

This author finds this approach beneficial for individuals with:

- Poor thoracic posture combined with poor abdominal strategies that are creating excessive intra-abdominal pressure with or without symptoms of urinary incontinence, pelvic organ prolapse or pelvic pressure.

- The classic low diaphragm, pericardial vector posture (Fig. 3.71A–C).

The Integrated Systems Model integrates very well with Low Pressure Fitness™. Drivers and their underlying

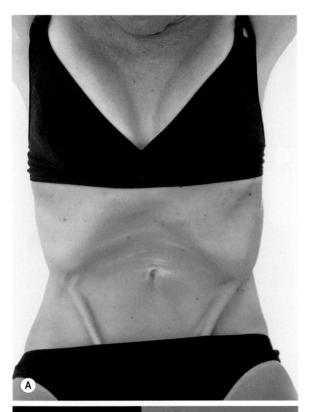

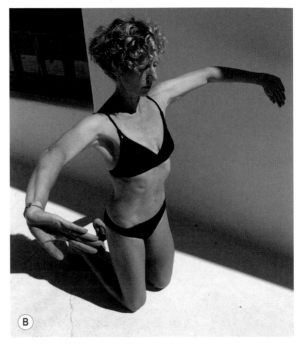

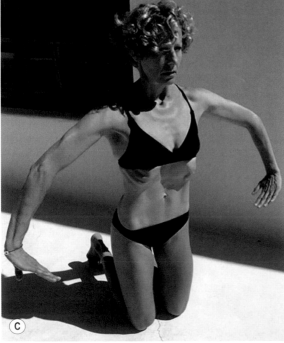

Figure 7.50

Low Pressure Fitness™ exercises. (A) Profile of the rib cage and abdomen during an apnea (or false inhalation with a closed glottis). Trista is in four-point kneeling here. (B) Lateral costal breath training in high kneeling prior to performing a false inhalation. (C) Addition of the apnea to the high kneeling posture.

system impairments are treated first to restore optimal postural alignment and control of the trunk. Integral to this treatment is the training of lateral costal breathing in inverted postures (four-point kneeling on elbows and knees). This position loads the diaphragm since gravity displaces the abdominal viscera superiorly. It is important that the exhale is not forced and does not recruit the abdominals excessively.

After two to four weeks of treatment, a false inhalation, or apnea, is added to the lateral costal breathing practice in inversion. At the end of three 'rest breaths,' the glottis is closed to avoid air entering the lungs on the next inhale. The central tendon of the diaphragm cannot descend if air is not allowed to enter the lungs. The diaphragm contraction results in elevation of the anterior rib cage and hollowing of the abdomen. This reduces the intra-abdominal pressure. Further cuing to lengthen the posterior thorax with the false inhalation reduces the intra-abdominal pressure further. Over time the patient can sustain the apnea for up to 20 seconds thus building diaphragm strength and endurance. Upright postures are then added to the patient's program.

While the underlying mechanisms for improved pelvic organ position have yet to be validated scientifically, clinical experience suggests that this method has merit for those whose symptoms are derived from excessive intra-abdominal pressure, combined with poor thoracopelvic posture and muscle recruitment strategies. Improvements in the classic pericardial vector posture have also been noted.

Summary

The thorax plays a critical role in multiple conditions since it is part of many integrated and interdependent systems, including the musculoskeletal, nervous, respiratory, cardiovascular, digestive, and urogynecological systems – all parts of the whole body or person. The biomechanics of the thorax are fundamental to the function of these systems and therefore relevant to all forms of treatment across multiple conditions. How movement patterns of the thorax are interpreted depends on one's understanding of optimal biomechanics in this region. The assessment and treatment of a whole person (body, mind, and spirit) requires an understanding of the relationship between, and the contribution of, various body regions and systems that are ultimately manifesting as cognitive, emotional or sensorial dissonance with variable sensitization of the nervous system. Ultimately, conservative care should consider and address the role of each system and body region on an individual basis.

The Integrated Systems Model is an evidence-informed, clinical-reasoning, biopsychosocial approach. It is a framework, not a classification, that considers all three dimensions of the patient's experience (sensorial, cognitive, emotional) and the barriers that each may present to the recovery process for both acute and persistent conditions. The body or person can no longer be considered as individual parts or problems in either assessment or treatment. Most tasks involve the whole body; therefore, assessment must include an analysis of the relationship between the body regions and the impact and interplay of each.

Finding drivers requires the skill to not only interpret a finding, but to find it reliably. For therapists, visual and kinesthetic perceptions are foundational tools for assessing the human form in function. Understanding our individual strengths, weaknesses, accuracies, and misperceptions enhances our reliability and the skills necessary to find a finding. Clinical reasoning then determines the finding's relevance to the clinical picture, which subsequently directs management of the individual patient. While clinical reasoning can be taught through texts and online media, there will always be a need for hands-on practical courses; this is the art and skill of physiotherapy that is so difficult to measure with science. For more information on further training in the Integrated Systems Model please visit the online education platform at www.learnwithdianelee.com.

REFERENCES

Andersson E A, Nilsson J, Ma Z and Thorstensson A (1997) Abdominal and hip flexor muscle activation during various training exercises. European Journal of Applied Physiology and Occupational Physiology 75 (2) 115–123.

Andriacchi T, Schultz A, Belytschko T and Galante J (1974) A model for studies of mechanical interactions between the human spine and rib cage. Journal Biomechanics 7 (6) 497–507.

Axer H, Keyserlingk D G and Prescher A (2001a) Collagen fibers in linea alba and rectus sheaths. Journal of Surgical Research 96 (2) 239–245.

Axer H, Keyserling D G and Prescher A (2001b) Collagen fibers in linea alba and rectus sheaths I: General scheme and morphological aspects. Journal of Surgical Research 96 (1) 127–134.

Barral J P (2007) Visceral Manipulation II. Seattle: Eastland Press.

Becker R E (2000) The Stillness of Life: The osteopathic philosophy of Rollin E. Becker. Portland: Stillness Press.

Beer G M, Schuster A, Seifert B et al. (2009) The normal width of the linea alba in nulliparous women. Clinical Anatomy 22 (6) 706–711.

Beyer B, Sholukha V, Dugailly P M et al. (2014) In vivo thorax 3D modelling from costovertebral joint complex kinematics. Clinical Biomechanics 29 (4) 434–438.

Bialosky J E, Bishop M D and Cleland J A (2010) Individual expectation: An overlooked but pertinent factor in the treatment of individuals experiencing musculoskeletal pain. Physical Therapy 90 (9) 1345–1355.

Bogduk N L T (1997) Clinical Anatomy of the Lumbar Spine and Sacrum, 3rd ed. New York: Churchill Livingstone.

Brown S H M and McGill S M (2008) An ultrasound investigation into the morphology of the human abdominal wall uncovers complex deformation patterns during contraction. European Journal of Applied Physiology 104 (6) 1021–1030.

Brown S H M and McGill S M (2009) Transmission of muscularly generated force and stiffness between layers of the rat abdominal wall. Spine 34 (2) 70–75.

Butler D S (2000) The Sensitive Nervous System. Adelaide: NOI Group Publications.

Butler D S and Moseley G L (2003) Explain Pain. Adelaide: NOI Group Publications.

Carmichael, J P (1987) Inter- and intra-examiner reliability of palpation for sacroiliac joint dysfunction. Journal of Manipulative Physical Therapy 10 (4) 164–171.

Cyriax J (1954) Textbook of Orthopaedic Medicine. London: Cassell.

Delancey J O L and Ashton-Miller J (2004) Pathophysiology of adult urinary incontinence. Gastroenterology 126 (Supplement 1) S32.

Delphinus E M and Sayers M G L (2013) The interrelationship of the thorax and pelvis under varying task constraints. Ergonomics 56 (4) 659–666.

Dickey J P and Kerr D J (2003) Effect of specimen length: Are the mechanics of individual motion segments comparable in functional spinal units and multisegment specimens? Medical Engineering & Physics 25 (3) 221–227.

Doidge N (2007) The Brain that Changes Itself: Stories of personal triumph from the frontiers of brain science. New York: Penguin Books.

Dorey G (2006) Pelvic Dysfunction in Men. Diagnosis and Treatment of Male Incontinence and Erectile Dysfunction:

A textbook for physiotherapists, nurses and doctors. West Sussex: John Wiley & Sons Ltd.

Dreyfuss P, Dryer S, Griffin J, Hoffman J and Walsh N (1994) Positive sacroiliac screening tests in asymptomatic adults. Spine 19 (10) 1138–1143.

Edmondston S (2004) Clinical biomechanics of the thoracic spine including the rib cage. In: J Boyling and G Jull eds, Grieve's Modern Manual Therapy, 3rd ed. Edinburgh: Elsevier.

Edmondston S J, Aggerholm M, Elfving S et al. (2007) Influence of posture on the range of axial rotation and coupled lateral flexion of the thoracic spine. J Manipulative Physiol Ther 30 (3) 193–199.

Edmondston S J, Ferguson A, Ippersiel P et al. (2012) Clinical and radiological investigation of thoracic spine extension motion during bilateral arm elevation. Journal of Orthopaedic & Sports Physical Therapy 42 (10) 861–869.

Edwards I and Jones M A (2007) Clinical reasoning and expert practice. In: G M Jensen, J Gwyer, L M Hack and K F Shepard eds, Expertise in Physical Therapy Practice, 2nd ed. St Louis: Saunders, pp. 192–213.

Ehara S (2010) Manubriosternal joint: Imaging features of normal anatomy and arthritis. Japan J Radiology 28 (5) 329–334.

Falla D and Hodges P W (2017) Individualized exercise interventions for spinal pain. Exercise and Sport Sciences Reviews 45 (2) 105–115.

Fitts P M and Posner M I (1967) Human Performance. Belmont: Brooks/Cole.

Garner G (2016) Medical Therapeutic Yoga. Edinburgh: Handspring Publishing.

Giles L G F and Singer KP eds (2000) The Clinical Anatomy and Management of Back Pain Series. Volume 2: Clinical Anatomy

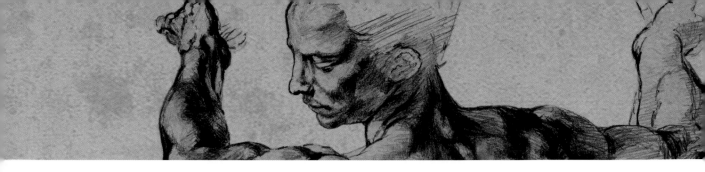

and Management of Thoracic Spine Pain. Woburn: Butterworth-Heinemann, pp. 17–33.

Gräßel D, Prescher A, Fitzek S et al. (2005) Anisotropy of human linea alba: A biomechanical study. Journal of Surgical Research 124 (1) 118–125.

Guimberteau J-C (2005) Strolling under the skin. [Online video] Available: https://www.youtube.com/watch?v=eW0lvOVKDxE [Feb 20, 2018].

Guimberteau J-C and Armstrong C (2015) Architecture of Human Living Fascia. Edinburgh: Handspring Publishing.

Gunn C C (1996) The Gunn approach to the treatment of chronic pain. Intramuscular stimulation for myofascial pain of radiculopathic origin. New York: Churchill Livingstone.

Hartman L S (1996) Handbook of Osteopathic Technique. London. Chapman & Hall.

Hebb D O (1949) The organization of behavior: A neuropsychological theory. New York: John Wiley & Sons.

Henegan N R and Rushton A (2016) Understanding why the thoracic region is the 'Cinderella' region of the spine. Manual Therapy 21 274–276.

Herzog W, Read L, Conway P J W et al. (1989) Reliability of motion palpation procedures to detect sacroiliac joint fixations. Journal of Manipulative and Physical Therapy 12 (2) 86–92.

Hewitt J D, Glisson R R, Guilak F and Parker Vail T (2002) The mechanical properties of the human hip capsule ligaments. Journal of Arthroplasty 17 (1) 82–89.

Higgs J and Jones M (2000) Clinical reasoning in the health professions. In: J Higgs and M P Jones eds, Clinical reasoning in the Health Professions, 2nd ed. Oxford: Butterworth-Heinemann, pp. 3–17.

Hodges P W (2015) The role of motor control training. In: G Jull, A Moore, D Falla et al. eds, Grieve's Modern Musculoskeletal Physiotherapy. Edinburgh: Elsevier, pp. 482–487.

Hodges P W and Smeets R J (2015) Interaction between pain, movement and physical activity: Short-term benefits, long-term consequences and targets for treatment. Clinical Journal of Pain 31 (2) 97–107.

Hodges P W, Pengel L H M, Herbert R D and Gandevia S C (2003) Measurement of muscle contraction with ultrasound imaging. Muscle & Nerve 27 (6) 682–692.

Hodges P W, Cholewicki J and van Dieen J H (2013) Spinal Control: The rehabilitation of back pain. State of the art and science. Edinburgh: Elsevier.

Hodges P W, Ferreira P H and Ferreira M L (2016) Lumbar spine treatment of motor control disorders. In: D J Magee, J E Zachazewski, W S Quillen, R C Manske eds, Pathology and Intervention in Musculoskeletal Rehabilitation, 2nd ed. Elsevier, pp. 520–560.

Hsu C J, Chang Y W, Chou W Y et al. (2008) Measurement of spinal range of motion in healthy individuals using an electromagnetic tracking device. Journal of Neurosurgery: Spine 8 (2) 135–142.

Hungerford B, Gilleard W and Hodges P W (2003) Evidence of altered lumbopelvic muscle recruitment in the presence of sacroiliac joint pain. Spine 28 (14) 1593–1600.

Hungerford B, Gilleard W and Lee D (2004) Altered patterns of pelvic bone motion determined in subjects with posterior pelvic pain using skin markers. Clinical Biomechanics 19 (5) 456–464.

Hungerford B A, Gilleard W, Moran M and Emmerson C (2007) Evaluation of the ability of physical therapists to palpate intrapelvic motion with the Stork test on the support side. Physical Therapy 87 (7) 879–887.

Ishii S and Yamamoto S (2008) Kinematic analysis of screw home movement with active knee extension in the non-weight bearing position. Journal of Physical Therapy Science 23 (1) 11–16.

Jones M A and Rivett D A (2004) Introduction to clinical reasoning. In: M A Jones and D A Rivett eds, Clinical Reasoning for Manual Therapists. Edinburgh: Elsevier, pp. 3–24.

Junginger B, Baessler K, Sapsford R and Hodges P W (2010) Effect of abdominal and pelvic floor tasks on muscle activity, abdominal pressure and bladder neck. International Urogynecology Journal 21 (1) 69–77.

Kapandji I A (1964) Illustrated physiology of joints. Med Biol Illus 14 72–81.

Kent P and Hartvigsen J (2015) Clinical reasoning and models for clinical management. In: G Jull, A Moore, D Falla et al. eds, Grieve's Modern Musculoskeletal Physiotherapy. Edinburgh: Elsevier, pp. 242–249.

Kleim J A and Jones T A (2008) Principles of experience-dependent neural plasticity: Implications for rehabilitation after brain damage. Journal of Speech, Language and Hearing Research 51 (1) S225e39.

Lee D (1994) Manual Therapy for the Thorax – A biomechanical approach. Delta: Diane G. Lee Physiotherapist Corporation.

Lee D (2001) Imagery for Core Stabilization. VHS. Delta: Diane G. Lee Physiotherapist Corporation.

Lee D (2003) The Thorax – An integrated approach. Delta: Diane G. Lee Physiotherapist Corporation.

Lee D (2011) The Pelvic Girdle: An integration of clinical expertise and research. Edinburgh: Elsevier.

Lee D (2016) Highlights from an integrated approach to the treatment of pelvic pain and dysfunction. In: D J Magee, J E Zachazewski, W S Quillen, R C Manske eds, Pathology and Intervention in Musculoskeletal Rehabilitation, 2nd ed. Elsevier, pp.:612–650.

Lee D (2017a) Assessment of the abdominal wall. In: D Lee (2011) Diastasis Rectus Abdominis: A clinical guide for those who are split down the middle. Surrey: Learn with Diane Lee, pp. 65–128. www.learnwithdianelee.com [April 4, 2018].

Lee D (2017b) Diastasis Rectus Abdominis: A clinical guide for those who are split down the middle. Surrey: Learn with Diane Lee. www.learnwithdianelee.com [April 4, 2018].

Lee D and Hodges P W (2016) Behavior of the linea alba during a curl-up task in diastasis rectus abdominis. An observational study. Journal of Orthopaedic & Sports Physical Therapy 46 (7) 580–589.

Lee D and Lee L-J (2011a) Techniques and tools for addressing barriers in the lumbopelvic-hip complex. In: D Lee (2011) The Pelvic Girdle. An integration of clinical expertise and research, 4th ed. Edinburgh: Elsevier, pp. 283–321.

Lee D and Lee L-J (2011b) Techniques and tools for assessing the lumbopelvic-hip complex. In: D Lee (2011) The Pelvic Girdle: An integration of clinical expertise and research, 4th ed. Edinburgh: Elsevier, pp. 174–254.

Lee D G (1993) Biomechanics of the thorax: A clinical model of in vivo function. Journal of Manual and Manipulative Therapy 1 (1) 13–21.

Lee D G (1996) Rotational instability of the mid-thoracic spine: Assessment and management. Manual Therapy 1 (5) 234–241.

Lee D G (2015) Biomechanics of the thorax – research evidence and clinical expertise. Journal of Manual & Manipulative Therapy 23 (3) 128–138.

Lee D G and Jones M A (2018) Postpartum thoracolumbar pain associated with diastasis rectus abdominis. In: M A Jones & D A Rivett eds, Clinical Reasoning in Musculoskeletal Practice, 2nd ed. Elsevier [in press].

Lee D G, Lee L-J and McLaughlin L (2008) Stability, continence and breathing: The role of fascia following pregnancy and delivery. Journal of Bodywork and Movement Therapies 12 (4) 333–348.

Lee L-J (2003a) Thoracic stabilization & the functional upper limb: Restoring stability with mobility. Course Notes [Unpublished].

Lee L-J (2003b) Restoring force closure/motor control of the thorax. In: D Lee (2003) The Thorax. Delta: Diane G. Lee Physiotherapist Corporation.

Lee L-J (2004–2013) Discover Physio courses developed individually or co-developed with Diane Lee [Unpublished].

Lee L-J (2016) The thoracic ring approach: A whole person framework to assess and treat the thoracic spine and rib cage. In: D J Magee, J E Zachazewski, W S Quillen, R C Manske eds, Pathology and Intervention in Musculoskeletal Rehabilitation, 2nd ed. Elsevier, pp. 436–470.

Lee L-J and Lee D (2011) Clinical practice – the reality for clinicians. In: D Lee (2011) The Pelvic Girdle: An integration of clinical expertise and research, 4th ed. Edinburgh: Elsevier, pp. 147–171.

Lee L-J, Coppieters M W and Hodges P W (2005) Differential activation of the thoracic multifidus and longissimus thoracis during trunk rotation. Spine 30 (8) 870–876.

Lee L-J, Coppieters M W and Hodges P W (2009) Anticipatory postural adjustments to arm movement reveal complex control of paraspinal muscles in the thorax. Journal of Electromyography and Kinesiology 19(1) 46–54.

Lee L-J, Chang A T, Coppieters M W and Hodges P W (2010) Changes in sitting posture induce multiplanar changes in chest wall shape and motion with breathing. Respiratory Physiology & Neurobiology 170 236–245.

Lee L-J, Coppieters M W and Hodges P W (2011) En bloc control of deep and superficial thoracic muscles in sagittal loading and unloading of the trunk. Gait & Posture 33 (4) 588–593.

Lowcock J (1990) Thoracic joint stability and clinical stress tests. Orthopaedic Division of the Canadian Physiotherapy Association Newsletter 15.

MacConaill M A and Basmajian J V (1977) Muscles and movements: A basis for human kinesiology, 2nd ed. New York: Krieger.

MacIntosh J E and Bogduk N (1991) The attachments of the lumbar erector spinae. Spine 16 (7) 783–792.

Maitland G D (1986) Vertebral Manipulation, 5th ed. Oxford: Butterworth Heinemann.

Masharawi Y, Rothschild B, Dar G et al. (2004) Facet orientation in the thoracolumbar spine: Three-dimensional anatomic and biomechanical analysis. Spine 29 (16) 1755–1763.

Meijne W, van Neerbos K, Aufdemkampe G and van der Wurff P (1999) Intraexaminer and interexaminer reliability of the Gillet test. Journal of Manipulative Physiological Therapeutics 22 (1) 4–9.

Melzack R (1990) Phantom limbs and the concept of a neuromatrix. Trends in Neurosciences 13 (3) 88–92.

Melzack R (2001) Pain and the neuromatrix in the brain. Journal of Dental Education 65 (12) 1378–1382.

Molnár S, Manó S, Kiss L and Csernátony Z (2006) Ex vivo and in vitro determination of the axial rotational axis of the human thoracic spine. Spine 31(26) 984–91.

Moseley G L (2003) A pain neuromatrix approach to patients with chronic pain. Manual Therapy 8 (3) 130–140.

Moseley G L (2007) Reconceptualising pain according to modern pain science. Physical Therapy Reviews 12 (3) 169–178.

Moseley G L and Butler D S (2015) Explain Pain Handbook. Protectometer. Adelaide: Noigroup Publications.

Moseley G L and Butler D S (2017) Explain Pain Supercharged. Adelaide: Noigroup Publications.

Moseley G L, Gallace A and Spence C (2012) Bodily illusions in health and disease: Physiological and clinical perspectives and the concept of a cortical 'body matrix'. Neuroscience and Biobehavioral Reviews 36 (1) 34–46.

Mota P, Pascoal A G, Carita A I and Bø K (2015) The immediate effects on inter-rectus distance of abdominal crunch and drawing-in exercises during pregnancy and the postpartum period. Journal of Orthopaedic & Sports Physical Therapy 45 (10) 781–788.

O'Sullivan P, Dankaerts W, O'Sullivan K and Fersum K (2015) Multidimensional approach for the targeted management of low back pain. In: G Jull, A Moore, D Falla et al. eds, Grieve's Modern Musculoskeletal Physiotherapy. Edinburgh: Elsevier, pp. 465–470.

Oxland T R, Lin R M and Panjabi M M (1992) Three-dimensional mechanical properties of the thoracolumbar junction. Journal of Orthopaedic Research 10 (4) 573–580.

Pak N, Patel S G, Hashemi Taheri A P et al. (2016) A reappraisal of adult thoracic and abdominal surface anatomy in Iranians in vivo using computed tomography. Clinical Anatomy 29 (2) 191–196.

Paoletti S (2006) The Fasciae: Anatomy, dysfunction and treatment. Seattle, WA: Eastland Press Inc.

Panjabi M M (1992) The stabilizing system of the spine: Part II. Neutral zone and instability hypothesis. Journal of Spinal Disorders 5 (4) 390–396.

Panjabi M M, Brand R A and White A A (1976) Mechanical properties of

the human thoracic spine as shown by three-dimensional load-displacement curves. Journal of Bone and Joint Surgery 58 (5) 642–652.

Pascoal A G, Dionisio S, Cordeiro F and Mota P (2014) Inter-rectus distance in postpartum women can be reduced by isometric contraction of the abdominal muscles: A preliminary case-control study. Physiotherapy 100 (4) 344–348.

Peng, Q Jones R, Shishido K and Constantinou C E (2007) Ultrasound evaluation of dynamic responses of female pelvic floor muscles. Ultrasound in Medicine and Biology 33 (3) 342–352.

Pettman E (1981) The Quadrant Courses. Orthopaedic Division of CPA [Unpublished].

Pettman E (1984) The Functional Shoulder Girdle. IFOMT Vancouver.

Pettman E (2011) Sternoclavicular joint. In: C Fernández-de-las-Peñas, J Cleland, P Huijbregts eds, Neck and Arm Pain Syndromes. Edinburgh: Elsevier.

Potter N A and Rothstein J (1985) Intertester reliability for selected clinical tests of the sacroiliac joint. Physical Therapy 65 (11) 1671–1675.

Richardson C A, Jull G A, Hodges P W and Hides J A (1999) Therapeutic exercise for spinal segmental stabilization in low back pain – scientific basis and clinical approach. Edinburgh: Churchill Livingstone.

Sackett D L, Straus S, Richardson W S et al. (2000) Evidence-Based Medicine. How to Practice and Teach EBM. New York: Elsevier.

Sahrmann S and van Dillen L (2015) Movement system impairment syndromes of the low back. In: G Jull, A Moore, D Falla et al. eds, Grieve's Modern Musculoskeletal Physiotherapy. Edinburgh: Elsevier, pp. 474–482.

Sancho M F, Pascoal A G, Mota P and Bø K (2015) Abdominal exercises affect inter-rectus distance in postpartum women: A two-dimensional ultrasound study. Physiotherapy 101 (3) 286–291.

Scholten P J M and Veldhuizen A G (1985) The influence of spine geometry on the coupling between lateral bending and axial rotation. Engineering in Medicine 14 (4) 167–171.

Schuenke M D, Vleeming A, van Hoof T and Willard F H (2012) A description of the lumbar interfascial triangle and its relation with the lateral raphe: Anatomical constituents of load transfer through the lateral margin of the thoracolumbar fascia. Journal of Anatomy 221 (6) 568–576.

Schultz A B, Belytschoki T B and Andriacchi T P (1973) Analog studies of forces in the human spine: Mechanical properties and motion segment behavior. Journal of Biomechanics 6 (4) 373–383.

Setchell J, Costa N, Ferreira M et al. (2017) Individuals' explanations for their persistent or recurrent low back pain. A cross-sectional survey. BMC Musculoskeletal Disorders 18 (1) 466–475.

Siegel D (2010) Mindsight. New York: Bantam Books.

Singer K P and Goh S (2000) Anatomy of the thoracic spine. In: L G F Giles and K P Singer eds, The Clinical Anatomy and Management of Back Pain Series. Volume 2: Clinical Anatomy and Management of Thoracic Spine Pain. Woburn: Butterworth-Heinemann, pp. 17–33.

Sizer P S, Brismée J M and Cook C (2007) Coupling behavior of the thoracic spine: A systematic review of the literature. Journal of Manipulative and Physiological Therapeutics. 30 (5) 390–399.

Smeets R J E M, Vlaeyen J W S, Kester A D M and Knottnerus J A (2006) Reduction of pain catastrophizing mediates the outcome of both physical and cognitive-behavioral treatment in chronic low back pain. Journal of Pain 7 (4) 261–271.

Snijders C J, Vleeming A and Stoeckart R (1993a) Transfer of lumbosacral load to iliac bones and legs. Part 1: Biomechanics of self-bracing of the sacroiliac joints and its significance for treatment and exercise. Clinical Biomechanics 8 (6) 285–294.

Snijders C J, Vleeming A and Stoeckart R (1993b) Transfer of lumbosacral load to iliac bones and legs. Part 2: Loading of the sacroiliac joints when lifting in a stooped posture. Clinical Biomechanics 8 (6) 295–301.

Snodgrass S J, Heneghan N R, Tsao H et al. (2014) Recognising neuroplasticity in musculoskeletal rehabilitation: A basis for greater collaboration between musculoskeletal and neurological physiotherapists. Manual Therapy 19 (6) 614–617.

Stafford R E, Ashton-Miller J, Constantinou C et al. (2015) Pattern of activation of pelvic floor muscles in men differs with verbal instructions. Neurourology and Urodynamics 35 (4) 457–463.

Standring S ed. (2008) Gray's Anatomy: The Anatomical Basis of Clinical Practice, 40th ed. London: Elsevier.

Stecco C (2015) Functional Atlas of the Human Fascial System. Edinburgh: Elsevier.

Sueki D G, Cleland J A and Wainner R S (2013) A regional interdependence model of musculoskeletal dysfunction: Research, mechanisms, and clinical implications. Journal of Manual & Manipulative Therapy 21 (2) 90–102.

Theodoridis D and Ruston S (2002) The effect of shoulder movements on thoracic spine 3D motion. Clinical Biomechanics 17 (5) 418–421.

Tsao H and Hodges P W (2007) Immediate changes in feedforward postural adjustments following voluntary motor training. Experimental Brain Research 181 (4) 537–546.

Tsao H and Hodges P W (2008) Persistence of improvements in postural strategies following motor control training in people with recurrent low back pain. Journal of Electromyography and Kinesiology 18 (4) 559–567.

Tsao H, Druitt T R, Schollum T M and Hodges P W (2010) Motor training of the lumbar paraspinal muscles induces immediate changes in motor coordination in patients with recurrent low back pain. Journal of Pain 11 (11) 1120–1128.

Urquhart D M, Barker P J, Hodges P W et al. (2005) Regional morphology of transversus abdominis and obliquus internus and externus abdominis. Clinical Biomechanics 20 (3) 233–241.

van Dieën J H, Flor H and Hodges P W (2017) Low-back pain patients learn to adapt motor behavior with adverse secondary consequences. Exercise and Sport Sciences Reviews 45 (4) 223–229.

van Wingerden J P, Vleeming A and Snijders C J (1993) A functional-anatomical approach to the spine-pelvis mechanism: Interaction between the biceps femoris muscle and the sacrotuberous ligament. European Spine Journal 2 (3) 140.

Vleeming A, Stoeckart R and Snijders C J, (1989a) The sacrotuberous ligament: A conceptual approach to its dynamic role in stabilizing the sacroiliac joint. Clinical Biomechanics 4 (4) 201–203.

Vleeming A, van Wingerden J P, Snijders C J et al. (1989b) Load application to the sacrotuberous ligament: Influences on sacroiliac joint mechanics. Clinical Biomechanics 4 (4) 204–209.

Vleeming A, Volkers A C W, Snijders C J and Stoeckart R (1990) Relation between form and function in the sacroiliac joint. Part II: Biomechanical aspects. Spine 15 (2) 133–136.

Watson L and Dalziel R (1996) Conservative treatment of thoracic outlet syndrome by scapula strengthening techniques. In: A P Skirving ed, Shoulder Surgery: The Asian Perspective, Volume 2. Perth: Asian Shoulder Association, pp. 219–222.

Watson L A, Pizzari T and Balster S (2009) Thoracic outlet syndrome part 1: Clinical manifestations differentiation and treatment pathways. Manual Therapy 14 (6) 586–595.

Webb A L, O'Sullivan E, Stokes M and Mottram S (2018) A novel cadaveric study of the morphometry of the serratus anterior muscle, one part, two parts, three parts, four? Anatomical Science International 93 (1) 98–107.

Wetzler G and Lee D (2015) Active and passive listening techniques – definition. ISM Series Intensive Clinical Mentorship Program. California [Unpublished].

Willard F H, Vleeming A, Schuenke M D et al. (2012) The thoracolumbar fascia: Anatomy, function, and clinical considerations. Journal of Anatomy 221 (6) 507–536.

Willems J, Jull G and Ng J K (1996) An in vivo study of the primary and coupled rotations of the thoracic spine. Clinical Biomechanics 11 (6) 311–316.

Williams P L (1995) Gray's Anatomy, 38th ed. New York: Churchill Livingstone.

Wilson T A, Legrand A and De Troyer A (2001) Respiratory effects of the external and internal intercostal muscles in humans. The Journal of Physiology 530 (Pt 2) 319–330.

Wurff P, Hagmeijer R and Meyne W (2000) Clinical tests of the sacroiliac joint. A systematic methodological review: Part 1: Reliability. Manual Therapy 5 (1) 30–36.

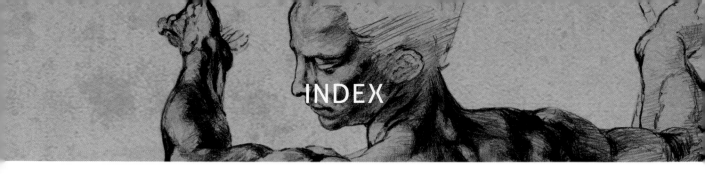

INDEX

Note: Page numbers followed by f or t indicate figures or tables, respectively.

Also available from Handspring Publishing…

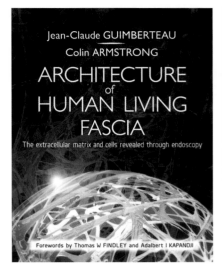

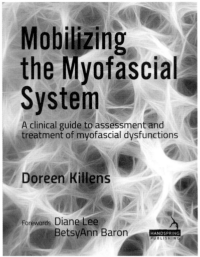

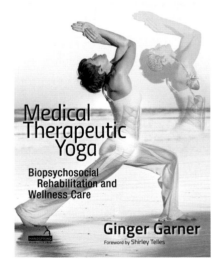

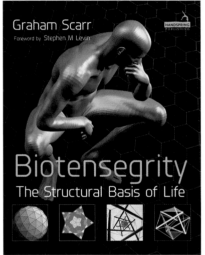

USA/Canada orders: e-mail hpl.orders@aidcvt.com
Telephone 855 375 7304 • **Fax** 802 864 7626

UK/Europe/Asia/Australasia orders: e-mail orders@booksource.net
Telephone +44 (0)845 370 0067 • **Fax** +44 (0)845 370 0068

Full details at **www.handspringpublishing.com**

Register for news of forthcoming books. E-mail info@handspringpublishing.com

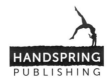

HANDSPRING
PUBLISHING